HEAD INJURY

DATE DUE

JUL 16 1992	FEB 2 5 1998
OCT 6 1992	JAN 27 1999
OCT 2 3 1992	MAR- 3 1999
JAN 1 8	MAR - 4 1999
OCT 1 5 1993	APR - 7 1999
NOV 2 4 1993	JUL 1 4 1999
JAN 3 1 1994	Jul 27
FEB 2 7 1994	Aug 9
MAR 3 0 1994	Aug 23
APR 1 3 1994	OCT 2 2 1999
APR 2 5 1994	NOV 1 5 1999
APR 1 5 1995	MAR - 4 2000
OCT 1 0 1996	DEC - 9 2000
OCT 2 5 1996	MAR 4 2002
NOV. 6	JUN 1 7 2002
NOV. 21	MAR 0 5 2003
OCT 2 3 1997	MAR 1 9 2003
NOV 1 8 1997	JAN 0 5 2004

HEAD INJURY

A FAMILY MATTER

EDITED BY

JANET M. WILLIAMS, M.S.W.
Beach Center on Families and Disability
Bureau of Child Research
University of Kansas
Lawrence, Kansas

AND

THOMAS KAY, Ph.D.
Director of Research
Department of Rehabilitation Medicine
Research and Training Center
on Head Trauma and Stroke
New York University Medical Center
New York, New York

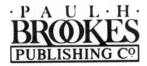
·P A U L·H·
BROOKES
PUBLISHING C<u>O</u>

Baltimore • London • Toronto • Sydney

Paul H. Brookes Publishing Co.
P.O. Box 10624
Baltimore, Maryland 21285-0624

Typeset by The Composing Room of Michigan, Inc., Grand Rapids, Michigan.
Manufactured in the United States of America by
The Maple Press Company, York, Pennsylvania.

Library of Congress Cataloging-in-Publication Data

Head injury : a family matter / [edited by] Janet M. Williams, Thomas
   Kay.
       p.   cm.
   Includes bibliographical references.
   ISBN 1-55766-063-8
   1. Brain damage—Patients—Family relationships.   2. Brain damage—
Patients—Rehabilitation.   I. Williams, Janet M., 1960–   .   II. Kay, Thomas,
1951–
   [DNLM: 1. Family.   2. Head Injuries—rehabilitation.   WE 706 H4315]
RC387.5.H43   1990
362.1'97551044—dc20
DNLM/DLC
for Library of Congress   90-2344
                                                                               CIP

CONTENTS

ABOUT THE EDITORS

JANET M. WILLIAMS

Janet M. Williams, M.S.W., has worked with people with disabilities and their families since 1981. She received a Bachelor of Arts degree from Providence College, and a Master of Social Work from Boston College. She began her career with Family Service America in Boston working as a family therapist with families of people with disabilities and chronic illnesses. She then became Director of Social Services at a head injury rehabilitation center in Boston, continuing her work with families in family therapy, family counseling, case management, and support groups. Before moving to Kansas in 1990, she was Director of Family and State Services at the National Head Injury Foundation (NHIF) in Framingham, Massachusetts. During her 4-year tenure at the NHIF, she developed programs for providing support and information to families. Additionally, she served as Project Director of a national public education program on head injury, Project TAP, funded by the Department of Education. She has traveled to more than 43 of the United States and several provinces in Canada, working with families and professionals to create innovative support programs. Additionally, she recently completed a study visit through a fellowship from the World Institute on Disability on how families in Denmark, Norway, the Netherlands, and Germany care for people with head injuries at home.

Currently Ms. Williams is in the doctoral program in Family Studies and Disability at the University of Kansas while working at the Beach Center on Families and Disability. The Beach Center on Families and Disability is a rehabilitation research and training center devoted to supporting the inherent strengths of families over the lifespan. The Center is funded by the National Institute of Disability and Rehabilitation Research, Office of Rehabilitation Services, United States Department of Education; and by various academic and research units at the University of Kansas.

THOMAS KAY

Thomas Kay, Ph.D., received his Bachelor of Arts degree in English Literature from Dartmouth College, his Master of Arts degree in English Literature from the University of Rochester, and his Doctorate of Philosophy in Clinical Psychology from Emory University. He did his clinical internship in psychology at the University of Washington Medical Center in Seattle, and a postdoctoral fellowship at the Rusk Institute of Rehabilitation Medicine at New York University Medical Center.

Since 1983 Dr. Kay has coordinated research studies in recovery from traumatic brain injury at N.Y.U. He currently serves as Director of Research at the N.Y.U. Research and Training Center on Head Trauma and Stroke and is Coordinator of Psychology Research within the Department of Rehabilitation Medicine. Dr. Kay is clinically involved in the rehabilitation of persons with head injuries and their families; his research interests include minor head injury, return to work after head injury, and the impact of head injury on the family system. Dr. Kay is on the Boards of Directors of the New York State Head Injury Association and the National Head Injury Foundation and has produced a federally funded educational videotape on minor head injury in collaboration with the National Head Injury Foundation. His presentations and publications have been primarily in the area of traumatic brain injury.

CONTRIBUTORS

Anastasia Barrett, M.S., C.R.C.
Head Trauma Program
New York University Medical Center
400 East 34th Street
New York, New York 10016

Marty Beaver, R.N.
1491 Timberland Road
Lawrenceville, Georgia 30245

Maureen Campbell-Korves
185 West End Avenue, #4-L
New York, New York 10023

Robert R. Carter, Ed.D.
Castleton State College
Castleton, Vermont 05735

Marie M. Cavallo, M. A.
Behavioral Science Department
Rusk Institute of Rehabilitation
  Medicine
New York University Medical Center
400 East 34th Street
New York, New York 10016

**Roberta DePompei, M.A., CCC
  SLP/A**
Department of Communicative
  Disorders
University of Akron
Akron, Ohio 44325

Lynn Grahame, M.S.W.
Drucker Brain Injury Center
Moss Rehabilitation Hospital
12th and Tabor
Philadelphia, Pennsylvania 19141

Hope Hardgrove
Route 4, Box 183
Winder, Georgia 30680

Bradley Hutchins, M.A., CCC-SLP
Marianjoy Rehabilitation Center
P.O. Box 795
Wheaton, Illinois 60189

Harvey E. Jacobs, Ph.D.
Associate Research Psychologist
Department of Psychiatry and
  Behavioral Sciences
Neuropsychiatric Institute
UCLA Medical Center
Westwood, California 90024

Thomas Kay, Ph.D.
Director of Research
Research and Training Center
  for Head Trauma and Stroke
New York University Medical Center
400 East 34th Street, Room RR811
New York, New York 10016

**Sally Kneipp, Ph.D., C.R.C.,
  C.I.R.S.**
Community Skills Program
Counseling and Rehabilitation, Inc.
1616 Walnut Street, #800
Philadelphia, Pennsylvania 19103

JoAnn Kramer, M.A.
6315 Sage Road R#3
Waterloo, Iowa 50703

Jeffrey S. Kreutzer, Ph.D.
Medical College of Virginia
Department of Rehabilitation Medicine
MCV Box 677
Richmond, Virginia 23298-0677

Edward A. Maitz, Ph.D.
Clinical Neuropsychology Associates
117 South 17th Street
Suite 1700
Philadelphia, Pennsylvania 19103

Joseph Maurer
2307 Silver Ridge Avenue
Los Angeles, California 90039

Heidi Hansen McCrory, B.F.A.
135 Chester Turnpike
Auburn, New Hampshire 03032

Patricia L. Price, M.Ed., C.R.C.
Mentor Head Injury Services
53 Cummings Park
Woburn, Massachusetts 01801

Mitchell Rosenthal, Ph.D.
Rehabilitation Institute
Wayne State University School of
    Medicine
261 Mack Boulevard
Detroit, Michigan 48201

Ronald C. Savage, Ed.D.
Professor
Castleton State College
Castleton, Vermont 05735
Program Director
New Medico–Capital District

Saralyn M. Silver, M.S., C.R.C.
Head Trauma Program
New York University Medical Center
400 East 34th Street
New York, New York 10016

Ann P. Turnbull, Ed.D.
Beach Center on Families and
    Disability
3111 Haworth Hall
Lawrence, Kansas 66045

**H. Rutherford Turnbull III, LL.B.,
LL.M.**
Beach Center on Families and
    Disability
3111 Haworth Hall
Lawrence, Kansas 66045

Janet M. Williams, M.S.W.
Beach Center on Families and
    Disability
Bureau of Child Research
University of Kansas
4138 Haworth Hall
Lawrence, Kansas 66045

John J. Zarski, Ph.D.
Director, Clinic for Child Study and
    Family Therapy
Carroll Hall, Room 128
University of Akron
Akron, Ohio 44325-5007

Nathan D. Zasler, M.D.
Brain Injury Rehabilitation Services
Department of Rehabilitation Medicine
Medical College of Virginia
Virginia Commonwealth University
Box 677, MCV Station
Richmond, Virginia 23298

FOREWORD

The title of this book says it straight out—head injury is a family matter! Where there is no commitment to support family caregiving, there is minimal chance for optimal return of function. This is a fact that must be appreciated by families, intervention professionals, and policymakers. Families are an integral partner in the rehabilitation process.

Having spent the past 15 years deeply involved with all aspects of head injury concerns as a parent, friend, advocate, and professional, I have no question that the family is the focal point in the long recovery process of the loved one with a head injury. However, families must recover their own emotional and physical well-being before they can function effectively as caregivers. This process frequently requires and benefits from professional intervention. I am particularly pleased that the editors of this book have chosen to focus on this timely and important subject. There is tribute to be paid to both Janet M. Williams and Thomas Kay, as they exemplify in their own work the importance of family in the recovery process. I worked closely with Janet Williams for a number of years. In 1985 I made a good decision to hire her to manage a growing and stressed family service system for the National Head Injury Foundation (NHIF). At the time, my fear was that her young age would be a detrimental factor. I thought that maturity of years and life experience were essential assets for the manager of this department. I knew that families value having a person who can relate to them from an experiential point of view. A mature professional must be able to control her or his own emotions while giving empathetic, sincere, and honest support and information. My concern dissipated as I worked with and watched Janet emerge as a responsive, knowledgeable, and caring professional, and she, in turn, was awed by the resilience, courage, and tenacity of so many grieving and overwhelmed families. Yes, there were those families who fit the dysfunctional model, but with appropriate help and direction, many families learned to become quite functional, and they began to participate in the recovery of their loved ones and in their own recovery process. In time, many became advocates for others when they had information and knowledge—and in that way, healed themselves. With Janet's and her staff's help, they gained more control of their lives, and over the years, they became knowledgeable consumers.

I also had the privilege of getting to know Thomas Kay and his outstanding colleagues as we cooperated on programs and projects sponsored by the New York University-Rusk Rehabilitation Research & Training Center and the NHIF. I admired and respected his commitment, his genuine concern, and his expertise as a friend to me and the NHIF. His admiration of persons with head injury and of their family members as they struggled to meet the challenges before them influenced and inspired his work.

The authors of the chapters of this book walk in like paths; they are strong and caring as they give of themselves to a movement. They believe in and spread the concept that head injury, as well as all disabilities and chronic illnesses, are truly a family matter.

It was an honor to be asked to contribute to this book which is so meaningful to me. This foreword is written at a special point in my family's life. It was just 10 years ago, April/May 1980, that the NHIF was conceived—out of our *need,* frustration, grief, and anger. The *need* was our own and that of our daughter, Deborah—the need to regain control of our lives as individuals and as a family after her head injury. I knew my husband Martin (Deborah's stepfather), my older daughter Lisa, my mother (now deceased), and I could not be Deborah's family first, then her therapists, caregivers, support system, and friends for the rest of her life in an isolated environment. Her life and ours could not be confined in this manner for the next 40–60 years. Our dreams and goals could not be shattered any further. Deborah was too precious to be further disabled by this impending isolation and lack of opportunity. She had her unique qualities and fantastic personality. She needed a structure to recreate goals and the support systems to allow her to attain them. We too needed to rebuild our own lives, to regain our focus on a brighter and fulfilling future. We needed to be the decision-makers again and not accept what appeared to be a devastating destiny. Our family's grief and frustration needed to be turned to positive action that would ultimately change environments and attitudes and create opportunities for Deborah and the thousands of people each year who sustain head injuries. We knew that there was also a need to establish networks of supports, services, and resources for families, caregivers, and providers. We also knew how hard it was to network with others who had similar experiences, and what it was like to feel as if we were the only family in Massachusetts with a daughter with such a critical injury.

In 1980 the NHIF was created. This was 5 years after Deborah's accident, 4 years after my son's death, and 1 year after their father's death—all were violent injuries that were jolting, catastrophic, and preventable.

In 1980, we faced a dead end in services and options. There were no programs or services that were appropriate for persons who sustained traumatic brain injury (TBI). "Injuries" were ignored as a public health crisis. We were determined to effect a change. First, our need was to advocate for systems of care and services, and then to promote the education of professionals working with individuals with TBI. Medical advances in technology and management were saving lives, but attempting to restore and rehabilitate persons with TBI was a new challenge for the field of rehabilitation. There was a need to establish TBI as a category of disability that deserved its place in medical care and rehabilitation services, in basic science and biomedical research, in professional training and education, in special education systems, in vocational rehabilitation services, and in many other programs in the vast array of human/social service systems.

There was a clear necessity to convince the private and public sectors within the established reimbursement systems that payment for services and programs was required. Unique post acute rehabilitation and extended programs are critical and ultimately cost-effective for decreasing dependency and economic burden public and private sectors. From my point of view, reduction of depe decreasing financial burden on the family and, more important, on the person who sustained the injury can stabilize families and keep them united.

Through the process of building the NHIF as a national advocacy organization, we—as families, individuals with head injuries, and professionals—joined forces in the development of these goals. Ten years later, many of the original goals have been reached and surpassed, but the job is not yet done! The progress of the head injury movement is clear within these pages. Each author has made a contribution to the movement by bringing recognition of the family as an integral component of the support and rehabilitation systems. At the time of the catastrophic event the family must be nourished and cared for. The education process should begin as soon as possible; it should be determined by the ability and receptiveness of the individual family and primary caregiver. The family's receptiveness is often determined by the compassion and communication skills of the involved professionals.

The chapters of this book provide the reader with objective, analytical, and well-documented professional approaches to interventions that can help families regain their balance, accept new roles and new realizations, and ultimately adapt to new dreams. Within these chapters readers will be touched by subjective accounts of courageous and special people. Their statements provide the depth and dimension of the real impact on caregivers in the family system—on the person with an injury, and on the family system as an entity. This book is of special value as it provides the reader with a broad perspective on how head injury is understood and perceived in the hearts and minds and experiences of persons with head injuries, families, and professionals.

Early intervention with families who have been traumatized by a catastrophic event such as TBI can make the significant difference in an array of outcome potentials. Both medical and rehabilitation professionals now acknowledge the importance of family for chronic illness and disability management, but the training required and identification of the discipline responsible are still vague. Even the established disability systems recognize the fragmentation and lack of resources and training for therapeutic and support systems for persons with head injuries.

It is easy for professionals in the field of head injury to adopt the paternalistic attitudes that pervade the community of professionals in all health care disciplines. Giving information and providing education is done with deliberate caution. Sharing resources and referrals and further networking are not within the established and traditional counseling systems. However, some hospital and rehabilitation administrators are recognizing the importance of family systems; they are encouraging their staffs to provide education and information along with sponsorship of family and patient support groups. Administrative support and professional commitment can make a vast difference!

Head injury, indeed, is a family matter—it is a family affair not entered into by choice, desire, or design. It is a matter not terminated except by death—or divorce.

This book clearly documents the uniqueness of each family in their capacity, abilities, goals, and commitment to their members. The values, rules, and roles may vary—each family has its own set of crises, burdens, fears, and challenges at the time of injury. No family is the same as another.

Tolstoy ref?

No one is prepared and ready; no family can sweep away existing issues to clear the deck for this monumental consuming event that presents complex and devastating problems. The family is often not fully matured or financially stable. Those that are may have the difficulties of coping with aging parents or may have other family members with chronic illnesses or disabilities. Many families are not prepared to cope with the social stigma and prejudices they may encounter from extended family, friends, and the community in response to the disabilities of their loved one. Negative attitudes and fear of disability still pervade our society. Also, family members must meet their own fears regarding their own aging process while worrying about their loved one who may require a lifelong support system as she or he also ages with increased disability.

With the passage of the Americans with Disability Act (ADA), the 1990s may well see changes in public attitudes toward disability. ADA will lead to improved regulations and ensure the civil rights of people with disabilities, including access to employment, public accommodations, and transportation.

As we move toward the year 2000 we will see more cooperation and unification. But we must strive for strong public and private partnerships to enhance the quality of life of persons with head injuries and their families. ADA should create an influential force on the delivery of rehabilitation services and on the development of support systems so that these opportunities may be realized and enhanced.

Again, my appreciation to the editors and the contributing authors of this book for turning their dreams into accomplishments that inspire all of us to continue to work together to reach common goals.

Marilyn Price Spivack
Founder, Past President
National Head Injury Foundation
Framingham, Massachusetts

PREFACE

Head injury happens not only to the person who sustains the injury, but to the entire family system. The injured person's process of "recovery" and redefinition of self is both paralleled by, and embedded in, the family's "recovery" and redefinition of itself as an altered family system. From a purely pragmatic point of view, understanding and dealing effectively with families' responses to head injury (and they are multiple and diverse) are essential for rehabilitation professionals, since the injured person's functional potential is largely defined by the family context, values, expectation, and relationships. The best-laid rehabilitation plans can flounder on the hidden rocks of unseen family issues.

The purpose of this book is to provide the first comprehensive consideration of the impact of head injury on the family system, from the dual perspectives of families who have experienced head injury and professionals who work with families. In addition, it provides an understanding of how families work—and how to work with families—to achieve a successful outcome during and after the formal provision of rehabilitation services.

Section I sets the stage by giving voice to six individuals who describe the issues facing the family from their own personal experience. They are unique by virtue of their ability to both communicate their experiences eloquently, and to reflect with sensitivity and intelligence on the meaning and implications of those experiences. Their range of experience is both diverse and representative. One lives in the heart of New York City, another on a rural farm in Iowa. One is the identical twin of a man with a head injury, another is the adolescent daughter of a man who sustained a head injury 11 years ago. One is married to a man with a severe head injury; another experienced an apparently "minor" head injury herself, and describes with humor and a voice of determination the struggles of the other side of marriage. In a way these stories all provide a counterpoint to the usual theme of family suffering and tragedy; these families have found a way to transcend the tragedy and teach us to appreciate the qualities of families that not only survive, but unromantically move on and flourish.

Section II provides an overview of a family systems perspective on families who have a member with a disability. Turnbull and Turnbull describe the revolutionary implications of conceptualizing the family system as the focus of intervention, rather than the person with the disability, and illustrate this perspective with commentary on the personal accounts of Section I. The chapter by Maitz applies this perspective specifically to families of persons with head injury, articulating the specific issues these families face. In her chapter on family reactions to head injury, Williams utilizes an episodic loss reaction framework to explore two models of family reaction to head injury. The practical assessment of these family reactions is described in the chapter by DePompei and Zarski, and Kay's and Cavallo's chapter on evolutions both explores the way families have been described in the research literature and suggests some parallels between the changes experienced by persons with head injury, individual family members, and family systems.

Section III is devoted to describing family needs in all phases of service delivery. It integrates earlier concepts of loss and realignment, helping people understand and deal with these issues on a day-to-day basis in each stage of rehabilitation. Grahame's chapter on the acute phase emphasizes the family's need for information, education, family assessment, and the development of an "ecologically valid" plan—one that is compatible with the individual family's needs, capacities, and value system. The community reintegration chapter by Kneipp vividly illustrates with clinical examples the importance and value of conducting family based assessments and interventions within the real-life setting of the person with head injury. The chapter by Silver, Price and Barrett charts the turbulent course of vocational rehabilitation as it involves the values, expectations, and fragile cooperation of families emotionally invested in the work and social status of the person with a head injury. And finally, Savage's chapter provides guidelines for supporting families for a successful transition back to a school system that may not understand, or be equipped to cope with, the profound changes a child and family experience after head injury.

Section IV presents special issues that are frequently encountered by families after a family member sustains a head injury. Young children encounter special problems that are different from those of young adults because they have not yet reached specific developmental milestones; these issues are dealt with by Williams and Savage. Helping families learn to cope with behavioral problems is one of the most difficult and controversial issues facing families; Jacobs's chapter presents a model for training families to deal directly with these problems. Perhaps the most troublesome and least discussed family issue after head injury is sexuality; Zasler and Kreutzer present a straightforward and practical perspective on dealing with these issues.

Section V, the final section, provides the resources and tools to provide the family intervention and support necessary to optimize family outcome after head injury. Levels of intervention for the rehabilitation team are described by Rosenthal and Hutchins. Williams describes the need for long-term informal support networks for families across the life cycle, and what form this support might take. Finally, we acknowledge and describe the resources available to families through the National Head Injury Foundation, and the powerful advocacy force that the family-professional partnership has generated to support people with head injuries and their families.

Throughout this book we have tried to conform to the guidelines for writing about people with disabilities, adopted by the Research and Training Center on Independent Living at the University of Kansas. We believe that persons with head injuries are persons first, and secondarily persons who have sustained head injuries.

We hope that this book—a documentation of experiences personal and professional—provides a resource to professionals and families. To professionals used to the medical model, we hope to convince you of the crucial importance of the family system in outcome. To professionals already convinced, we reaffirm your beliefs. To families, we hope to validate your experiences and reinforce your role as the primary support system—but also as a network of people whose relationships and selves have been altered as a result of one person's injury. The challenge to all of us is to help prepare for the lifelong commitment families make to a loved one with a head injury.

ACKNOWLEDGMENTS

All books are the result of hours of hard work and dedication (and sometimes coercion) by many people. This book is no different. We would like to thank all who made the book possible. First, we thank all of the families who have supported and tolerated our learning about the impact of head injury on the family through their experiences—including the countless families we have met individually and in support groups, especially Maureen Campbell-Korves, Doug Korves, JoAnn Kramer, Marty Beaver, Joseph Maurer, Hope Hardgrove, Opal Hardgrove, Beth O'Brien, Jane Dean, MaryPat Beals, Jean and Gerry Bush, Cindy Hutzler, Judy Ferguson, and Ginger Krueger. And most especially we thank Marilyn Price Spivack and Martin Spivack, the leaders and pioneers of the family movement, and Denise, whose creativity and sensitivity were inspirational. Sharing your experiences has given more than you will know.

Second, we thank all of the contributors who were friends and colleagues before the book and, thankfully, remain friends and colleagues after the book. We look forward to future collaborations with you.

Third, we thank all of the people who have done the behind-the-scenes work. Thanks to Kirsten Johnson, Jeanette Thomes, Barbara Koppetsch, Elise Herz, Melissa Berenson, and Claudia Jensen at the NHIF who provided the initial resources, and to Heidi Hansen McCrory and Gary Wolcott, for years of team work.

Fourth, we remember with appreciation Mary Romano. Mary was an enthusiastic supporter of and initial contributor to the book but was unable to complete her chapter before her death. She was a pioneer in understanding families, and we and her colleagues mourn her loss. Her contributions, her involvement, and her spirit remain with us.

Finally, we thank our mentors and editors. Ann P. Turnbull told us we could do it in the beginning and was the first to say she was not surprised when we did. Her constant belief, humor, and vision are an inspiration. Leonard Diller and Yehuda Ben-Yishay provided the mentorship, guidance, challenge, and belief to instill a sense of integrity and purpose. Vice President Melissa Behm and Production Editor Natalie Tyler coached us from the initial outline through the final copy; their encouragement, patience, cajoling, and cool deadlines worked wonders.

HEAD INJURY

I

FIRST
PERSON ACCOUNTS

Section I sets the tone of the book by expressing how a head injury in the family affects all members throughout the life span of the family. The entire book stresses the concept that the family system necessarily includes the person with a head injury. The perspectives of family members from diverse areas of the country with the experience—a person who has experienced head injury, a parent, a spouse, a sibling, and a child—are provided in their own words. Unlike traditional presentations of family situations, these chapters give a perspective over time rather than a snapshot of the family at any one point. The perspective of each member is clearly described and serves as a point of reference throughout the book and as a reminder that families change and adapt over time.

1

SPECIAL ISSUES
FOR A PERSON
WITH A HEAD INJURY

MAUREEN CAMPBELL-KORVES

What I was, I am not.

What I was, I am never going to be again.

The struggle to be what I have become and live with it is almost equal to the struggle involved in getting well after my head injury. It requires as much professional care, family love, and self-motivation. That sense of self, so easily defined pre-head injury, has to be redefined with a new understanding that does not come without much soul searching. Because the easy thing is to want the me I was one second before the accident and to make everyone's life hell around me because I cannot have this.

My mother has a saying, "God never closes a door that He doesn't open a window." In 1977 I started to feel those doors close, and it was a number of years before I realized the windows had opened. At that time I was attending Columbia University. The year before I had made a major change in my life by leaving a well-paid executive position at a Fortune 500 company to return to school to fulfill a dream of becoming a lawyer. I was tremendously self-motivated and disciplined. This person knew what she wanted and how to achieve those goals.

On a clear autumn afternoon I was in a taxi accident. As a result several bad things happened, but also several good. *Bad:* the accident. *Good:* no coma. *Bad:* my speech and language centers were my biggest problems. *Good:* the neurosurgeon contacted a speech pathologist who had a special feel for dealing with adult patients, and I started speech therapy 3 days after my accident. *Bad:* I was not considered injured enough to qualify for the then existing rehab programs. *Good:* My husband Doug got in touch with the Dean of Students at Columbia University, explained the situation, and within a few months the Head of the Mathematics Department volunteered to create a program to patiently reteach math to me. Doug, an architect, was very creative; we lived with a series of charts taped to mirrors and cabinets—anything that could help me remember was utilized. *Bad:* I could not remember a lot of things about the kitchen and cooking. I would put a pot on the stove to cook, walk out of the room, and forget about it until the smell of the burning pot filled our apartment. *Good:* Doug, who had not even known where the pots were kept, took over the cooking and has become a gourmet cook.

My speech pathologist was an extraordinary young woman who looked liked a china doll and acted like a boot camp drill instructor. For this I will be forever grateful. I was very dysphasic and had many problems with understanding basic English language functions. The first rule she laid down had to do with Doug and everyone I would come in contact with. "No one was to help me with words. No one was to finish my sentences, no matter how much time it required. And most of all I was not to act like I needed them to do it for me." When I look back to the 10½ months I was in intensive speech therapy, that one rule brought highs and lows.

I remember one day Doug took me shopping but made me do all the talking—my stuttering was very bad. The saleswoman never responded to me; she acted as though I was not there, asking Doug if I was retarded. That was definitely a low. But even now, years later, I can still smile when I recall my high. The first time I went grocery shopping by myself, Doug had made a list for me. He had drawn pictures of the fruits and vegetables with each name next to them. I had sat in front of the mirror practicing each word and trying to look confident. When I got to the supermarket I discovered I had lost the magic list, but I was out on my own and ready to try anything. I picked up a tomato, walked over to the young woman at the scales and said, "lemon." She smiled back at me and in a stage whisper said conspiratorially, "You dun speak English, right? I teach you." She then walked me up and down the aisle identifying fruit and vegetables. When she was finished she confided, "I been here awhile. I speek good now, you wheel too." I was so happy that I was all the way home before I remembered I hadn't bought anything. But it didn't matter; she didn't think I was retarded—she just thought I was foreign.

I thought I was doing great. I was working hard on my speech, but apparently not hard enough to put some of my friends at ease. One person literally bolted from my room not to be heard from again for years. Another person told people, "that it would be best not to call me because it was painful for me to speak." As a couple, if people dropped me, they also dropped Doug. There was also the sense that since I was beginning to look physically alright I must be alright. I was being made to feel that I was somehow letting the side down.

Five months after my accident I walked into the reflecting pool in front of the Vivian Beaumont Theater at Lincoln Center. I do not remember going into the pool, but with certainty I do remember the water seeping into my boots. Only in New York City could a fully dressed woman stand in a reflecting pool, in March, without attracting attention.

Shortly after my accident I started to complain about losing time. I could not remember whole mornings or afternoons passing by; but it was nothing that would lead me to think I had a seizure condition. After my wading debut at Lincoln Center I was finally told all about seizures and what I might expect.

I have a neighbor who happened to be in the lobby of our apartment building the day I came back wet from Lincoln Center; since that day she has never gotten on the elevator alone with me. In fact, if we are both coming out of our apartments, she will make believe she is going back inside. I live with a fantasy that because of her stupidity she is late for all important appointments.

One year after the accident I returned to school. Ever the optimist, I took a complete course load. A month after starting I knew I was in big trouble. I dropped all but one course. I worked as hard for that one course as I used to for a whole semester's work. I told the doctor (I had now been switched from a neurosurgeon to a neurologist) the problem was reading; I just did not retain what I was reading. The doctor counseled patience—I just needed to get back into it again. For the next couple of semesters I stopped and started watching my grades get worse and worse, all the while continuing to complain to the doctor, who continued to tell me how smart I was and that nothing was wrong.

In the summer of 1980, I was coming down a pool slide and had a seizure. By the time I finally hit the water I had bounced off the side of the pool and fractured all the bones in my left side from the shoulder to the waist. I spent the summer in the hospital, but that September found me back in school still trying and getting more and more depressed.

By 1981 I had started to withdraw. I doubted my sanity. Why couldn't I get things to work right? I was losing control. Try as hard as I could, I could not make things right. Decision-making was a severe problem. Simple shopping at the supermarket was painful. I now knew the names of everything, but confronted with so many choices I would cry and leave. I told my neurologist how I felt; he suggested I be less introspective and just try to get on with life. I felt I had failed miserably. I no longer left our apartment; some days I never even got dressed.

When I think back now to my first appointment with the psychiatrist I almost cringe. I was convinced that Doug and the psychiatrist were in cahoots to have me institutionalized. This was no chi-chi—because it is the latest thing to do—visit to a shrink; this was a woman hiding in the bedclothes being told she must see a psychiatrist. And I was scared. But I was finally in the right place, this man found nothing I said absurd.

In March of 1983, Jane Brody's Personal Health column in the *New York Times* was devoted to head injury. For the first time since 1977 I felt I was not alone. I now knew there were thousands of people out there like me. I showed the article to my psychiatrist and he set up an appointment for me with two neuropsychologists for testing. My neurologist completely discounted their work. He felt the whole thing was unnecessary, but they vindicated me. I was not going crazy—there was something definitely wrong with my reading abilities. I did reading therapy for the next year. Problems did not and have not completely disappeared, but things got better and I am now equipped with a new set of learning tools I can use.

By August of 1983 when the first head injury support group meeting for the New York City region was held, I was desperate. I wanted—and needed—this meeting so badly. But it is not fair to put all one's desperate expectations on someone else's shoulders. That meeting did not answer my needs, but I came back to the next meeting and all the meetings after that. I found people going through pain on all levels and I found hope. I have met wonderful people willing to share what they went through and how they are coping with their ordeals.

The most important thing the New York City Regional Head Injury Association offered me was the ability to start rebuilding a sense of myself. The more involved I became, the more I had to leave my apartment. I also started to question my neurologist about my drug therapy. I had never been able to take Dilantin, so I was taking large doses of two other drugs. With the help of Donna Whitam, a nursing specialist in head and spinal cord injuries at New York University Hospital, I got an appointment with a seizure specialist at Columbia Presbyterian Hospital. I have been able to drastically reduce my medications, but most important I found out I had become addicted to one of the drugs I was using and spent 3½ months in slow, painful withdrawal.

This created a sense of outrage that acted as a cathartic experience for me. Here I had been the perfect patient; I did everything I was told to do and still look what happened. What eventually happened was, when I finally got off my heavy drugs, I was a fiestier, more verbal person bent on not letting this happen to anyone else.

I have had to relearn patience; but there are still times when situations get the better of me. A few years ago for Head Injury Awareness month my local group had gotten permission from different hospitals to set up tables in their lobbies to distribute information. In one of the hospitals a doctor came by to look over the exhibit. He said he had never heard of us before and I launched into the merits of the Head Injury Association. We must have talked for more than 15 minutes when he asked me where I had received my training. I laughed and said I had done intimate on-the-job-training—I was head injured.

He then said, quite slowly, "Do you find day-to-day living difficult?" There was a pregnant pause and then I answered, just as slowly, "Only when I have to deal with assholes." He stood there smiling at me and then walked away. He didn't get it! Ten seconds before we had been peers, but now I was to be treated like a moron.

I was trying to take back more of the life I had handed over to Doug. I started to do some of the cooking again, but Doug would either hover just out of sight or over my shoulder. "Stir this more; lower the heat on that." I started to do a slow burn and we really had to talk it out. What was happening was that I had now become the interloper. The kitchen had become Doug's province, and I was going to have to prove I was not going to poison us or burn the house down. It has taken time, but we are now creating some memorable meals together.

The next step was asking (to be honest, I think I demanded in a loud voice) for a greater participation in the day-to-day decision-making of our married life. Since 1977 Doug and I have learned that head injury can redefine a marriage. Unless the two people involved are willing and flexible enough to change, the marriage does not stand a chance. We have sometimes gone from hero worship to hatred in a single day, but we have always come around to love. Seeking counseling to protect our marriage was important. Therapy was not a sign of weakness but rather a reaffirmation of our faith in each other.

Therapy was also the only way to get a handle on the rage inside myself. I had gone from being a partner to a nonparticipant in our marriage. And now I wanted full partner status back again. When Doug did not respond fast enough, my temper was not a pleasant thing. I only saw Doug's holding back as a lack of trust in me. I never understood his fears or need to protect me. But nothing as important as re-establishing a marriage is given to you; each of you has to reshape and earn your new role.

My final step was going back to work. Doug now had his own architectural office staffed and in place. I started going in a few hours a day and then a few days a week. In the beginning I felt so lost; I couldn't remember the day-to-day functions of running an office. Where was I supposed to fit in or what was I supposed to do? What I did do was clean the bathrooms. I think the reason I picked this work was because I still did not have a lot of confidence, and it offered a job with a place to hide. I don't know what Doug's other employees thought, but I do know we had the cleanest bathrooms of any architectural office in New York City. Slowly I did other things. I answered the telephone; I typed; I filed; I started to keep product information. It has taken a while, but I am now Office Manager.

From 1977 to now is a long time. We have come so far in our knowledge and understanding of head injury. Many of the things that happened to me then would not—please God—happen now. Through the different head injury associations we have all learned to ask more questions and demand better quality care. The founding of the National Survivors' Council has offered a strong voice for we who are head injured. If we want to see things change then we have to be willing to become involved. We cannot sit back, complain, and then expect someone else to do for us. We must become our own best advocates, and the Survivors' Council offers this opportunity.

So in retrospect, I am not the person I was pre-head injury, but I have learned something very important, "Head injury does not mean being bad. It just means being different from who you were before. Not good, not bad, just different."

2

SPECIAL ISSUES
FOR A PARENT

JOANN KRAMER

Our family experienced a very permanent change in our lives in December of 1975—2 days after Christmas to be exact—when our 10-year-old daughter Jennifer suffered a severe brain stem injury in a fall from a horse on our family farm. We have been living with the changes precipitated by that tragic event for 14 years.

The day of the accident was what Midwesterners refer to as an "open winter"—very little snow on the ground and milder temperatures on sunny days than one normally expects in Iowa. My husband Jerry had stayed home with our two children while my cousin and I had gone antiquing in the morning. We had stopped at a grocery store around noon, and I had just started down the aisle with a grocery cart mentally sorting through a menu that I had planned for a Sunday dinner for aunts and uncles the following day. The radio was playing out into the store and a news commentator interrupted the music and said that a 10-year-old girl named Jennifer Kramer had been taken to the hospital and was in serious condition after a fall from a horse. I couldn't believe what I was hearing, and in disbelief I went to a telephone and called my mother. She was not aware of the event, so my cousin and I left the store and drove to my home about 20 miles away; I was still imagining that I had been hearing things. The people that were boarding their horses at our home were there because they had heard the same report on the radio that I had. They confirmed the news report, and drove me to the hospital where I joined my husband and 8-year-old son Nate. Details were blurry, but a doctor came out and told us that she was a very sick girl and that if she did recover she would probably be aphasic. (I didn't know what that meant at the time!) It must be recognized that at the time of Jennifer's injury we did not have a neurosurgeon in our town and a general surgeon was called in. The hospital did not have a CAT scanner, or an intracranial pressure measure at that point in time either.

A National Guard helicopter pilot came in eventually to the emergency area and asked if we were the girl's parents. She had to be air lifted to a major university hospital in Iowa City 100 miles away for intensive care. We were told that we were unable to ride in the helicopter, so we drove home as the helicopter was taking off from the hospital lawn. My parents came over to our home and stayed with our son. We packed our bags and took off about 10:00 at night. The night seemed darker than usual, and the 100-mile drive seemed like a journey through a long tunnel. We arrived at the hospital and found our way to the intensive care unit. The nursing staff and the night chaplain gave us support and information. After a visit to Jennifer's bedside with the tubes and machines dominating, we were encouraged to get a motel room down the hill from the hospital. We methodically drove there and checked in. After we had gotten into bed, my body began to shake uncontrollably. My husband held me; we cried together and eventually fell into an exhausted sleep, praying for life for our seemingly lifeless daughter just up the hill.

That was the beginning of what was supposed to be a relaxing holiday vacation. Time took on a new meaning—every hour was life or death—we weren't sure which way the pendulum would swing. It was comforting when professionals including nurses, residents, and clergy were concerned with our emotional needs from the onset. They encouraged us to get out of the hospital for meals and breaks between intensive care visits. One nurse even offered us her apartment while she was going to be away so that we could go to a home-like atmosphere and watch television. However, it was very difficult to leave the hospital, and the emotional closeness to Jennifer helped us through the child-in-coma frustration that all parents feel regardless of the age of the child. A few close friends, family members, and our pastor came to visit us in the intensive care waiting area over the next couple of days. The weirdest time was spending New Year's Eve in the hospital with hardly anyone around, feeling numb to festivity.

Jerry had to go back to school the day after New Year's, but I was able to arrange emergency medical leave. The time from December 27 lengthened into 3 weeks, with a series of crisis times. We were never quite certain if Jenny would live or die in this time period, and we learned early on to take life an hour at a time. Jerry found it even more difficult to be 100 miles away from the hospital scene, but he had to return to work and also maintain the home atmosphere for our son.

Fortunately, grandparents kept our household organized so that our son could carry on his life in the absence of his parents. His life as a sibling of a person with head injury began on the day of the accident when he maturely waited at the end of our farm lane for the ambulance to arrive. He remembers the "very fast" ride in the deputy sheriff's car as they led the way to the hospital.

Telephone calls, telegrams, and cards from friends arrived constantly. Our family physician called the University Hospital frequently to check on Jennifer's condition, and the nursing staff always communicated his concern to us. We were encouraged to talk to Jennifer even though she could not respond, and I resorted to reading to her from a Laura Ingalls Wilder book that she had been reading prior to her accident. I found a great deal of comfort from the sound of my voice, but the sentences carried little meaning as I helplessly kept vigil at her bedside without any response from her.

We had a tremendous mentor for modeling communication with physicians from the patient advocate provided in the intensive care unit. The patient advocate was a retired physician whom I had known from Student Health Services when I was a student at the University of Iowa. We were supported and coached by this compassionate person to make appointments with specific doctors and address questions to them personally, even "busy" neurosurgeons. We developed bonds with other individuals and families in the intensive care area. The financial stress was obvious, and for those individuals unable to afford lodging and food to be near their loved one, the hospital provided room and board in an area of the nurses' dorm. Today a Ronald McDonald House is within walking distance of the hospital.

Jerry and I had a stable marriage relationship before we were thrust into the injured family environment. We share similar values, and work diligently at parenting. In the hospital we were with some families that were not intact, and the guilt feelings could be observed in the numbers of people reuniting in the intensive care waiting room. Some family members had not seen the critically injured person for years, and individuals were attempting to reunite over the comatose person. A counselor provided as a service later in acute rehab helped us deal with guilt feelings that we might have had so that we could go on with the business at hand, and that was to adjust to the new person who had resulted from the injury.

I have vivid memories of Jenny receiving a basketball as a Christmas present the day before her accident. The agile, aggressive, little bubbly blond girl dribbled that ball all over our farm house and was so excited. Twenty-four hours later she was lying in intensive care, eyes closed and decerebrate. This is where the new and different Jenny began. I cried every day for at least a year out of frustration, and at intermittent times later. It took me 5 years to truly accept the personality change and to totally convince myself that I could handle this new person in my mind.

Another stressful time for families in recovery is when the patient is moved from one level of care to another. The cycle begins anew with building trust in other health professionals. A family with a person with a head injury often faces a long period of hospitalization. Family members get tired and in time may address some of their latent anger for the situation that they have been thrust into with the nursing staff or other health professionals. If professionals are aware of the possibility of prolonged stress on a family and its manifestations, they can attempt to help the family rather than take the criticism personally.

Jenny improved enough after 5 weeks to be moved back to our local hospital. We were relieved to be home, but Jenny remained in acute rehab for 2 months. I returned to work half time as a result of having an understanding employer. My husband's school district would not allow him to teach half time, so we were fortunate that at least one of us could modify our work schedule for a period of time. Jerry and I were able to split up the hospital visits and also include our son in his sister's recovery process. We were exhausted emotionally, but mustered strength to comfort others who came to see Jenny. The therapists and medical staff gave us support and educated us on how to help with Jenny's care. We are eternally grateful to our family physician who networked us to the appropriate professionals, but at the same time kept knowledgeable of Jenny's progress and supportive of our family.

Jenny's speech returned spontaneously one day in February, and this seemed like a miracle because we were living with the fear that she could be aphasic. A new world opened—we could again begin to communicate in words! At first the rehab plan was to allow Jenny to come home when she was able to walk again, but the plan was changed when Jenny did not seem to progress as quickly as hoped. The doctor felt that she would get stronger in her home environment, so we brought her home at the end of March. She could only crawl for mobility, and physically was skin and bones. The staff had coached us on how to help her. We forced her to crawl upstairs to bed every night, rather than carrying her, even though she would whine and cry most of the way. We put her mattress on the floor so she could crawl into her bed as well. Our parents helped us with care the days I worked, and as I reflect on the emotional pace we kept, I think we operated day-to-day on sheer visceral fortitude.

An in-home tutor was provided by the area education agency as soon as she came home. We continued to take Jenny to out-patient physical therapy. In May it was determined to try a half day of school with a full-time aide in the classroom. It was difficult for Jenny's classmates to deal with a new person who wasn't able to be an aggressive playground buddy. She was confined to a wheelchair, and didn't even look like the same person because her head had been shaved and she was unusually thin. That summer she made physical progress and was able to walk with a brace. We took part in a summer Vacation Ventures program for other kids with special needs, arranged through the area education agency. The program provided stimulation and socialization for Jenny, as well as parent education. I was involved in summer school at the

University, so Jerry was the parent who accompanied Jenny to school. He was the only man in the parent class, but was glad that teaching offered him the summer to be involved in Jenny's rebuilding process.

Re-entry into the school and community seemed like a nightmare for the next 3–4 years. Most of Jenny's friends gradually quit coming to visit her, and her brother became increasingly embarrassed by her inappropriate behavior. An alert school psychologist counseled us the first fall post-injury to seek a more structured school setting outside of our home community to provide for her needs as well as to have Jenny and her brother in separate schools for his sake. She attended a parochial school for a year and a half, and then went to a regular junior high with resource room support in seventh grade. This was a setting in a community 15 miles from our home, chosen for the teacher, not the label of the program. Jenny was not successful academically or socially in the mainstream and was placed in a self-contained classroom for emotionally disturbed students in a temporary classroom across the street from the junior high. She was somewhat successful, but sometimes would refuse to go to school, or would run away from the school and come back later. The principal knew where she was on these occasions and she always returned for the ride home. The principal counseled us to seek a more structured school setting for grades 10–12.

When we were at our wits' end in this stage of re-entry, we made an appointment to talk with our family physician about consultation through the University Hospital system. He arranged for an outpatient evaluation with a psychiatrist and a pediatric neurologist. The staff neurosurgeon who took care of Jennifer in acute care told us at discharge that if we ever felt that we needed psychiatric services to be sure and come back to that source. I thought that was a strange piece of advice, and it wasn't until a period of time post-injury that I understood his savvy. The result of that visit was that we were encouraged to seek family counseling at a local mental health clinic to help manage Jenny's behavior and our response to her as a family. We were not mentally ill, and neither was Jenny, but we needed counseling support. We were counseled on how to help guide her through resistance to school and how to gain a better degree of management in the home. She received individual counseling as well to help her deal with her low self-concept. One morning we had to physically pull her out from under the bed and state that we would take her to school in her pajamas if she didn't get dressed. Many mornings were a long, stressful wait because Jenny had become progressively more manipulative. Work was therapy for both Jerry and me because managing teenagers in our work was a relief compared to living with a child with a head injury. Our children grew further apart rather than together. Jenny felt so inferior and responded with a negative attitude. Nate found her increasingly frustrating and was embarrassed to bring friends home. They actually hated each other for several years. Social visits as a family were often uncomfortable, too. Our friends who stuck with us through those difficult times will eternally be appreciated. Without them, we would have felt even more isolated.

Jenny would have dropped out of high school and our family would have been very stressed had we not found a private residential school for students with learning disabilities in Colorado. Jenny lived with boarding parents in a home-like atmosphere, and we had weekly contact with Jenny and her boarding parents on the telephone. Most parents could not understand how we could "send" our daughter off to school so far from home, but most also could not empathize with the stress that her recovery put on our entire family. We rationalized the situation by the belief that she would not have remained in school, and her future was at stake. There was just not anything close by that seemed a possibility for meeting her needs. No one knew what to do, so as parents we took charge of the situation and went after the funding.

The cost for the private school was shared. The education agency paid for her tuition and we paid board and transportation expenses. We were fortunate that we both had jobs and could help finance the costs. We were desperate, and we viewed the school as essential for her future. There were no other appropriate options in our state.

After graduation Jenny spent over a year at home because she had determined that she wanted to work and be near home for awhile. She had never worked prior to injury, so she had no work experience to draw from. In retrospect, we believe that she would have progressed better vocationally if we had had a structured vocational program for her to make a transition into immediately after high school. She professed wanting to work, but even after Jerry had educated an employer who was willing to give her a chance, she was not successful. She could drive, so she went to work independently. At least we thought she was going to work, but we later learned that she left early the first day and never showed up again. She led us to believe that she was going to work 3 half days per week, and it wasn't until Jerry followed up with the employer a couple of weeks later that we learned she had been faking.

We were frustrated that Jenny could lie to us so skillfully. Our next idea was to encourage her to do volunteer work at a hospital or nursing home. She tried both, but was never able to sustain the interest in either over a period of time. Her self-worth was increasingly depleted, so we arranged for a private counselor to help her see the possibilities for moving on with her life. Jerry and I began to explore the options for adult services and programs in our state. We convinced Jenny to meet with DVR (Department of Vocational Rehabilitation). She walked out on the first interview, but we remained and discussed options. An evaluation at the DVR center in Des Moines was arranged after Jenny kept a couple of other appointments with the DVR counselor. We simultaneously applied for SSI (supplemental security income) once she was approved for DVR services—we didn't realize she was eligible for this funding until DVR made us aware of it.

We had learned of a semi-independent living program in Minnesota specifically for persons with head injury through an NHIF (National Head Injury Foundation) contact we had worked with at the national level. DVR was willing to fund the vocational component, but we were on our own to obtain funding for the residential part. We contacted the State Department of Human Services for funding options, and a social worker went with us to a County Board of Supervisors' meeting where we requested support for 6 months for the program for Jennifer. They listened politely, but turned us down by not bringing the issue to a vote. There was a long pause at the meeting—we again felt the isolation of dealing with head injury. One supervisor spoke up and said that she felt that they should study the issue. The others agreed. We helped the compassionate supervisor with research, and about a month later they voted to fund Jennifer. Jenny had entered the program a month before the funding was approved, but we had determined that we would borrow the money for 3 months if necessary because she had to take the spot available in the program or lose the opportunity.

Jenny moved to Minnesota with mixed emotions. Many setbacks occurred in the vocational program because it took place in a facility with persons with mental retardation, and she was not comfortable in that environment. Community placements were attempted, but not successful. She has been in the semi-independent living program for 3½ years and is now a legal resident of Minnesota. She is ready to move into an apartment without 24-hour supervision but with case management and support available through a county funded program. However, there are no vacancies at present in the low-income housing.

Jenny did not date in high school, although she really would have liked a boyfriend like her peers. Her social immaturity was not likely to attract young men her age. She was usually most comfortable talking to elderly people because they would listen to her. Sex issues surfaced when Jenny moved into her own apartment in Minnesota. She may have repressed her interests when she was living at home, as she did not have the opportunity to meet many young people and was not working. The public health nurse provided by the county that Jenny lives in has been dealing with birth control issues. Jenny has personally decided to have a tubal ligation because she believes that she could not deal with bearing and raising a child and is opposed to abortion. As parents we are relieved and very supportive of her decision and can appreciate why it has taken her a couple of years to reach her decision.

This summer Jenny applied for low-income housing in a town near our farm. Once there is an opening she would like to move back to Iowa to be closer to her family. We believe that we will be ready for that when the time comes if we have a third party to provide service coordination for her. She will always need some support, and we know that we would be burned out in a short time helping Jenny manage her daily living. We believe that it is important to her future for her to continue developing her self-advocacy skills.

Four years post-injury we received a letter from our rehab physician calling families together who had experienced head injury. We attended the initial meeting and were amazed that some people had driven over 100 miles to attend. The 20 or so of us who were present provided the nucleus of the present Iowa Head Injury Association. The support group provided us with people with similar needs, and this beginning gave us access to state and national advocacy networks as well as friends all over the U.S. with whom to share information. We were fortunate to have a rehab physician so tuned into the needs of families and willing to share his time. We still attend support group meetings, as they have helped us adjust to changes in the stages of life in living with a person with head injury. As parents we still feel pain that Jenny's quality of life will never be what it could have been without the trauma of head injury. We deal with our sadness by working diligently in advocacy and support groups at the state and national levels. We believe that our volunteer work will assist others in gaining access to systems and supports in a more concise manner. We are thankful for Jennifer's life, and we celebrate the opportunity that God has given us to help others through her life.

As I reflect on the course of life after head injury for our family, I have identified five issues that keep surfacing as we move with time:

Grieving—Initial and life stages—We first grieve over the loss of the child that was. After time we begin grieving through life stages because our child is not experiencing those stages in a normal progression or at a level that he or she might have.

Communication—Families must learn to communicate with professionals and each other. With knowledge comes understanding and gradual acceptance and wisdom to deal with the lifelong changes. Emotional support also is a result of communication with family and friends.

Family stability—The entire family is injured. The marriage relationship is threatened because of the emotional and physical demands of care for a person with head injury. Counseling may be necessary to guide families through rough times in the recovery process. Marriage partners need respite away from the family—"Honeymoon Weekends."

Dealing with the system—Obtaining financial support for needed services taxes time and energy. NHIF support and advocacy is now available for help. Transition from educational to adult services is a tense time because parents sometimes have difficulty accepting the reality of an adult child with reduced abilities and responses.

Permanency planning—Parents need help to give the adult with head injury the dignity of risk. Many persons with head injury will need lifetime support, and in a sense the parents have to give up the parenting role to a third party to help the person achieve more independence. Wills and trusts must be carefully planned so as not to deprive the person with head injury of necessary benefits.

3

SPECIAL ISSUES
FOR A SPOUSE

MARTY BEAVER

Marriage was always a childhood dream for me. I always wanted to be a wife and have children. This possibility began in 1966 when I met John. He had just gone through a very traumatic divorce and needed a friend. He was hurt and very depressed. He said that he could never again trust another person. Our friendship grew and I fell in love. For John love did not come easy or soon. Over time love grew and matured between the two of us. Over the next 3 years we spent a lot of time together. John was committed to getting debt free prior to our marriage and worked two jobs for more than 9 months. During this time I graduated from nursing school, began my career, and lived on my own. After 5 years of dating my dream came true as John and I were married in March of 1971. Plans for our future together were made and prioritized and we worked toward a home of our own. Ours was a special relationship, we were best friends and shared everything with each other. We both enjoyed snow skiing, water skiing, rafting, and entertaining our friends. Although I tried, I could not really share John's love for deer hunting. We complemented each other and I was emotionally very dependent upon him to provide that listening ear, support, concern, and objectivity that I needed. I was not financially dependent upon him, as I had a profession of my own.

After 3 years of marriage and moving into our own home on the lake, we were blessed with the birth of our son Mark. Three and a half years later we had a beautiful daughter, Nicole. After 7 years of marriage we were on top of the world. We had grand dreams for the future, ours was a marriage many couples envied.

Suddenly our dream was shattered. John was injured in a work-related accident and was in a coma with little hope for survival. When faced with this crisis I was numb. This just couldn't be happening to us, the ideal family.

During this crisis period, my faith in God and support from family and friends provided me with a great deal of strength. Because I was at the hospital so much I spent very little time with our children, now ages 3½ years and 6 months. They needed me more than ever, but I didn't realize that at the time. This is a mistake many care providers make during the crisis and rehabilitation period. Children in the family need to be given love and attention. They are not as flexible as you might think.

Following a week in a coma, John began his physical recovery. I was elated that my husband was going to live and felt that he would be "normal" in a matter of weeks. After 6 weeks in acute care he was transferred to a local rehabilitation facility for another 6 weeks. Little was known about head injury in 1978, and, without any physical limitations, John was the only walking patient at this rehab center. The staff had no idea of what to do when John pulled the fire alarm twice during his first 24 hours. When John was moved to this rehab facility it was very difficult for me to let go, for I had been with John almost all of the time, and now I could only visit in the evening. I did not know it was best for all of us.

John's rehabilitation was little more than an evaluation, and we were quickly at home to deal with John's cognitive deficits with little assistance. I had been told that John would reach his "full" recovery at 6 months. As this time drew closer I became more and more anxious. I needed and wanted some answers. The "not knowing" what the immediate future would bring was hard for me to deal with. After all, I was a health care professional and my business was that of making people well. Why couldn't something be done for John? Those months at home were exhausting, as I aimed toward providing structure and therapy for John along with balancing my role as mother for two young children. The responsibility of disciplining and teaching our children became a problem because their father was more difficult to manage than the kids.

We had suffered a great loss, and it was as though we were not given an opportunity to grieve. I had lost my best friend, my lover, my husband, and the father of my children, but because he was physically present, that loss was not readily recognized by anyone. I missed the friendship, intimacy, and sexual fulfillment that our marriage had held.

Although some improvement was noted, John became more and more depressed and I grew more and more concerned that he would have some long-term problems. We began our search for a specialized head injury rehab facility, but no center was found. I needed more family help and support, so we moved closer to John's family. John was unable to handle a different environment, and due to his anxiety and agitation, he had to be admitted to a psychiatric facility. This was certainly not in John's best interest, but we had no other choice at that time.

After a few months of inappropriate treatment, John was sent up north to a large rehab center for an extensive work up and evaluation. During these 3 months, having finally found professionals who knew what they were doing, I began to accept that John had serious deficits and began to think of the future for my children and me. At this time I was given some of my options for the future, being told of the seriousness of John's injury.

I was young, had become the sole head of our household, and had two preschool-age children to raise and a dependent husband. There was tremendous frustration as I searched for help for John and our family. No one knew very much about those who survived a severe brain injury. The cognitive and behavioral consequences were more than most could imagine. The trials and tribulations of running a household, raising children, and being responsible for everything put me under a great deal of pressure. I was used to having a husband who shared all the "family" responsibilities. I wished for someone else to make a decision, or pay a bill, or answer a question, but the reality was—it was left up to me. The constant and total responsibility for two children was ever present, even when a member of the family helped by keeping them. I was not sure how I could go another day with these burdens and responsibilities. Only by having faith in God and living one day at a time did I mentally and physically survive.

Because John's behavior was adversely affected by continuous interaction with family, John was returned to our home town to live in an apartment with 24-hour attendants. Without the proper psychological support and management, this plan was doomed to fail. These 9 months were some of the most difficult, as John's behavioral problems soared. Again we had to move John out of state to find a treatment facility for persons with behavioral problems associated with head injury. This move was much easier, as I was becoming more and more aware of John's problems. I wanted the best for him and was ready for anything that sounded optimistic.

With John away from home, my children and I became very close. We only had each other, and I worried about the fact that they could not be raised in a two-parent household. I knew that a young boy needs a male role model. Members of our families filled in as that male figure, but I knew it just was not the same. I grieved for both of my children as I remembered how much my father meant to me as a child. I also grieved for John as I realized how much he had lost—he lost everything short of his life.

Behaviorally, John showed much improvement in his new treatment environment. Otherwise, he was still unable to care for himself without many prompts and cues. He had no short-term memory and had a very short attention span. He knew and remembered everything prior to the accident but nothing since.

It was during this time that I learned of the National Head Injury Foundation (NHIF), a newly formed organization for persons with head injuries and their families. I sent in my membership and shared my trials of lack of resources and understanding. I attended a conference on head injury and, after meeting Marilyn Price Spivack, the founder, came back to Georgia with the commitment to begin an NHIF chapter. I was soon put in touch with two other family members who shared my frustrations. Together we started the Georgia Head Injury Foundation (GHIF). I poured myself into the organization and had little time to think of myself or socialize. When not working full time, caring for two children, or visiting my husband, I was talking to individuals and groups and sending out information about head injury and its consequences. With the help of many caring professionals and family members we were able to see a lot of growth in our infant organization. It was easy to see that I was not alone; there was a head injury epidemic in the nation. I was in the minority as a spouse, though.

Ever since John's accident I had wanted so much to meet another wife and mother who was in a similar situation. I felt it would be good to be able to share some of my feelings with someone who really understood. After 3 years I met Opal, who more than met my expectations. Her understanding, role modeling, and support have meant so much to me over the last 9 years.

After a year in rehab John was making little improvement, and it was time to make some long-term decisions. I wanted so much for John to be well enough to come home to live with me and our children. After all, he was my husband and their father. He needed full-time attendant care and his behavior was still a problem. Decisions had to be made with everyone in mind, not just John. I knew that John would want his children to be given every opportunity to develop in a happy and secure environment.

What would happen if John came home? How would our children respond? How could I manage? It took my closest friend to help me see what had to be done. She brought me into reality and helped me to realize the decisions that had to be made. John's family was very supportive and agreed that a lifelong care facility for him would be in the best interest of the whole family.

Many spouses make a decision for their husband or wife to come back into the home environment. I had to choose another direction. Either way, the decisions are difficult and usually meet with resistance or negativism from friends and family. I know that my decision for long-term care was made easier because I had cared for John at home for 9 months prior to extensive rehabilitation. I doubt I would have made the decision without that experience. I was also very fortunate in that John's care and rehabilitation were covered by workers' compensation. I know many other spouses who struggle to get necessary therapies approved by private insurance that will not provide for lifelong care. The financial burdens of most families with persons with head injury are staggering. This is especially true when the person with the injury is the husband. Those wives who care for their head injured husbands are often unable to work outside the home due to the attention and care their loved one requires. This places undue stress on the caretaker and other family members. My profession was a life saver for our family, as I became the sole provider.

Being married without a partner placed additional stresses on me. Socially I was in limbo (Lezak, 1978), not fitting with any group—couples, singles, divorcees, or widows. Even spouses with their husband/wife at home may also have to deal with this feeling because of the social/behavioral problems that the spouse with a head injury often displays. I know that when John was at home, going out with another couple was just not the same as before his accident. His behavioral and social problems were embarrassing to me.

When John and I married it was for "better or for worse, in sickness or in health." These vows, when taken as a lifelong commitment, are very important and extremely difficult to break. The opportunity to discuss the option of divorce, along with appropriate understanding and guidance, needs to be provided to both the spouse and person with a head injury. Emotional and ethical concerns, as well as financial, legal, social, and religious issues must be taken into consideration.

Eleven years following John's accident my children and I are satisfied with our life as it is now. I still grieve for John and his losses and look back at the shattered hopes and dreams, but with a strong Christian faith I face each day with optimism and hope. Who knows what the future will bring? John shows little cognitive improvement but seems content and is well cared for. Our children are typical teens. Mark just turned 16, is driving, and loves basketball. Nicole, at 11, enjoys being with her friends and cares much too much about how she looks. Me, I enjoy my work coordinating special projects for the Nursing Department at the hospital where I have worked for 18 years. I am very involved in my church family; I stay involved with my children and after many years have not yet totally gotten over the emptiness I feel without John.

REFERENCES

Lezak, M.D. (1978). Living with the characterologically altered brain injured patient. *Journal of Clinical Psychiatry, 39*, 592–598.

4

SPECIAL ISSUES
FOR A CHILD

HOPE HARDGROVE

One tragic day, just a few weeks before I turned 5, my life was shattered just like a crystal glass being dropped on a hard surface. I did not realize then what had happened. My dad, whom I loved and adored, was lying in a hospital bed with a brain injury, and whether or not he would live only God knew.

August 10, 1979, began, I suppose, as any other day. My mom and dad got up, got ready for work and got me up and ready for school, then we each went our separate ways. That afternoon I was told my dad had been in an accident. As I recall, I was concerned, but I didn't really know what to do. And besides that, what does a child of 4 comprehend of an "accident?" For weeks I was "left out in the cold" not knowing how to act or what to do; I didn't even know what was going on. I suppose I was told, but it never was explained until I was older what had happened. All I knew was my mom would go to work, and I would go to school. After school I would go to a nursery or to my grandmother's, and after my mom got home from work, she would run in just long enough to see how my day was and then she was gone again to see Daddy. This was repeated for days and weeks. During this time I really missed my mom and dad. I missed their love and attention. I was looking so forward to the day things would return to "normal." Little did I know things would never be normal for our family again.

The months of rehabilitation are a blur. I have no idea what went on. All I remember is for weeks at a time I wouldn't see either Mom or Dad, not any. I remember, though, the first time I saw Dad after the injury; even though his face was really messed up, I was ecstatic. I knew things were going to return to normal soon.

When Mom finally brought Dad home, I was so happy. Dad was home again and everything was normal. This feeling continued for about a day or so after he got home. See, I was never told until Dad got home that he wasn't normal anymore, that his injury took away the part of his brain which controlled whether he was upset and angry, or whether he was happy and content. Weeks passed and I realized this was the same man that was my father, but he was very different. He functioned on my level, and although he was an adult and my father, I treated him as a 5-year-old. Well, of course, he really didn't appreciate the above reaction; therefore, he would get mad. Dad's anger wasn't just a little bit of a raised voice. On an anger scale of 1–10, he would hit a 100. When he got mad I had best go to my room and let him cool down to at least a 10, which usually took about 10 minutes, and then within 5 minutes he was happy and whistling away.

Dad has not hit the all time high of 100 anytime recently, but he still hits a 20–25 sometimes, but within a minimal amount of time he is perfectly happy again. I would say over the past 10 years Dad has improved a lot. He has been in a behavioral modification program, which really benefited us all. Thanks to this, Daddy is usually very, very happy. He is constantly singing, humming, talking, etc. Although the change from being almost constantly angry to continually happy may seem better to you, the singing etc. gets very annoying. Have you ever had to stay in a house with someone who 90% of the time is singing, whistling, etc., while you are studying, reading, or talking on the telephone? I will admit, though, after 8 years of this it really gets very amusing sometimes, but it gets old fast too. These are just a few of the things I have had to accept as part of Dad's injury.

When I was 6, about 2 years after Dad's injury, I became a Christian. Even though I was a Christian, I developed a very strong hate and became very angry towards my father. When I realized God had let this happen to my wonderful father, I also began to hate God. This continued for about 8 years until almost a year ago. I realized God let this happen for a purpose in my life, and that I need to be thankful for it. Now I still struggle, especially when Dad gets mad, but I am learning to accept and be thankful for this abnormal life.

Dad has been home almost 9½ years now, and I have had to accept his behavior and everything else due to his injury. This includes giving up things most families and adolescents can do, such as having a friend over to spend the night or playing a game with the family, because Dad can't emotionally take things like this. To me, the hardest thing to accept about a parent with a brain injury is their behavior. I constantly wonder what people think of me when they see me with my dad and he gets mad because he drops something in public, for example. I get totally embarrassed, but I am learning that it is not me he is embarrassing; it's himself. It is not me that people think is strange; it is him. It is not me people are blaming for his unusual behavior; all eyes are on him.

Head injury is a horrible thing to go through, and there is no support whatsoever for 13–19-year-olds with parents who have had head injuries. I just really wish there was some way we could have the support of each other and talk about our circumstances and hear others so maybe ours wouldn't be so bad. I am sure, depending on the extent of the injury the parent sustains, a son or daughter will respond and feel differently. I have presented the way I have felt as the daughter of a dad with a severe head injury.

5

SPECIAL ISSUES
FOR A SIBLING

JOSEPH MAURER

The sibling of a person who has experienced a head injury faces a number of challenging, if not unique, issues within the family. To the extent that my own experiences can shed light on the experiences of other siblings, I relate them briefly here.

Like most siblings of individuals with a head injury, I knew nothing about head injury when my identical twin Ed had a near-fatal motorcycle accident 5 years ago. Ed, 31 at the time of his injury, had been a sometimes rebellious, always spirited outdoorsman in Seattle, Washington with a fledgling general contracting business to finance his real passions. Our own paths had diverged dramatically over the years, with me pursuing a career in the entertainment business in Los Angeles. I had often considered, with some envy, his more mellow life-style—one that allowed unscheduled hang gliding expeditions to Mt. Ranier or a late afternoon sail around Lake Washington. Despite our separate paths, we had remained close, with the special intimacy of twins that even our older sister Maryann, though close to us both, could not share.

Into each family experiencing head injury comes a life-changing telephone call. Mine came from my parents, who had already arrived in Seattle from their home in San Jose, California. They had been trying to reach me for several hours. The message was chilling. Ed's motorcycle had skidded on a wet road and slammed into a tree. He had taken the full impact on his unhelmeted head. He had then been thrown some 25 feet down a cliff onto a concrete jogging path along Lake Washington. He was comatose. The prognosis was not good. They hoped I could get to Seattle before he died. Dumbstruck, I took the next plane from Burbank.

The first few days there were a blur, with Ed's broken body wired to a snakelike tangle of life support equipment at Harborview Medical Center's intensive care unit. For me, as his brother, the days were fraught with emotional upheaval of every type. There was the first look horror and disbelief at his condition. There were the confusing, jargon-laden emergency conferences with neurosurgeons, and the absolute uncertainty that, if Ed lived, he would have any brain functions left. There was the stark confrontation with my own mortality. I had experienced a potent premonition of his accident—and continued to sense (even, I think, before the doctors) his waxing and waning condition. There was the unsettling immersion into his world, his friendships, his history—as the waiting room filled up with friends and the curious (many of whom I had never met).

My parents, Mary and Ed, are strong, likable people. But I felt, and would continue to feel, a particular stab of sorrow when I looked into their careworn faces. The strain on them, on me, on my brother's girlfriend, and on my sister (who flew in from her home and family in West Virginia), was acute. Ed's girlfriend, Laurie, a lovely woman I had known as well since childhood, was good enough to put us all up in the small house she and my brother owned together. There were tensions here, though, as she and Ed had recently separated. Laurie needed solace too, and we had descended on her and her life, upsetting all that was familiar and private. None of this, during those first few weeks, mattered. We had circled the family wagons to survive a nightmare.

Siblings, I think, even in the first days of trauma, undergo sweeping changes. I found myself on some subtle levels becoming the caregiver, the parent, to my own family. In those first early mornings—when you awaken to the crushing weight of what has happened, when you race to the telephone to see if your brother has survived the night, when you strategize the family's plans for the day, spelling each other at the hospital—the sibling takes on a new role. It's a role for which there are no guidelines—just instinct and gut feeling. And one begins to live moment by moment—taking baby steps to avoid shattering altogether. I found myself becoming suddenly protective of all our emotions—trying to buffer my parents and sister (and myself) from unwanted visitors, unnecessary long-distance telephone calls, a callous meeting with a social worker who had not acquainted herself adequately with my brother's condition, but felt compelled to share her worst case scenarios with us. The sibling (and I have seen this even with younger siblings) finds himself playing new roles during this time—often taking the lead with doctors and nursing staff, gaining a higher profile than what had been traditionally the role within the family structure. It is, I recall well, a disorienting time.

Ed, miraculously, survived. My sister returned to her young boys and husband, grieving at her inability to be a more active participant in Ed's slow recovery. I, too, grieved over that impossibility of time, distance, and financial imperatives. My parents, as is so often the case in other families with head injuries, became Ed's primary caregivers during those first few months that became years. My mother rented a house in Seattle for a time and brought my brother there after his 8-week stay in various hospitals. His HMO had determined that, since he was ambulatory, he was no longer in need of rehabilitation—just one of the many incongruous medical realities my family and brother have faced since this phase in our lives began. The sibling learns an Olympian patience, or goes mad, I suppose.

The sibling often wrestles with deep frustrations at not being able to provide direct care. As older siblings particularly, we are often just starting families or businesses, launching our own lives when the trauma occurs. And there is a tangle of guilt attached to returning to those lives and obligations when our sibling is so imperiled.

The tension between parents and sibling mounts as well. Despite my own family's general openness and ability to discuss our problems, I witnessed the literal decay of my mother's health (and my father's temperament) during those early months of family-based rehabilitation. I felt resentment toward my brother. How dare he drive (perhaps intoxicated) on a motorcycle and bring all this down upon us? How dare he become so dependent that he dragged down my mother's, and then my father's health in his consuming need for attention and care? Irrational, perhaps, but real feelings nonetheless. Almost in the same breath, I would recognize his own titanic problems—and eventually his own sadness at needing so much help even though he knew on some level what a toll it exacted on our parents. This tangle of emotions, though certainly not the unique domain of siblings, is frequently a factor in the family's recovery.

I noticed, when I was able to visit Seattle (and later my parents' San Jose house, where Ed lived for over a year), that I could play a certain valuable, if limited, role in Ed's rehabilitation. As one who was not his primary caregiver, I could be lighter with him, prod him into old sibling games, push him to pick up the guitar again, recall intimate family moments that helped him recapture his memory, needle him good-naturedly to lift weights (a painful and mind-tiring process for him), force him to reclaim what remained of his old self. I could also provide needed respite for my parents, who ultimately did a remarkable job of helping Ed regain first his legs, then his speech, and eventually much of his old self (and some new as well).

These days my parents, sister, and I continue to refine our complex interdependence where Ed is concerned. As his brother, and the one who perhaps understands him best of all, I begin, delicately, to shoulder the responsibility for Ed's later years—and all of the financial, legal, and medical details attached to that stewardship. It is a role siblings (and their parents) could use considerable help in addressing. Never a great track star, I find the baton-pass a challenge.

My relationship with Ed, too, is changing. We are, in many ways, more dependent on each other than before. It is a delicate transition which allows me to sometimes be "the older brother," and other times forces me to "know my place." There is much Ed does *not* need me for. And the dance, as his brother, I am learning, involves equal steps forward and back. I am proud of the independence he exercises. It will help us both survive in the long run.

Today Ed lives in a group home in a northern Seattle suburb. He is unemployed, has not been able to stay with any of the handful of jobs the Department of Vocational Rehabilitation has helped drum up. The reasons are many—need perhaps for more structured work environments, better preparation beforehand, more realistic expectations (certainly on Ed's *and* the employers' parts). I feel, as his brother, the nagging frustration of not being close enough to interact more frequently with his limited support network. We do not give up hope. Nor does Ed. He is an optimist. The care at his group home is good, if, at best, maintenance-level. The great sibling struggle of the past few years, for me, has been just how involved to become in Ed's day-to-day life. He relishes his autonomy, and there is so little left that he can truly call his own. My own measuring tools for what I would find acceptable, I learn, are not his—and perhaps never were. My family and I have agitated over whether or not Ed should move closer to one of our communities. (My parents are now retired and in Arizona.) But to what benefit for Ed? For us? For each other? He says he is happy right where he is. This, I find, is the great sibling conundrum: How much is enough, (in rehabilitation, communication, intervention), and when do you simply embrace what is and live?

In the past few years, my brother, his old girlfriend, my sister, my parents, and I have matured in many ways. The old Norman Rockwell image of a perfectly healthy family around the holiday table has been sometimes replaced by violent outbursts of medication-hazed frustration. We have been surprised to find humor in heartbreak. We have adjusted our expectations and are thankful mostly. Having shared Ed's struggle, we are thankful to the many doctors, nurses, speech pathologists, orderlies, and others in the medical profession who have helped along the way. Their contributions are not lost on families or siblings, though we are often too burdened by our own problems to show the appreciation we feel.

I have aged, I think, many years in just 5. This, I am certain, is the purview of all siblings of head injury. But despite the hard days, there have been remarkable moments too. The one I carry with me is the first day I returned to Seattle, after many weeks, having last seen Ed still deep in coma. This day my brother stood up like Lazarus when I entered his room, reached his impossibly frail arms around me, and embraced me. I heard for the first time his bruised, beautiful voice after months of silence. He whispered, "Joe," and I was flooded with a sensation of love and triumph. I had been witness to a resurrection. There are gifts, odd and dark though they may be, for the sibling of a person with a head injury, if only we have courage and grace enough to accept them.

II

THE FAMILY SYSTEM

Section II provides various theoretical frameworks to understand the family as a system that is at the center of a person's life after head injury. The various frameworks stress the need to understand head injury from the perspective of the impact on the individual as well as the changes that may take place in his or her family, community, and support system. Drawing examples from the experiences shared in Section I, the frameworks emphasize the need to understand the family system over time from the perspective of the family's strengths.

6

UNDERSTANDING FAMILIES FROM A SYSTEMS PERSPECTIVE

ANN P. TURNBULL

H. RUTHERFORD TURNBULL III

A revolution is occurring in the field of disability in the recognition that the basic unit of consideration in policy and services is the individual and family, rather than solely the individual with a disability. From the perspective of the field of special education, which has traditionally had an emphasis on parent involvement, the revolution can be characterized as follows:

> The term parent involvement sums up the current perspective. It means we want parents involved with *us*. It means the service delivery system we helped create is at the center of the universe, and families are revolving around it. It brings to mind an analogy about the old Ptolemaic view of the universe with the earth at the center. . . .
>
> Copernicus came along and made a startling reversal—he put the sun in the center of the universe rather than the Earth. His declaration caused profound shock. The earth was not the epitome of creation; it was a planet like all other planets. The successful challenge to the entire system of ancient authority required a complete change in the philosophical conception of the universe. This is rightly termed the "Copernican Revolution."
>
> Let's pause to consider what would happen if we had a Copernican Revolution in the field of disability. Visualize the concept: The *family* is the center of the universe and the service delivery system is one of the many planets revolving around it. Now visualize the service delivery system at the center and the family in orbit around it. Do you see the difference? Do you recognize there is a revolutionary change in perspective. We would move from an emphasis on parent

involvement (i.e., parents participating in the program) to family support (i.e., programs providing a range of support services to families). This is not a semantic exercise—such a revolution leads the authors to a new set of assumptions and a new vista of options for service. (Turnbull & Summers, 1987, pp. 295–296)

Translating the Copernican Revolution in the field of disability to the area of head injury could be described as the family becoming the center of the rehabilitation process. Rather than families being required to conform to the medical model of discrete diagnosis and prescription and the schedules and protocols of traditional rehabilitation, putting the family at the center of the process means that the system tailors its support and services to the unique strengths and needs of each family unit. Accomplishing such individualization, however, entails the prerequisite of a keen understanding of each family in terms of its own set of characteristics, interactions, functions, and life cycle.

In order to accomplish such an understanding, the authors and colleagues have synthesized family theory and related literature into a conceptual framework that helps us understand families as a system (Turnbull & Turnbull, 1990). This framework serves as a basis for understanding the particular strengths and needs of each family as a first step in providing relevant support. This framework leads to a revolutionary new set of assumptions about families and a new vista of options for supporting them.

This framework comprises four major components:

1. *Family Characteristics* consist of the descriptive elements of the family, including the characteristics of the exceptionality, characteristics of the family, and personal characteristics, including special challenges. Within a systems framework, characteristics can be thought of as the *input* into family interaction.
2. *Family Interaction* refers to the relationships that occur within subgroups of family members on a daily and weekly basis. Within a systems framework, family interaction is considered the *process* of responding to individual and collective family needs.
3. *Family Functions* represent the different categories of needs for which families generally assume responsibility. Within a systems framework, carrying out family functions represents the *output* of family interaction in response to fulfilling the needs of family members individually and collectively.
4. *Family Life Cycle* represents the sequence of developmental and non-developmental changes that affect families. Within a systems perspective, these changes alter family resources and family functions; in turn, these changes influence how the family interacts.

The four sections of this chapter address each of these components. The discussion of each component includes: 1) vignettes drawn from the first

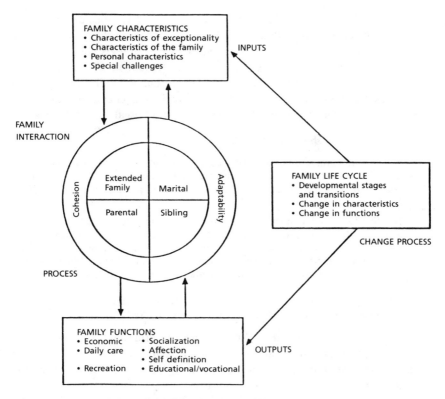

Figure 1. Family systems conceptual framework. From: Turnbull, A.P., Summers, J.A., & Brotherson, M.J. (1984). *Working with families with disabled members: A family systems approach.* Lawrence, Kansas: The University of Kansas, Kansas University Affiliated Facility, p. 60. Adapted by permission.

person accounts in Section I of this book and 2) related family research from areas of the disability field other than head injury.

FAMILY CHARACTERISTICS

> In the past few years, my brother, his old girlfriend, my sister, my parents, and I have matured in many ways. The old Norman Rockwell image of a perfectly healthy family around the holiday table has been sometimes replaced by violent outbursts of medication-hazed frustration. We have been surprised to find humor in heartbreak. We have adjusted our expectations and are thankful mostly. (Joseph Maurer, brother)

Traditionally many people have had a nostalgic image of families fitting the Norman Rockwell image of holiday celebration; however, the truth is that few American families, whether or not one of their members has had head injury, actually transform this image into reality. All families differ tremendously in the characteristics they possess and the resources they have available to address the needs of their members. Since every family is unique, a beginning point in "placing families in the center of the universe" is to recognize the tremendous variety among families. This section on family characteristics addresses three major types of variations, including characteristics of the exceptionality, characteristics of the family, and personal characteristics.

Characteristics of the Exceptionality

> To me, the hardest thing to accept about a parent with a brain injury is their behavior. I constantly wonder what people think of me when they see me with my dad and he gets mad because he drops something in public, for example. (Hope Hardgrove, child)

> By 1981 I had started to withdraw. I doubted my sanity. Why couldn't I get things to work right? I was losing control. Try as hard as I could, I could not make things right. Decision-making was a severe problem. Simple shopping at the supermarket was painful. I now knew the names of everything, but confronted with so many choices I would cry and leave. I told my neurologist how I felt; he suggested I be less introspective and just try to get on with life. I felt I had failed miserably. I no longer left our apartment; some days I never even got dressed. (Maureen Campbell-Korves, person with a head injury.)

Characteristics of the disability will greatly influence the family's reaction to it. There are many aspects of disability, but those briefly addressed in this section include the nature of the disability, the severity of the disability, and the demands of the disability on others.

In terms of the nature of the disability, there are many issues to consider regarding the particular type of impairments present, age of onset, stage in the recovery process, and capability of the family to respond to the specific impairment. In the two vignettes above, the nature of the exceptionality differs greatly in terms of concern about behavior versus concern about life support, and how the particular impairments of the individual with a head injury affect that individual and other family members. Although these differences exist, it is also important to recognize similarities such as dealing with uncertainty and ambiguity in daily living, the typical severe drain on family financial resources, and the need for a break from caregiving.

In addition to the nature of disability, the severity of the disability creates differences in family impact. Often it is tempting, but simplistic, to assume that a more severe disability will always mean a more intense reaction. The effects of different levels of severity may be qualitatively different but not necessarily easier or more difficult to deal with. In some situations it may be easier to obtain services for a person with a severe disability than for a person with a mild one. Also, milder disabilities may be invisible, which may cause greater concerns for siblings about whether they might have the same type of problem (Powell & Ogle, 1985). Also the family may go through a roller-coaster of expectations, with hopes for the future raised and dashed as the family member goes through periods of progress and crisis (Wadsworth & Wadsworth, 1971).

Finally, the family must examine very carefully the demands of a person with a disability in order to understand its impact. Beckman (1983) found that 66% of the variance in mothers' stress could be accounted for by unusual caretaking demands of infants with disabilities, including dealing with irritability and fussiness. The issue of behavioral control is crucial with families and can vary greatly depending upon the nature of the disability. For example, families of youth with autism may go out in public less frequently because they fear tantrums or episodes of aggression may occur (Bristol & Schopler, 1983).

Characteristics of the Family

Families have many different characteristics. The characteristics of size and form and cultural background are briefly highlighted here. Each of these characteristics shapes responses to a disability of a family member.

In terms of family size and form, some research on families with members with disabilities suggests that larger families tend to be less stressed by the presence of a member with a disability than smaller families. One possible explanation is that in families with a larger number of members there may be more people to help share caretaking responsibilities (Trevino, 1979).

In addition to the size of the family overall, the number of parents can make a difference in a family's reaction to a child with a disability. An important predictor of a mother's ability to cope with the child with a disability is the presence of a supportive partner even if he does not participate in child care (Friedrich, 1979; Kazak & Marvin, 1984). Two-parent families in which both parents participate in the childcare role seem to make a smoother adaptation to a child with a disability (Trute & Hauch, 1988). Also, it is important to consider families in which one or both of the parents in the original family have new partners, so that there are more than two parents. Currently, approximately one out of five children is a stepchild. Albert (1988) predicts that, if current trends continue, stepfamilies will be the most common family structure in the future. Thus, it is imperative that services take into consideration the needs and perspectives of different types of families.

A second consideration in terms of family characteristics is cultural background. The cultural background of the family can substantially influence its reaction to the needs of all of its members. A major component of cultural background is ethnicity, which McGoldrick (1982) describes as follows:

> Ethnicity patterns our thinking, feeling, behavior in both obvious and subtle ways. It plays a major role in determining what we eat, how we work, how we relax, how we celebrate holidays in rituals, and how we feel about life, death, and illness. (p. 4)

The shift of demography in the United States is very important to consider in terms of recognizing the importance of family culture. In 1987, public school enrollment was characterized as being composed of 16% white students, 10% Hispanic-American students, and 3% students of Asian and Pacific Island origin (DBS Corporation, 1987). By the turn of the century, it is projected that one out of three Americans will be nonwhite (Rodriquez, 1987).

Many professionals and service providers in the disability fields represent the majority rather than minority cultures. Although it is important not to stereotype different ethnic groups, there are ethnic trends that have been identified by family theorists that are important in understanding professional and family perspectives. For example, McGoldrick (1982) contrasts the values of white Anglo-Saxon Protestants as emphasizing self-reliance, self-control, achievement, and self-determination; whereas the values identified in the Mexican-American population are cooperation, interdependence, collectivism, and cohesiveness. These different values can vastly influence a family's reaction to disability and the dynamics of relationships between families and professionals.

Personal Characteristics

In addition to considering the characteristics of the exceptionality and the family, it is also necessary to consider the idiosyncratic personal characteristics of each family member. These could be described in a number of ways, but for the purposes of this chapter the focus is on mental and physical health and coping styles. The health needs of family members other than the person with a disability must be taken into consideration. Parents of children with disabilities have reported having headaches, lower back pain, depression, and other stress-related problems (Bristol & Schopler, 1983; McAndrew, 1976). Another major issue to consider is the aging of the caretakers within a family and their own declining health as they continue to maintain a supportive environment for the family member with a disability.

The coping styles of individual family members vary greatly both within and across families. Coping is defined as any strategy a person may choose to reduce feelings of stress (Pearlin & Schooler, 1978). It is characterized primarily by taking some positive action to reduce feelings of stress or to solve a problem. One way to conceptualize family coping is to look at it in terms of the strategies of passive appraisal, reframing, spiritual support, social support, and formal support (Olson et al., 1983; Turnbull & Turnbull, 1990).

Passive appraisal involves ignoring a problem or "setting it on the back burner," either on a temporary or permanent basis. Family members use passive appraisal when they decide to not worry about particular aspects of a disability because they may feel they can do nothing about them.

The second coping style of reframing represents a more active approach of redefining a situation so that a problem may be solved or may be viewed in a less stressful way. Problem-solving involves learning to identify needs, prioritize needs, generate workable alternatives, select the most appropriate alternative, take action, and evaluate the consequences of the action (Goldfarb, Brotherson, Summers, & Turnbull, 1986). Redefinition, however, involves thinking about a stressful situation in a way so that the positives rather than the negatives are emphasized:

> But despite the hard days, there have been remarkable moments too. The one I carry with me is the first day I returned to Seattle, after many weeks, having last seen Ed still deep in coma. This day my brother stood up like Lazarus when I entered his room, reached his impossibly frail arms around me, and embraced me. I heard for the first time his bruised, beautiful voice after months of silence. He whispered, "Joe," and I was flooded with a sensation of love and triumph. I had been witness to a resurrection. There are gifts, odd and dark though they may be, for the sibling of a person with a head injury, if only we have courage and grace enough to accept them. (Joseph Maurer, sibling)

A third coping strategy is spiritual support. The perspectives of mothers of children with Down syndrome concerning the role of religion in helping them cope indicated that 37% of the mothers reported seeking help and guidance from members of their church or clergy for problems associated with the disability and 66% responded that religion had helped them to understand and accept their child (Fewell, 1986). This point is illustrated also by the experiences of Hope Hardgrove:

> I realized God let this happen for a purpose in my life, and that I need to be thankful for it. Now I still struggle, especially when Dad gets mad, but I am learning to accept and be thankful for this abnormal life. (Hope Hardgrove, child)

The fourth coping style, social support, is the assistance the family receives from other family members, friends, and the community at large. Formal support, the fifth coping style, is the assistance provided from professionals. Maureen Campbell-Korves described her experience with formal support, "My speech pathologist was an extraordinary young woman who looked like a china doll and acted like a boot camp drill instructor. For this I will be forever grateful" (Maureen Campbell-Korves, person with a head injury). However, families have often characterized interactions with professionals as not being sensitive enough to their needs (Turnbull & Turnbull, 1985).

Conclusion—Family Characteristics

Even the brief discussion in this section indicates that families differ in many ways, including differences in terms of the characteristics of the exceptionality, characteristics of the family, and personal characteristics. Despite these variations, a major point is that all families have strengths and resources to draw upon from their particular constellation of characteristics. Applying a family systems framework requires recognition of the unique and special characteristics of each family.

FAMILY INTERACTION

Family interaction refers to the networks of relationships that exist within families and the multiple ways in which a family member with a disability influences those relationships and is influenced by them. The family is a unit of many simultaneous interactions, and what has been overlooked for too long in the disability field is that any event that affects any one member of the family has an impact upon all members (Carter & McGoldrick, 1980; Minuchin, 1974). Within a systems perspective, the different relationships that exist within families are referred to as subsystems. The four subsystems addressed in this section are the marital, parental, sibling, and extended family subsystems.

Marital Subsystem

> I had lost my best friend, my lover, my husband, and the father of my children, but because he was physically present, that loss was not readily recognized by anyone. I missed the friendship, intimacy, and sexual fulfillment that our marriage had held. (Marty Beaver, spouse)

> Since 1977 Doug and I have learned that head injury can redefine a marriage. Unless the two people involved are willing and flexible enough to change, the marriage does not stand a chance. We have sometimes gone from hero worship to hatred in a single day, but we have always come around to love. Seeking counseling to protect our marriage was important. Therapy was not a sign of weakness but rather a reaffirmation of our faith in each other. (Maureen Campbell-Korves, person with a head injury)

The marital subsystem consists of interactions between husbands and wives. When one of the spouses is the member with the disability, the family is affected as Marty Beaver described.

The marital subsystem is affected in a different way when a couple has a child with a disability. There are reports of disproportionately high rates of divorce, marital disharmony, and husbands' desertions in marriages where there is a child or youth with a disability (Gath, 1977; Murphy, 1982; Reed & Reed, 1965). However, some husbands and wives have reported that their relationship is closer and stronger as a result of dealing with a child with a disability (Kazak & Marvin, 1984). These conflicting results may suggest that the impact on the marriage is influenced very much by the nature of the marriage before the disability occurred. A strong marriage may be made stronger and a marriage with problems may be made more vulnerable.

Parental Subsystem

> Weeks passed and I realized this was the same man that was my father, but he was very different. He functioned on my level, and although he was an adult and my father, I treated him as a 5-year-old. (Hope Hardgrove, child)

The parental subsystem is composed of interactions between parents and their child or children. The presence of a parent with a disability such as a brain injury will affect parental roles in multiple ways, and the parent-child relationship will be shaped accordingly. A major issue for both parents and children is learning new roles and expectations in developing support systems to deal with the losses that occur in the relationships. Some of these losses are compensated for by the other spouse, who must assume double responsibility:

> I wished for someone else to make a decision, or pay a bill, or answer a question, but the reality was—it was left up to me. The constant and total responsibility for two children was ever present, even when a member of the family helped by keeping them. (Marty Beaver, spouse)

Another type of impact on the parent-child interaction occurs when the child is the person with a disability in the family. In a comparison of mothers and fathers of children with mental retardation, mothers were found to be significantly more affected than fathers by emotional family strain, additional child care time, and efforts to maintain family harmony. Fathers showed a higher degree of concern about their children's activities away from the family than for those with the family (Gumz & Gubrium, 1972). Other researchers found that fathers with children with disabilities experience lower self-esteem, particularly when the child is the first-born, a namesake, or a male (Cummings, 1976).

Sibling Subsystem

> I found myself on some subtle levels becoming the caregiver, the parent, to my own family. In those first early mornings—when you awaken to the crushing weight of what has happened, when you race to the telephone to see if your brother has survived the night, when you strategize the family's plans for the day, spelling each other at the hospital—the sibling takes on a new role.

> I witnessed the literal decay of my mother's health (and my father's temperament) during those early months of family-based rehabilitation. I felt resentment toward my brother. How dare he drive (perhaps intoxicated) on a motorcycle and bring all this down upon us? How dare he become so dependent that he dragged down my mother's, and then my father's health in his consuming need for attention and care?

> As one who was not his primary caregiver, I could be lighter with him, prod him into old sibling games, push him to pick up the guitar again, recall intimate family moments that helped him recapture his memory, needle him good-naturedly to lift weights (a painful and mind-tiring process for him), force him to reclaim what remained of his old self.

As his brother, and the one who perhaps understands him best of all, I begin, delicately, to shoulder the responsibility for Ed's later years—and all of the financial, legal, and medical details attached to that stewardship. . . . Never a great track star, I find the baton-pass a challenge. (Joseph Maurer, sibling)

These quotes aptly exemplify the multiple impacts on and roles of siblings of a person with a disability. Joseph Maurer has described the critical roles that brothers and sisters play in responding to the crisis of disability, including the anger and resentment that occurs because of the negative impact on family members, the role of socialization in creating a context for skill development, and the long-term responsibilities that must be addressed in dealing with future concerns. The particular reaction of siblings depends upon all of the components of the family systems framework.

One of the most well-known early sibling studies was conducted by Grossman (1972) among 83 college-age brothers and sisters of persons with disabilities. Approximately 45 of the siblings reported they had benefited from having a brother or sister with a disability, and 45 reported negative experiences. The benefits included more tolerance and compassion, greater understanding of other people, increased awareness of prejudice and its consequences, and greater appreciation of their own health and intelligence; the negative experiences included resentment and guilt, fear that they might also have a disability, shame, and a sense of being neglected by their parents. Older sisters of a child with a disability have been found to be the most vulnerable for increased responsibilities (Cleveland & Miller, 1977; Farber, 1960; Gath, 1974).

The topic of future roles is prominent in the minds of many siblings. In a survey of parents and siblings of the child with a disability concerning future plans, 41% of parents reported that their sons or daughters without disabilities would assume at least partial care for their sibling with a disability at some point in the future, while 68% of the brothers and sisters reported that they would assume such responsibility (McCullough, 1981).

Extended Family Subsystems

Fortunately, grandparents kept our household organized so that our son could carry on his life in the absence of his parents. . . . We had a tremendous mentor for modeling communication with physicians from the patient advocate provided in the intensive care unit. . . . Our friends who stuck with us through those difficult times will eternally be appreciated. Without them, we would have felt even more isolated. (JoAnn Kramer, parent)

The extended family subsystem is composed of family or individual interactions with relatives, friends, and professionals. All of these different relationships are illustrated above by JoAnn Kramer in terms of the contributions made to the family by grandparents, family friends, and a patient advocate. Families vary tremendously in the size and richness of their support system network.

Support programs are beginning to emerge to help extended family members. In a support group program for grandparents, approximately half of the grandparents reported that they had never visited a medical professional or an educational professional regarding their grandchild's disability and/or specific needs. Approximately two-thirds reported that they understood some of their grandchild's needs, but they had many questions that needed to be answered such as:

> How can we help him in therapy? What is the earliest program we can find? What kinds of programs are most effective? What is his potential? What can we do to develop her talents? How can we avoid sheltering the child too much? (Vadasy, Fewell, & Meyer, 1986, pp. 14–15)

One of the greatest family needs in terms of relationships with people outside of the family concerns the person with a disability and his or her own relationships. People with disabilities have been found to have minimal contact with people in the neighborhood (Salzberg & Langford, 1981) and to spend very little time in community activities (Crapps, Langione, & Swaim, 1985).

JoAnn Kramer provides insight on this issue:

> Re-entry into the school and community seemed like a nightmare for the next 3–4 years. Most of Jenny's friends gradually quit coming to visit her, and her brother became increasingly embarrassed by her inappropriate behavior.

> Jenny did not date in high school although she would have liked a boyfriend like her peers. Her social immaturity was not likely to attract young men her age. . . . Sex issues surfaced when Jenny moved into her own apartment in Minnesota.

In the field of disability there is emerging recognition of the importance of concentrating on how to foster relationships between people with and without disabilities so that the natural helping networks are available. One example is an effort with the Sigma Alpha Epsilon fraternity at the University of Kansas, which has a young man with mental retardation as an honorary member (Knowlton, 1989). The friendship, social opportunities, and recreation that are available through chronological age peers are a vital resource for ensuring a good quality of life.

Cohesion and Adaptability

After considering the four different types of family subsystems, it is also important to recognize some of the rules families have for interaction. Two important elements of interaction are cohesion and adaptability (Olson, Russell, & Sprenkle, 1980).

Family cohesion represents both the close emotional bonds that members have with each other, as well as the level of independence or autonomy that individuals experience within the family system (Olson et al., 1980). Family cohesion can be considered along a continuum with high disengagement on one end and high enmeshment on the other. In disengagement, families have rigid subsystem boundaries (Minuchin, 1974), and interactions are often characterized by under-involvement, few interests or friends in common, excessive privacy, and extensive time apart. Examples of disengagement between subsystems are parents becoming distanced from the extended family in their effort to support a child with a brain injury or emotional distance between siblings.

Enmeshment occurs when the boundaries between subsystems become blurred or weak (Minuchin, 1974). In such families, interactions are often characterized by over-involvement and over-protection, with little privacy provided to individual family members. Families who are highly enmeshed may organize all of their interactions around the issue of disability as though it were the focal point of the family. The goal in supporting families within a family systems framework is to establish balance and avoid extremes of enmeshment or disengagement in order to promote cohesion.

Family adaptability refers to the family's ability to change in response to situational and developmental stress (Olson et al., 1980). Adaptability helps families plan and work out differences, respond to changes, forge new ways of interacting, and formulate new goals. At one end of the adaptability continuum, a family who demonstrates a high degree of control and structure might be characterized as rigid. In such families, rules might be strictly enforced and there likely would be specifically delineated roles related to participation in their power structure. At the other end of the continuum, some families have a low degree of control and structure and have interactions characterized by ever-changing rules and commitments. This kind of family life is often referred to as chaotic. Though all families go through periods of chaos, constantly changing patterns of interaction within families usually produce high levels of stress. Again, as in cohesion, the goal with adaptability is to seek balance in relationships.

Conclusion—Family Interaction

This section has described the four family subsystems and how these subsystems form a network for the interactions within the family. An essential point to remember is that any change or major need in one subsystem will have an effect on all other subsystems in the family. The interactions among the subsystems influence how the family is able to carry out its functions. These functions are discussed in the next section.

FAMILY FUNCTIONS

In this society, families are expected to meet the individual and collective needs of their members (Caplan, 1976; Leslie, 1979). The tasks that families carry out to meet their needs can be characterized as family functions. Within the family systems framework, seven broad categories of family functions have been delineated: economic, daily care, recreation, socialization, affection, self-definition, and educational/vocational (Turnbull & Turnbull, 1990).

Economic Needs

> I was also very fortunate in that John's care and rehabilitation were covered by workers' compensation. I know many other spouses who struggle to get necessary therapies approved by private insurance that will not provide for lifelong care. The financial burdens of most families with persons with head injury are staggering. (Marty Beaver, spouse)

More accurate data are needed in assessing the economic impact on families caring for a member with a disability. A national evaluation of services for children and adolescents using ventilators found that 47% of the parents reported "serious financial problems" for their families during periods of hospitalization (Aday, Aitken, & Wegener, 1988). Expenses and adjustments included lost income from work, transportation, extra telephone calls, lost vacation time, child care for siblings, meals in motels, accumulated back debts, medications, increased utility bills, and foregoing luxuries, in addition to the usual family expenses.

Families have also reported sacrificing careers to care for a child or to relocate to another area with appropriate services. In one study 27% of the families believed that their work performance was affected by having a child with a disability (Lonsdale, 1978).

Daily Care Needs

> I was trying to take back more of the life I had handed over to Doug. I started to do some of the cooking again, but Doug would either hover just out of sight or over my shoulder. "Stir this more; lower the heat on that." I started to do a slow burn and we really had to talk it out. What was happening was that I had now become the interloper. The kitchen had become Doug's province, and I was going to have to prove I was not going to poison us or burn the house down. It has taken time but we are now creating some memorable meals together. (Maureen Campbell-Korves, person with a head injury)

> Jerry and I were able to split up the hospital visits. . . . We were exhausted emotionally, but mustered strength to comfort others who came to see Jenny. (JoAnn Kramer, parent)

The daily care demands that are created when a family member has a disability depend greatly on the characteristics of exceptionality, including the nature, severity, and special demands as discussed earlier. The tremendous difference between the daily care needs of primarily attending to emotional problems and the daily needs surrounding acute medical care in the hospital is reflected in the examples above.

A key aspect in family coping is the chronicity of caregiving over prolonged periods of time. The chronicity of responsibility takes a toll on the well-being of caregivers, especially females who have maintained much of the responsibility for meeting family care (Willer, Intagliata, & Wicks, 1981). The chronicity of caregiving for individuals with disabilities has been related to increased parental stress (Quine & Paul, 1985; Ventura & Boxx, 1983) and family burnout (LePontois, Moel, & Cohn, 1987).

A major response to supporting families in daily care needs is the provision of respite care services. Respite care provides temporary assistance for persons with disabilities for the purpose of providing a break from responsibility for the family or primary caregiver (Cohen & Warren, 1985). Twenty states have reported the availability of publicly sponsored respite service (Slater, Bates, Eicher, & Wikler, 1986).

Recreation Needs

> Dad has been home almost 9½ years now, and I have had to accept his behavior and everything else due to his injury. This includes giving up things most families and adolescents can do, such as having a friend over to spend the night or playing a game with the family, because Dad can't emotionally take things like this. (Hope Hardgrove, child)

Although a major function of the family is to encourage the relaxation and recreation of its members, fulfillment of recreation needs is sometimes limited by a family member with a disability. Families have reported having greater difficulty enjoying family outings because of the presence of problems that result from the disability (Dunlap & Hollingsworth, 1977; Lonsdale, 1978). Some people may consider recreation to be superfluous; however, a number of studies have identified a relationship between stress and family psycho-social functioning (Bristol, 1984). For example, Bristol (1984) found that well-adapted families of children with autism were able to engage in social and recreational activities outside the home, as well as to express their emotions and provide emotional support to each other. Increasingly, educational and rehabilitation programs are recognizing the importance of leisure and recreation and are developing support programs to teach skills and provide services in this important area (Schleien & Ray, 1988).

Socialization Needs

> Socially I was in limbo (Lezak, 1978), not fitting with any group—couples, singles, divorcees, or widows. Even spouses with their husbands/wife at home may also have to deal with this feeling, because of the social/behavioral problems that the spouse with a head injury often displays. I know that when John was at home, going out with another couple was just not the same as before his accident. His behavioral and social problems were embarrassing to me. (Marty Beaver, spouse)

Families are a basic unit in society and provide socialization both among family members and between the family and other members of society. However, many families with a member with a disability experience stress in attempting to meet socialization needs. In a study of 116 mothers of children with disabilities, one-third reported that their relationships with friends were adversely affected. They reported that friends were "frightened, embarrassed, and don't know how to approach us" (McAndrew, 1976, p. 229). Brotherson (1985) found that socialization options were the second greatest need, after residential options, identified by parents of young adults with mental retardation. However, families have reported a strong sense of social support from participating in programs such as the Parent-to-Parent model (Carter & Reynolds, 1984), which matches a trained "veteran" parent with one whose child was recently diagnosed as having a disability similar to that of the veteran's child. In this approach, families are able to develop social relationships with others who have "walked in their shoes." This same need for social support was expressed by Marty Beaver:

> Ever since John's accident I had wanted so much to meet another wife and mother who was in a similar situation. I felt it would be good to be able to share some of my feelings with someone who really understood. After 3 years I met Opal, who more than met my expectations. Her understanding, role modeling, and support has meant so much to me over the last 9 years. (Marty Beaver, spouse)

Social support can play a significant role in family coping. In a review of the role of socialization and the benefits of social support in illness, hospitalization, pregnancy, childbirth, unemployment, and bereavement, Cobb (1976) noted that in all cases, people with more social support experience greater adjustment to crises or life changes and less stress than those without.

Affection Needs

"I missed the friendship, intimacy, and sexual fulfillment that our marriage had held" (Marty Beaver, spouse). "Sex issues surfaced when Jenny moved into her own apartment in Minnesota" (JoAnn Kramer, parent).

Families provide a nurturing environment for meeting physical intimacy needs, as well as feelings of unconditional love by others. Some families report gaining a new understanding of unconditional love evolving out of their experiences in dealing with the challenges of disability, whereas other families experience isolation and alienation.

Rousso (1984), a social worker with a physical disability, highlights the important contribution that the family makes to meeting the affection needs of the member with a disability: "In particular, disabled children need to have their bodies, disability and all, accepted, appreciated, and loved, especially by significant parenting figures" (p. 12).

Issues of sexuality can pose tremendous conflicts for families. Families of females with a disability may fear that the need for acceptance may lead to sexual exploitation (Gardner, 1986); families of males may fear inappropriate sexual behavior such as public masturbation or advances to women (Haavik & Menniger, 1981). Some families do not realize that their member with a disability has sexual needs (Brotherson, 1985). Both educational and rehabilitation programs have responsibilities to provide quality sex education.

Self-Definition Needs

> We deal with our sadness by working diligently in advocacy and support groups at the state and national levels. We believe that our volunteer work will assist others in gaining access to systems and supports in a more concise manner. We are thankful for Jennifer's life, and we celebrate the opportunity that God has given us to help others through her life. (JoAnn Kramer, parent)

Families play a large role in helping their members establish their own identity and a perception of their worth. In many cases, family activities, such as advocacy efforts, revolve around issues of disability. The above quote describes how the Kramer family defines their own contributions and how they view the worth of their efforts.

The self-definition of family members has often been overlooked in rehabilitation programs. In the area of learning disabilities it has been reported that siblings may feel less important and less loved within the family because of the increased parental attention given to the member with a disability (Kronick, 1976). Brothers and sisters of children and adolescents with mild to moderate disabilities may have a more difficult time differentiating themselves from their siblings than those who have siblings with more severe disabilities (Tew, Payne, & Lawrence, 1974). All family members, including siblings, need specific information regarding the nature, severity, and special demands of the disability, and they need opportunities to discuss their feelings concerning self-identity (Seligman & Darling, 1989).

Educational/Vocational Needs

> We took part in a summer Vacation Ventures program for other kids with special needs, arranged through the area education agency. The program provided stimulation and socialization for Jenny, as well as parent education. (JoAnn Kramer, parent)

The educational family function can encompass academic learning, as well as informal instruction that the family provides in all of the functional areas—economic, daily care, recreation, socialization, affection, and self-definition. One of the goals of education is for children to take over gradual responsibility for meeting their own needs, given their own increased competence. When a disability exists in either a child or an adult member of the family, often more education than usual is needed over a longer period of time for achieving independence in each of the functional areas.

Families have had a significant role in the education of their children with disabilities, as exemplified by federal legislation. The Education of the Handicapped Children Act, PL 94-142, 1975, provides specific educational rights and responsibilities to families. The six major principles of that law include zero rejection, non-discriminatory evaluation, individualized education, least restrictive environment (LRE) placement, due process, and parent participation (Turnbull, 1990). Parents have specific duties related to each of the principles in ensuring that their child is provided with a free appropriate public education. Families must also address the vocational needs of their members. JoAnn Kramer describes the vocational experiences of her daughter Jenny:

> She professed wanting to work, but even after Jerry had educated an employer who was willing to give her a chance, she was not successful. She could drive, so she went to work independently. At least we thought she was going to work, but we later learned that she left early the first day and never showed up again (JoAnn Kramer, parent)

Another example of vocational implications is provided by Maureen Campbell-Korves:

> My final step was going back to work. Doug now had his own architectural office staffed and in place. I started going in a few hours a day and then a few days a week. In the beginning I felt so lost; I couldn't remember the day-to-day functions of running an office. Where was I supposed to fit in or what was I supposed to do? What I did do was clean the bathrooms. I think the reason I picked this work was because I still did not have a lot of confidence, and it offered a job with a place to hide. I don't know what Doug's other employees thought, but I do know we had the cleanest bathrooms of any architectural office in New York City. Slowly I did other things. I answered the telephone; I typed; I filed; I started to keep product information. It has taken a while, but I am now Office Manager. (Maureen Campbell-Korves, person with a head injury)

Increasingly, families are recognized as vital partners in vocational rehabilitation programs. Parents' attitudes towards work vary with the vocational aspiration of the youth, age of the youth, and degree of disability (Seyfarth, Hill, Orelove, McMillan, & Wehman, 1987). Turnbull and Turnbull (1988) have called for a family-professional partnership to promote great expectations for vocational opportunities.

Conclusion—Family Functions

Families have a variety of responsibilities related to the needs of all members. The impact of a member with a disability on family functions varies depending on the unique characteristics of the family and the patterns of family interaction. Life cycle stages and transitions through which the family has passed are also important considerations in family impact. The next section addresses these important issues.

FAMILY LIFE CYCLE

From our discussion thus far it is readily apparent that taking a snapshot of family life will give us some view of the complexity of the family in terms of family characteristics, family interaction, and family functions. On any given day, every family represents an interactive system in which these three components have distinctive elements and can be described in terms of both strengths and needs. Although this amount of complexity would be challenging enough to understand on its own, family life can never be accurately described as a snapshot because in reality it has more in common with a motion picture. Families are constantly changing and must be understood in terms of an appreciation of their past, present, and future.

Life cycle theorists have described life cycle stages of family life in many different ways, ranging from as many as 24 different stages to as few as 6 (Carter & McGoldrick, 1980). For the purposes of this discussion, the seven stages of the couple, birth and early childhood, school age, adolescence, young adult, post-parental, and aging (Turnbull & Turnbull, 1990) are highlighted.

Couple Stage

Typically, couples represent the initial stage of family life; however, in remarried families, the children from previous marriages may be brought into the new couple's relationship. During the couple stage there is a melding of values, priorities, and expectations of the two families of origin that are vastly influenced by the different family systems of the originating families. Couples strive to establish a new nuclear family and begin to form the characteristics of that nuclear family that will make it unique. These characteristics can be conceptualized in terms of the descriptive elements of the first component of the family systems framework discussed earlier in this chapter.

Disability affects the life of a couple in different ways. In some cases, one of the members of the couple will have a disability prior to the marriage and in other situations a disability might occur during the couple stage after the marriage. Furthermore, nonmarried couples can establish a pattern of family life:

> Ed's girlfriend, Laurie, a lovely woman I had known as well since childhood, was good enough to put us all up in the small house she and my brother owned together. There were tensions here, though, as she and Ed had recently separated. Laurie needed solace too, and we had descended on her and her life, upsetting all that was familiar and private. (Joseph Maurer, sibling)

Birth and Early Childhood Stage

The birth and early childhood life cycle stage includes the birth of one or more infants, who change the interaction patterns of the family and create new types of needs that must be met through family functions. Increasingly, infants with disabilities are diagnosed at birth, and even before birth through amniocentesis, and families are immediately launched into the world of early intervention and early childhood special education services. Federal legislation (PL

99-457, the Education of the Handicapped Act Amendments of 1986) was passed to stimulate states to provide these early services to infants, toddlers, and families. Such services are formalized through the development and implementation of an individualized family service plan (IFSP) (Johnson, McGonigel, & Kaufmann, 1989). The disability field places emphasis on family-centered services and intervention more during the early childhood life cycle stage than any other stage.

This stage can also be conceptualized in terms of the parent of a young child becoming disabled:

> Because I was at the hospital so much I spent very little time with our children, now ages 3½ years and 6 months. They needed me more than ever, but I didn't realize that at the time. This is a mistake many care providers make during the crisis and rehabilitation period. Children in the family need to be given love and attention. They are not as flexible as you might think. (Marty Beaver, spouse)

School-Age Stage

> Our family experienced a very permanent change in our lives in December of 1975—2 days after Christmas to be exact—when our 10-year-old daughter Jennifer suffered a severe brain stem injury in a fall from a horse on our family farm. We have been living with the changes precipitated by that tragic event for 14 years. (JoAnn Kramer, parent)

During the school-age stage, families generally focus a great deal of their time and attention on the education and socialization aspects of raising their children. When the onset of disability occurs during this stage, families are immediately plunged into a new service system of rehabilitation and special education. When a disability occurs in earlier life cycle stages, families usually have more experience in dealing with professionals and may be in a more comfortable position in negotiating for services from the educational system. As stated earlier, parents have prominent roles in educational decision-making regarding children with disabilities; these roles go far beyond those that are typical of parents whose children do not have disabilities. This additional responsibility for educational advocacy, as well as for teaching and reinforcing educational skills within the home, can add extra time demands and stress to family life.

Adolescence Stage

Adolescence is generally the time for rapid physical and psychological changes. Adolescence can certainly be a challenging time for family life when no special needs exist, but where issues of disability are present, adolescent issues can be exaggerated. Again, much depends on the role of the family member with a disability. Sometimes it is the adolescent within the family who has the disability. Different family dynamics exist when, for example, the parent has a disability and there is an adolescent in the family who must cope with this situation, as described by Hope Hardgrove:

> Head injury is a horrible thing to go through, and there is no support whatsoever for 13–19 year olds with parents who have had head injuries. I just really wish there was some way we could have the support of each other and talk about our circumstances and hear others so maybe ours wouldn't be so bad. (Hope Hardgrove, child)

When it is the adolescent in the family who has a disability, special issues can arise regarding sexuality, dealing with stigma, increased physical care needs, and developing self-advocacy skills. Although these issues can place major demands on the family system, it is important to realize that many of the services available to families primarily target the early childhood and school years. The lack of services for dealing with issues of adolescence leaves a major gap in support services.

Young Adult Stage

In many cultural groups of the United States, it is generally assumed that young adults will find employment, move away from the nuclear family, and begin a more independent life-style. Other cultural groups place greater value on family interdependence and continuing to live with the family. It is important to determine how different families define appropriate life-style during adulthood.

When adulthood does mean finding employment and moving away from the family, a major issue for families is creating additional support systems to enable the family member with a disability to obtain the highest level of independence and responsibility possible considering his or her individual circumstances. Although there is a mandate for public schools to serve students with disabilities in many states through age 21 or 22, there are no mandated services for adults with disabilities. Families often report experiencing high levels of stress when services for their adult member are unavailable.

Post-Parental Stage

Typically in this stage a couple lives together without their adult sons or daughters in their home. Their time and attention turns again to issues related to the couple without the responsibilities of addressing family functions for other members. This post-parenting stage, however, for many families with a member with a disability is a myth since they may continue to address the needs of their sons and daughters while simultaneously addressing needs of aging parents.

Many families provide care indefinitely for a son or daughter with a severe disability because of the lack of appropriate residential options outside of the family home (Seltzer, 1985; Zetlin & Turner, 1985). There is a trend of older parents reporting greater burnout, less support, less community acceptance, fewer formal services, and more isolation (Bristol & Schopler, 1983; Suelzle & Keenan, 1981).

Aging Stage

As parents age, there are implications for attending to their health and security needs, as well as considering the needs of a son or daughter with a severe disability. Families in such circumstances commonly are concerned about issues such as finances and who will care for the member with a disability when the parents die (Boggs, 1988). Joseph Maurer expressed his concern as follows:

> As his brother, and the one who perhaps understands him best of all, I begin, delicately, to shoulder the responsibility for Ed's later years—and all of the financial, legal, and medical details attached to that stewardship. It is a role siblings (and their parents) could use considerable help in addressing. Never a great track star, I find the baton-pass a challenge. (Joseph Maurer, sibling)

As parents age and face their own mortality, a clear need is to address strategies for making the "baton-pass" of family support. Siblings often take on caregiving roles, but not always with adequate preparation and attention to their own needs. Resources on life services planning (Parry, 1986; Stroud & Sutton, 1988; Turnbull, Bronicki, Summers, & Roeder-Gordon, 1989) need to be made available to families before they experience "baton-passing" crises.

Life Cycle Transitions

We have discussed briefly each of the seven life cycle stages, but an understanding of family cycle is incomplete unless we also address the periods of transition from one stage another. While stages can be thought of as the relatively stable plateau periods where family needs remain fairly constant, periods of transition are characterized by major adjustments in family characteristics and family functions, which, in turn, change family interactions. Transition periods are recognized as the time of greatest family stress because of the shifts in routines and patterns of interacting and carrying out responsibilities (Neugarten, 1976; Olson et al., 1983). Developmental and non-developmental transitions are considered briefly below.

Developmental Transitions   Transitions between stages are typically referred to as developmental transitions because they are expected at certain periods of time. An impact of disability on the family can be that transitions are delayed, such as in the situation of a young adult who is not able to become independent from his or her family. It is generally recognized that transitions that do not occur along society's generally expected time lines usually create greater stress for families.

A key to successful transitions for individuals with disabilities is development of a plan for the future based on the preferences of that individual, and then mobilization of family and professional support to implement that preferred plan (Mount & Zwernik, 1988; Turnbull, Turnbull, Bronicki, Summers, & Roeder-Gordon, 1989). It is stressful and time-consuming for families to consider future options when the present responsibilities might be overwhelming; however, transitions can be eased if a comprehensive array of services and supports is already in place prior to the experience of a crisis situation.

Nondevelopmental Transitions   Nondevelopmental transitions are not tied to life-cycle stages; thus, they are changes that can occur in families at any time. A prime example of a nondevelopmental transition is the occurrence of a head injury:

> One tragic day, just a few weeks before I turned 5, my life was shattered just like a crystal glass being dropped on a hard surface. I did not realize then what had happened. My dad, whom I loved and adored, was lying in a hospital bed with a brain injury, and whether or not he would live only God knew. (Hope Hardgrove, child)

> Into each family experiencing head injury comes a life-changing telephone call. . . . Ed's motorcycle had skidded on a wet road and slammed into a tree. He had taken the full impact on his unhelmeted head. He had been thrown some 25 feet down a cliff onto a concrete jogging path along Lake Washington. He was comatose. The prognosis was not good. They hoped I could get to Seattle before he died. Dumbstruck, I took the next plane from Burbank. (Joseph Maurer, sibling)

Such events in the lives of families can be characterized as nondevelopmental transitions because they can happen at any point and they profoundly change family life from that point on.

Another type of nondevelopmental transition can be geographic relocation. This sometimes occurs in families of a member with a disability for the purpose of gaining access to necessary services:

> Again we had to move John out of state to find a treatment facility for persons with behavioral problems associated with head injury. This move was much easier, as I was becoming more and more aware of John's disabilities. I wanted the best for him and was ready for anything that sounded optimistic. (Marty Beaver, spouse)

While it is true that a key to successful developmental transitions is planning for the future, it is often harder to plan for nondevelopmental transitions since their onset may be precipitous. The section on family interaction discussed the concepts of cohesion and adaptability. Families with more balanced levels of cohesion and adaptability are able to make changes more readily when transitions occur.

Summary of Family Life Cycle

One of the key elements of successful family life is the capability to grow and change with alterations in family characteristics, family interaction, and family functions. Family life can be conceptualized in terms of a number of developmental stages that are all connected by periods of developmental and nondevelopmental transitions. Although disability can complicate some of the adjustments and adaptations that are necessary in negotiating the family life cycle, services and supports from the formal and informal networks can greatly increase the probability that family challenges will meet with success.

SUMMARY

This chapter has advocated taking a systems perspective to understanding the unique strengths and needs of each family unit. The major assumptions of a family systems perspective and the implications for professionals are summarized below:

1. Every family can be described as having particular characteristics of the exceptionality, characteristics of the family, and personal characteristics of individual members; thus, it is necessary for professionals to individualize approaches to take into account family strengths and needs.
2. Families have a pattern of interaction that influences the way the members are arranged into subsystems and the way the subsystems interact to carry out family functions; thus, professionals need to respect the particular balance of relationships within a given family and to tailor services and supports according to their unique interactional pattern.
3. Families have multiple and sometimes competing responsibilities in meeting individual and collective needs within each of the seven functional categories; thus, professionals need to be sensitive to the family's priorities and help mobilize formal and informal services and supports to assist families in meeting their obligations.
4. Families progress through a number of different life–style stages and transitions as new members are born into the family and proceed through the developmental process; thus, professionals need to develop an awareness of the family's past, present, and future priorities and support them in making necessary changes.

The reader is encouraged to keep this framework in mind while reading the remaining chapters of this book and to consider how the information presented relates to one of the four components: family characteristics, family interaction, family functions, and/or family life cycle. The authors hope that this framework will be helpful in the development of a genuine appreciation of the uniqueness and diversity of family life.

REFERENCES

Aday, L.A., Aitken, M.J., & Wegener, D.H. (1988). *Pediatric homecare: Results of a national evaluation of programs for ventilator assisted children.* Chicago: Pluribus

Press, Inc. and the Center for Health Administration Studies, University of Chicago.

Albert, L. (1988). Strengthening stepfamilies. *Family Resource Coalition Report, 7* (1), 1–3.

Beckman, P.J. (1983). Influence of selected child characteristics on stress in families of handicapped infants. *American Journal of Mental Deficiency, 88,* 150–156.

Boggs, E.M. (1988). The changing roles of parents—Intergenerational perspectives. In J.L. Matson & A. Marchetti (Eds.), *Developmental disabilities: A life-span perspective* (pp. 67–87). Philadelphia: Grune & Stratton.

Bristol, M.M. (1984). The birth of a handicapped child—A wholistic model for grieving. *Family Relations, 33,* 25–32.

Bristol, M.M., & Schopler, E. (1983). Stress and coping in families with autistic adolescents. In E. Schopler & G.B. Mesibov (Eds.), *Autism in adolescents and adults* (pp. 251–278). New York: Plenum Press.

Brotherson, M.J. (1985). *Parents self report of future planning and its relationship to family functioning and family stress with sons and daughters who are disabled.* Unpublished doctoral dissertation, University of Kansas, Lawrence.

Caplan, P. (1976). The family as a support system. In G. Caplan & M. Killilea (Eds.), *Support systems and mutual help: Multidisciplinary explorations* (pp. 19–36). New York: Grune & Stratton.

Carter, E.A., & McGoldrick, M. (Eds.). (1980). *The family life cycle: A framework for family therapy.* New York: Gardner Press.

Carter, S., & Reynolds, K. (1984). *Parent to parent organizational handbook.* Athens, GA: University of Georgia University Affiliated Facility.

Cleveland, D.W., & Miller, N. (1977). Attitudes and life commitments of older siblings of mentally retarded adults: An exploratory study. *Mental Retardation, 14* (3), 38–41.

Cobb, S. (1976). Social support as a mediator of life stress. *Psychosomatic Medicine, 38,* 300–314.

Cohen, S., & Warren, R.D. (1985). *Respite care: Principles, programs, and policies.* Austin: PRO-ED.

Crapps, J.M., Langione, J., & Swaim, S. (1985). Quantity and quality of participation in community environments by mentally retarded adults. *Education and Training of the Mentally Retarded, 20*(2), 123–129.

Cummings, S.T. (1976). Impact of the child's deficiency on the father: A study of fathers of mentally retarded and chronically ill, and neurotic children. *American Journal of Orthopsychiatry, 46,* 246–255.

DBS Corporation. (1987, December). *1986 elementary and secondary school civil rights survey national summaries* (Contract Number 300-86-0062). Washington, DC: Office of Civil Rights, U.S. Department of Education.

Dunlap, W.R., & Hollingsworth, J.S. (1977). How does a handicapped child affect the family? Implications for practitioners. *The Family Coordinator, 26*(3), 286–293.

Farber, B. (1960). Family organizations and crisis: Maintenance of integration in families with a severely retarded child. *Monographs of the Society for Research in Child Development, 25*(1).

Fewell, R.R. (1986). Support from religious organizations and personal beliefs. In R.R. Fewell (Ed.), *Families of handicapped children: Needs and supports across the life span* (pp. 297–316). Austin: PRO-ED.

Friedrich, W.N. (1979). Predictors of coping behavior of mothers of handicapped children. *Journal of Consulting and Clinical Psychology, 47,* 1140–1141.

Gardner, N.E.S. (1986). Sexuality. In J.A. Summers (Ed.), *The right to grow up: An introduction to adults with developmental disabilities* (pp. 45–66). Baltimore: Paul H. Brookes Publishing Co.

Gath, A. (1974). Sibling reactions to mental handicaps: A comparison of the brothers and sisters of mongol children. *Journal of Child Psychology and Psychiatry and Allied Disciplines, 15*(3), 838–843.

Gath, A. (1977). The impact of an abnormal child upon the parents. *British Journal of Psychiatry, 130*, 405–410.

Goldfarb, L.A., Brotherson, M.J., Summers, J.A., & Turnbull, A.P. (1986). *Meeting the challenge of disability and chronic illness: A family guide.* Baltimore: Paul H. Brookes Publishing Co.

Grossman, F.K. (1972). *Brothers and sisters of retarded children: An exploratory study.* Syracuse: Syracuse University Press.

Gumz, E.J., & Gubrium, J.F. (1972). Comparative parental perceptions of a mentally retarded child. *American Journal of Mental Deficiency, 77*, 175–180.

Haavik, S.F., & Menniger, K.A. (1981). *Sexuality, law, and the developmentally disabled person.* Baltimore: Paul H. Brookes Publishing Co.

Johnson, B.H., McGonigel, M.J., & Kaufmann, R.K. (Eds.). (1989). *Guidelines and recommended practices for the Individualized Family Service Plan.* (Contract No. 300-87-0163). Washington, DC: U.S. Department of Education.

Kazak, A.E., & Marvin, R.S. (1984). Differences, difficulties and adaptation: Stress and social networks in families with a handicapped child. *Family Relations, 33*, 67–77.

Knowlton, E. (1989). *Natural ties.* Lawrence, Kansas: Beach Center on Families and Disability, University of Kansas.

Kronick, D. (1976). *Three families: The effect of family dynamics on social and conceptual learning.* San Rafael, CA: Academic Therapy Publications.

LePontois, J., Moel, D.I., & Cohn, R.A. (1987). Family adjustment to pediatric ambulatory dialysis. *American Journal of Orthopsychiatry, 57*, 78–83.

Leslie, G.R. (1979). The nature of the family. In G.R. Leslie (Ed.), *The family in social context* (4th ed., pp. 3–23). New York: Oxford University Press.

Lezak, M.D. (1978). Living with the characterologically altered brain injured patient. *Journal of Clinical Psychiatry, 39*, 592–598.

Lonsdale, G. (1978). Family life with a handicapped child: The parents speak. *Child: Care, Health and Development, 4*, 99–120.

McAndrew, I. (1976). Children with a handicap and their families. *Child: Care, Health and Development, 2*, 213–237.

McCullough, M.E. (1981). Parent and sibling definition of situation regarding transgenerational shift in care of a handicapped child (Doctoral dissertation, University of Minnesota) *Dissertation Abstracts International, 42*, 161B.

McGoldrick, M. (1982). Ethnicity and family therapy: An overview. In M. McGoldrick, J.K. Pearce, & J. Giordano (Eds.), *Ethnicity in family therapy* (pp. 3–30). New York: The Guilford Press.

Minuchin, S. (1974). *Families and family therapy.* Cambridge, MA: Harvard University Press.

Mount, B., & Zwernik, K. (1988). *It's never too early, it's never too late.* St. Paul: Metropolitan Council.

Murphy, A.T. (1982). The family with a handicapped child: A review of the literature. *Developmental and Behavioral Pediatrics, 3*(2), 73–82.

Neugarten, B. (1976). Adaptations and the life cycle. *The Counseling Psychologist, 6* (1), 16–20.

Olson, D.H., McCubbin, H.I., Barnes, H., Larsen, A., Muxen, M., & Wilson, M. (1983). *Families: What makes them work.* Beverly Hills: Sage Publications.

Olson, D.H., Russell, C.S., & Sprenkle, D.H. (1980). Circumplex model of marital and family systems II: Empirical studies and clinical intervention. In J.P. Vincent (Ed.), *Advances in family intervention assessment and theory* (Vol. 1, pp. 129–179). Greenwich, CT: JAI Press.

Parry, J. (1986). Life services planning for vulnerable persons. *Mental and Physical Disability Law Reporter, 10*(6), 516–522.

Pearlin, L.I., & Schooler, C. (1978). The structure of coping. *Journal of Health and Social Behavior, 19,* 2–21.

Powell, T.H., & Ogle, P.A. (1985). *Brothers and sisters—A special part of exceptional families.* Baltimore: Paul H. Brookes Publishing Co.

Quine, L., & Paul, J. (1985). Examining the causes of stress in families with severe mentally handicapped children. *British Journal of Social Work, 15,* 501–517.

Reed, E.W., & Reed, S.C. (1965). *Mental retardation: A family study.* Philadelphia: W.B. Saunders.

Rodriquez, F. (1987). *Equity education: An imperative for effective schools.* Dubuque, IA: Kendall-Hunt.

Rousso, H. (1984). Fostering healthy self esteem. *Exceptional Parent, 8*(14), 9–14.

Salzberg, C.L., & Langford, C.A. (1981). Community integration of mentally retarded adults through leisure activity. *Mental Retardation, 19*(3), 127–131.

Schleien, S.J., & Ray, M.T. (1988). *Community recreation and persons with disabilities: Strategies for integration.* Baltimore: Paul H. Brookes Publishing Co.

Seligman, M., & Darling, R.B. (1989). *Ordinary families, special children: A systems approach to childhood disability.* New York: The Guilford Press.

Seltzer, M.N. (1985). Informal supports for aging mentally retarded persons. *American Journal of Mental Deficiency, 90*(3), 259–265.

Seyfarth, J., Hill, J.W., Orelove, F., McMillan, J., & Wehman, P. (1987). Factors influencing parents' vocational aspirations for their children with mental retardation. *Mental Retardation, 25*(6), 357–362.

Slater, M.A., Bates, M.A., Eicher, L., & Wikler, L. (1986). Survey: Statewide family support programs. *Applied Research in Mental Retardation, 7,* 241–257.

Stroud, M., & Sutton, E. (1988). *Activities handbook and instructor's guide for expanding options for older adults with developmental disabilities.* Baltimore: Paul H. Brookes Publishing Co.

Suelzle, M., & Keenan, V. (1981). Changes in family support networks over the life cycle of mentally retarded persons. *American Journal of Mental Deficiency, 86,* 267–274.

Tew, B.J., Payne, E.H., & Lawrence, K.M. (1974). Must a family with a handicapped child be a handicapped family? *Developmental Medicine and Child Neurology, 16,* (Suppl.), 32, 95–98.

Trevino, F. (1979). Siblings of handicapped children: Identifying those at risk. *Social Casework: The Journal of Contemporary Social Work, 60,* 488–492.

Trute, B., & Hauch, C. (1988). Building on family strength: A study of families with positive adjustment to the birth of a developmentally disabled child. *Journal of Marital and Family Therapy, 14*(2), 185–193.

Turnbull, A.P., & Summers, J.A. (1987). From parent involvement to family support: Evolution to revolution. In S.M. Pueschel, C. Tingey, J.W. Rynders, A.C. Crocker, & D.M. Crutcher (Eds.), *New perspectives on Down syndrome* (pp. 289–306). Baltimore: Paul H. Brookes Publishing Co.

Turnbull, A.P., Summers, J.A., & Brotherson, M.J. (1984). *Working with families with disabled members: A family systems approach*. Lawrence, Kansas: University of Kansas, Kansas University Affiliated Facility.

Turnbull, A.P., & Turnbull, H.R. (1988). Toward great expectations for vocational opportunities: Family-professional partnerships. *Mental Retardation, 26*(6), 337–342.

Turnbull, A.P., & Turnbull, H.R. (1990). *Families, professionals and exceptionality: A special partnership*. Columbus: Charles E. Merrill.

Turnbull, H.R., & Turnbull, A.P. (1985). *Parents speak out: Then and now*. Columbus: Charles E. Merrill.

Turnbull, H.R., Turnbull, A.P., Bronicki, G.J., Summers, J.A., & Roeder-Gordon, C. (1989). *Disability and the family: A guide to decisions for adulthood*. Baltimore: Paul H. Brookes Publishing Co.

Vadasy, P.F., Fewell, R.R., & Meyer, D.J. (1986). Grandparents of children with special needs: Insights into their experiences and concerns. *Journal of the Division for Early Childhood, 10*, 36–44.

Ventura, J.N., & Boxx, P.G. (1983). The family coping inventory applied to parents with new babies. *Journal of Marriage and the Family, 45*, 867–875.

Wadsworth, H.G., & Wadsworth, J.B. (1971). A problem of involvement with parents of mildly retarded children. *The Family Coordinator, 28*, 141–147.

Willer, B., Intagliata, J., & Wicks, N. (1981). Return of retarded adults to natural families: Issues and results. In R.H. Bruininks, D.E. Meyers, B.B. Sigford, & K.C. Lakin (Eds.), *Deinstitutionalization and community adjustment of mentally retarded people* (pp. 207–216). Washington, DC: American Association on Mental Deficiency.

Zetlin, A.G., & Turner, J.L. (1985). Transition from adolescence to adulthood: Perspectives of mentally retarded individuals and their families. *American Journal of Mental Deficiency, 89*(6), 570–579.

√ 7

FAMILY SYSTEMS THEORY APPLIED TO HEAD INJURY

EDWARD A. MAITZ

The dramatic and often devastating effects of a traumatic brain injury on individual family members, and on the family as a whole, have become increasingly evident. Although the impact on the family is not always altogether negative (Mauss-Clum & Ryan, 1981; Sachs, 1985), families almost always report a period of turmoil and chaos. If the family system begins to break down under the strain associated with the injury, its ability to meet the needs of individual family members is jeopardized. This in turn causes stress and anxiety in the individual family members.

FAMILIES

Turnbull and Turnbull (1990) maintain that "families exist in order to meet the individual and collective needs" of family members in seven broad categories, including "1) economic, 2) daily care, 3) recreation, 4) socialization, 5) self-definition, 6) affection and 7) educational/vocational" (p. 79). Families typically are able to meet these needs through the organized and complementary contribution of individual family members. When the individuals in the system act in concert, the family system functions smoothly, and is able to meet the needs of the individuals. If one part of the system is removed or breaks down, the impact is felt throughout the system. The system must adapt if it is to remain intact and continue to meet the needs of the individual family members.

   The impact of a traumatic brain injury on family members has been eloquently described by Lezak (1976). She reports, "It is the symptoms of depression–the anxiety attacks, obsessive ruminations, disturbed sleep and eating habits, lethargy or agitation—that normally stable family members interpret as evidence of 'going crazy' " (p. 595). Lezak's clinical description is consistent with the empirical family studies. Rosenbaum and Najenson (1976) found that wives of men with head injury were more depressed than wives of men with spinal cord injuries, and men without injuries. Livingston, Brooks, and Bond (1985) reported significant anxiety in 45% of the relatives of men with head injuries. Given that the effect of the injury on the family is no longer in doubt, the question becomes: How can we best understand and conceptualize the impact on the family system and help the family function most effectively in order to meet the needs of individual family members?

INTERACTION MODEL

Typically, family studies have attempted to identify adjustment difficulties or emotional distress in individual family members. These studies have been extremely valuable in the sense that they have clearly identified the impact of a severe head injury upon relatives and have begun to untangle the complex interaction of variables that accounts for stress in individual family members. However, an individual does not exist in isolation. His or her feelings, attitudes, and behaviors are a function of the context in which the individual operates. Any approach that considers individual family members in isolation assumes a perspective that has inherent biases and limitations. The traditional individual approach tends to promote a pathology model. It identifies abnormal feelings, behaviors, and attitudes, but often neglects to consider the context in which these feelings and behaviors occur. It fails to take into account the disruption in family roles, alterations in the family system, changes in financial status, and social isolation that are relatively common after a family member sustains a traumatic brain injury. In their discussion of the "burden on caregivers," Livingston and Brooks (1988) recognize that family stress reflects the "interaction" of relationships among family members. With respect to subjective burden, they argue that "it is bound to reflect not only the effect one individual, the patient with brain damage, has on another, the caregiver, but also the nature of the interaction between these individuals and other family members" (p. 8). Making sense of what it means for a relative to be anxious or depressed after someone in the family sustains a head injury requires an understanding of these feelings within the context of a suddenly disrupted family system.

INTERVENTION ISSUES

The decision as to whether to consider the individual or family as the primary unit has significant intervention implications. From an individual perspective, should individual counseling be offered to each person in the family? If so, does that ensure that the family as a whole will operate more efficiently and effectively? Many of the adjustment issues and much of the emotional distress reported in the literature is attributable not to individual pathology, but to a sudden and dramatic disruption of family roles and role relationships. This is not to suggest that family members never have their own psychological problems. It does suggest that, before resorting to psychological diagnoses, it is important to understand family members' feelings and behaviors within the context of a suddenly disorganized family system. It may be that anxiety and depression represent very normal responses to a very abnormal family situation. Outcome studies have demonstrated consistently that the most effective approaches to intervention for family adjustment issues are those that conceptualize the family as a functional unit, and treat the family as a whole, rather than treating individual family members (Gurman & Kniskern, 1981).

A group of researchers and clinicians has suggested that the traditional individual model be supplemented with a family systems model that considers the family as a functional unit in which individuals affect, and are affected by, each other (Klonoff & Prigatano, 1987; Maitz, 1989; Rosenthal & Geckler, 1986; Zarski, Hall, & DePompei, 1987). While the family systems model has proven to be useful in gaining an understanding of and providing intervention for families, typically it has not been applied to families of individuals with traumatic brain injury.

FAMILY SYSTEMS THEORY

Family systems theorists regard the family, not the individual, as the primary unit of analysis. The family is defined as, "an arena of interacting personalities, intricately organized into positions, norms and roles" (Hill, 1958, p. 140). The family is defined not in terms of the individual members, but by the structural elements in the family system, which include positions, norms, roles, and the function and interaction of these elements. The theory recognizes that, while people are individuals, individuals are also part of a system, and that "the events in a system are interconnected, part of a constant process of reciprocal influence" (White, 1972, p. 59).

Family systems theory is an orientation that recognizes that a person's feelings and behaviors reflect his or her relationships with other people, including his or her family. It is especially useful for understanding the impact of a traumatic brain injury, given the effect of the injury on the entire family system. The principles of the family systems approach provide a theoretical foundation and a rationale for the shift in focus from the individual to the family system. The principles may appear complex, but they are inherent in any system.

The *principle of non-summativity* states, "the analysis of a family is not the sum of the analysis of its individual members. There are characteristics of the system, that is, interactional patterns that transcend the qualities of individual members" (Watzlawick, Beavin, & Jackson, 1967, p. 123). This suggests that in understanding the way in which a system operates, it is necessary to assess the system as a whole, not just the individual members. This applies not only to family systems, but to any organized functional system. For example, before investing money in a particular business, one would want to assess its overall efficiency and effectiveness and consider the company's policies, profit/loss statements, personnel turnover, and so forth. That is, one would want to go beyond an assessment of the individual employees, and consider the entire organization as a whole. The company may have extremely competent employees who may not be clear about their roles and/or their relationships with other employees. Also, the company may have average employees who communicate well and complement one another, and thereby enhance the overall operation of the system. Like a family system, the company is not the sum of the individual members. After a family member sustains a head injury, one needs to ask: What role did this person play in the family? How can the family system adapt its role structure in order to continue to function effectively?

The *principle of wholeness* states, "Every part of a system is so related to its fellow parts that a change in one part will cause a change in all of them and in the total system" (Watzlawick, Beavin, & Jackson, 1967, p. 123). Like the principle of non-summativity, the principle of wholeness applies to any system and is very familiar. Consider that when a car is driven the fan belt begins to stretch. It may become loose and slip on the pulley that turns the alternator, which charges the battery. One morning the driver attempts to start the car only to find that the battery is dead. The mechanic who did not recognize the principle of wholeness would simply replace the battery, since that was the defective part. Of course, in a few days the driver would once again try to start the car, only to discover another dead battery. As this example demonstrates, a change in one part of any system, be it a mechanical system or a family system, will affect all of the other parts of the system.

It is essential to recognize that any change, even a positive one, in the person with a head injury will have an impact on the family system. If the family is not involved in intervention planning, staff may develop an intervention plan that, while perfectly reasonable, is in conflict with the way in which the family functions. It is the intervention team's failure to recognize this conflict that often results in families being wrongfully accused of undermining treatment. An intervention team in one program believed they were helping a young man to become more independent by teaching him to cook and do his own laundry; he had never cooked or done laundry prior to his accident. The team perceived his parents as resistant because they did not implement his program at home. It eventually became apparent that the program was threatening to his mother, who feared that her role in the family was being eliminated. When the issue was clarified and his mother reassured that her role was not being usurped, the family was willing to implement the team's recommendations.

Finally, the *principle of homeostasis* suggests that systems strive to maintain balance or equilibrium. Balance, however, does not imply a static situation. The system is constantly evolving in order to meet the ever-changing needs of the system. The human body is a system made up of individual organs that operate in unison in order to maintain body temperature at 98.6°. Body temperature stays relatively constant even when a person comes into a warm house from subzero temperatures. The parts of the system work in concert to maintain the delicate balance of the body's temperature control system. Like the individual organs in the body, the individual members of a family operate in unison to maintain the delicate balance in the family system. If the system becomes unbalanced because one of the individuals is unable to fulfill his or her role, the family will seek a solution in order to re-establish the system's equilibrium.

Family homeostasis, or equilibrium, is enhanced when family members maintain clear, mutually agreed upon roles. Typically, family members know who is primarily responsible for maintaining the house, providing financial support, and disciplining the children. As long as each individual performs his or her role, the homeostasis, or balance, within the system is maintained. This delicate balance within the family system is susceptible to stress from outside the system, and from within the system itself. When this stress interferes with the role structure, homeostasis within the family is threatened, which causes tension both within the system and for the individual family members. A traumatic brain injury, which interferes with an individual's ability to fulfill family roles of, for example, wage earner, little league coach, or sex partner, threatens the equilibrium, or balance, in the family system. If this is understood and accepted as a given, then the stress in the family and in the individual family members following a traumatic brain injury becomes not only understandable, but predictable and, at least until the family re-establishes its equilibrium, unavoidable.

ROLE INTERACTION AND ROLE CHANGES

Typically, *role organization* is orderly. A dramatic change in the family system, as happens when an individual sustains a traumatic brain injury, produces changes in the manner in which family roles are organized and fulfilled. When a family member, especially an adult, sustains a serious injury, another member, typically a spouse, may attempt to assume all of the role responsibilities of the injured person in order to maintain homeostasis in the family.

If the number of roles becomes too great, the person assuming them will experience increased stress. It is important for the family system to adapt and share role responsibilities in order to guard against one person becoming overly responsible.

Another consideration is the issue of *role transition* or the relative ease or difficulty in moving from one role to another. Role transition generally is facilitated when an individual has some time to prepare for an unfamiliar role. A head injury is a sudden, traumatic event. It is unpredictable and does not allow family members time to prepare for the assumption of new and unfamiliar roles. Panting and Merry (1972) found that wives of individuals with traumatic brain injuries experience greater stress than mothers. It may be that mothers have less difficulty reverting to the caretaker role than spouses do acquiring the caretaker role.

Finally, *role strain* refers to the stress that is generated within an individual when he or she experiences difficulty meeting the demands of a particular role. When the wife of a man who sustains a traumatic brain injury says, "I just don't know how I can suddenly go back to work, care for my disabled husband, run the household, and be both father and mother to my children," she is describing the stress associated with the dramatic change of taking on new roles for which she feels unprepared.

Seen within the context of changes in roles, role interaction, and the family system, the nature of the personal and family stress that occurs after someone sustains a head injury becomes increasingly clear. Furthermore, the stress can be understood not only as a function of the injury or individual pathology but also as a function of a devastating disruption in the family system. The accompanying anxiety and depression may be reasonable and predictable responses to the disruption in the system.

CASE STUDY

The importance of helping families understand, and accommodate to, the impact of constantly shifting roles after a family member sustains a brain injury was evident in Mr. M's family. Mr. M, a 57-year-old European man, sustained a traumatic brain injury in a work-related accident in 1986. His wife, despite living in the United States for more than 20 years, never learned to speak English. They had three adult children who were married and living outside their home. Prior to his injury, Mr. M took responsibility for almost all of the household affairs, including managing the checkbook, banking, and buying property. Even his married children came to him with their problems and sought his advice.

While in the hospital, Mr. M was described as stubborn, but not aggressive or violent. During his weekends at home, however, he was uncharacteristically hostile and demanding. He stood in front of his daughter's car, vowing to allow himself to be run over if she did not return his car keys. On another occasion, he was brandishing a rifle and threatening suicide. The family was upset and felt unable to cope with Mr. M's sudden change in behavior. The family members themselves were described by the staff as difficult. When Mr. M was transferred to the outpatient unit, the author was told to expect frequent telephone calls and complaints about Mr. M's program.

It was apparent that this once stable family was disorganized and temporarily dysfunctional. Mr. M's case manager believed that his behavior was not solely a function of his head injury, but also reflected a disruption in the family system. The therapeutic issues were defined not in terms of Mr. M's difficult behaviors, but in terms of the changes in the family system subsequent to Mr. M's brain injury. It appeared that Mrs. M felt panic at the thought of suddenly needing to manage the home without her husband's support. The family's telephone calls were a reflection of their fear that the family system would crumble if Mr. M were unable to fulfill his previous roles in the family. Mr. M's behavior was a desperate attempt to re-establish his previous role as head of the family, in an effort both to support his wife and maintain his sense of self-worth. Regular weekly family sessions were initiated including the client, his wife, his two married daughters, the author, and a female co-therapist. With the help of the therapists, the family was able to identify alternative support structures that could be mobilized until Mrs. M gained more confidence in her ability to manage the house. Mrs. M was soon able to demonstrate to her husband that she could manage until he recovered, and his anxiety decreased. At the same time, the family was encouraged to identify roles that Mr. M could gradually begin to resume in the family. When he realized that his position in the family would not be undermined, Mr. M's anxiety, fear, and abusiveness abated. After just a few sessions, family equilibrium was restored. The family was able to rely on its inherent resources, and family meetings were held less frequently. As the family stress abated, Mr. M's daughters no longer called with complaints about their father's program.

The family did experience one subsequent crisis that required additional intervention. The family called the therapist and reported that Mr. M was once again suddenly becoming angry at his wife with no apparent provocation. During the session, the family casually mentioned that Mrs. M's confidence had improved to the extent that she was starting evening school to study English. The therapist was able to help the family recognize that this threatened Mr. M's still fragile position in the family. Once the problem was identified, Mr. M was reassured, and his anger again dissipated.

This family's experience demonstrates how a disruption in the family system contributes to personal and family stress in previously stable families. It also suggests that by re-establishing the equilibrium or balance in the family, individual and family functioning is enhanced. This does not suggest that the family re-establish roles as they existed prior to the injury. Families that attempt this solution experience continued frustration and disappointment. The family must redefine family roles, and continue to redefine them as the person with head injury continues to establish his or her new position in the family.

FAMILIES AND CATASTROPHIC EVENTS

Why do some families appear to cope with the stress associated with a catastrophic event, while other families remain chaotic and dysfunctional? Family systems theory provides a framework for understanding the variety of ways in which families respond to a catastrophic event such as a traumatic brain injury.

According to Hill (1958) there are at least three variables that combine to determine whether or not a family will experience a particular event as a crisis. These include: *the event* itself, *the family's crisis meeting resources,* and *the definition the family makes of the event.* In Hill's model "A (the event) interacting with B (the family's crisis-meeting resources) interacting with C (the definition the family makes of the event) produces X (the crisis). The second and third determinants—the family resources and definition of the event—lie within the family itself and must be seen in terms of the family's structure and values" (p. 141). Hill's insight helps to explain why families can react so differently to similar events. The event itself represents only one variable in the equation. It is also testimony to the fact that each family brings its own unique history and richness to life's challenges, the fabric of strengths and vulnerabilities needs to be understood, recognized, and respected.

With regard to A (the event), there is no doubt that some events are more stressful than others. Clearly, a traumatic brain injury that renders the individual unable to maintain his or her family roles is an extremely stressful event. Hill (1958) developed a system of classifying stressful events into three categories: stress associated with *dismemberment, accession,* and *demoralization.* Each of these is a potential problem in families of individuals with head injuries at different points in the process of reintegration into the family. In Table 1 the examples of dismemberment, accession, and demoralization are taken from Hill's work (1958, p. 142).

Table 1.   The three categories of stressful events

Dismemberment	Accession	Demoralization
Hospitalization of spouse	Unwanted pregnancy	Nonsupport
War separation	Deserter returns	Infidelity

Dismemberment refers to the loss of a family member. This can occur when a son or daughter leaves home to live independently from the parents. It also occurs when there is a death or serious illness in the family. Dismemberment may occur in a less obvious form when a person remains in the family but, because of serious physical or emotional illness, is unable to fulfill his or her role requirements. Dismemberment is universal in moderate or severe head injury when the person is hospitalized, and is unable, at least for some period of time, to fulfill his or her family roles. In order for the family to maintain its homeostasis, the roles of the person with injury must be reallocated, and redefined, as was done in Mr. M's family.

Accession refers to the addition to the family of an unplanned for family member. This may include an unexpected pregnancy or the addition to the household of an elderly parent or friend who stays for a protracted visit. Regardless of whether the family views the addition as positive or negative, it produces disequilibrium in the family system and requires a redefinition of family roles. Issues related to accession arise at the point when the person with head injury returns home. If he or she was living independently and returns to live with his or her parents, a couple that might have been anticipating retirement suddenly find themselves once again in the parental role. In some families, a friend or family member may move in to help the spouse or parents. While the help may be appreciated, the addition of a new person in the family system often obfuscates the family's existing roles, resulting in confusion and resentment in individual family members. This dilemma was clearly identified by McLaughlin and Schaffer (1985): "Spouses, on the other hand, find themselves in a confused role. While they may also vigorously engage in a caretaking role initially, a full marital relationship cannot be sustained under these conditions. Indeed, the spouse's role confusion can be intensified if the patient's parents are present and competing to be caretakers, a role with which they are more familiar" (pp. 15–16). The intervention team needs to be sensitive to these issues and maintain contact with families after the individual with a head injury is discharged, since these issues may not become obvious until he or she returns home.

Demoralization refers to the loss of morale or family unity. In its most extreme form demoralization leads to the total dissolution of the family. Hill maintains that prolonged stress associated with either accession or dismemberment can produce demoralization as family members are forced to give up their roles and assume new ones. This may explain the research that suggests that family stress does not abate simply with time after the injury. In fact, some families report increased stress as the strain and frustration build. In a 5-year longitudinal study of families of persons with head injury, Brooks, Campsie, Symington, Beattie, and McKinlay (1986) found an increase in family stress, with a rise in threats of personal violence from 15% to 54%. Reports of aggression and divorce in families of persons with head injury may reflect demoralization associated with the long-term effects of accession and dismemberment and the resulting breakdown in the family system. The intervention team should not assume that families will adjust with time. Many families may need continued support and consultation from the team as they seek to re-establish a sense of balance in the family system.

Another consideration with regard to variable A (the event) in Hill's model is the cumulative nature of stressor events. Family stress may linger from earlier unresolved events, leaving the family vulnerable to stress. However, families that have successfully adapted and coped with stress may actually become stronger as a result of the experience. It is important to recognize that after someone has a severe head injury, the family not only must cope with the physical trauma to the family member, but may also face social isolation, loss of income, limited opportunity for leisure activities, and a variety of other secondary issues (see Williams, 1987, and Williams, Chapter 8, this volume). If families are unable to successfully cope with these multiple events, the family's resources may be depleted, and the family is more likely to perceive an event as a crisis. The devastation experienced by a person who no longer receives understanding and support from a spouse due to his or her injury is an example of the depletion of family resources that can lead to crisis.

Variable B in the equation in Hill's model represents the family's crisis meeting resources. This reflects the family's level of organization and can be understood in terms of the concepts of *adaptability* and *cohesion*. First, adaptability is the extent to which the family system is flexible and able to change. It is defined as "the marital or family system's ability to change its power structure, role relationships and relationship rules in response to situational and developmental stress" (Olson et al., 1985, p. 4). The family's level of adaptability can be placed along a continuum from low to high, as represented in Figure 2.

According to Hill, families with very little adaptability are classified as rigid. Their role expectations or family rules are fixed, and the family finds it almost impossible to change these rules in response to changes within the family or the environment. These families appear to be immobilized by an injury to a family member and are unable to redefine family roles so that the system can continue to function efficiently. Families with moderately low levels of adaptability are labeled structured. They are more adaptable than

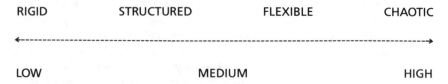

Figure 2. The continuum of family adaptability.

rigid families, but may still find it difficult to alter family patterns. Families with moderately high levels of adaptability are referred to as flexible. While these families have clear roles and role expectations, they are able to alter or redefine roles in response to internal or environmental demands. Finally, families with extremely high levels of adaptability are classified as chaotic. Family roles are so flexible that they are constantly changing in response to the slightest change in the environment. There is almost no consistency in the family, and no one in the family is clear about who is responsible for specific family functions. These families have difficulty carrying out tasks that are crucial to the effective operation of the family system. They require clear direction from the intervention team in order to secure medical equipment, arrange appointments, and manage the needs of the individual with the head injury. According to Hill's theory, family functioning is enhanced when families maintain a balanced position along this continuum. Families in which this occurs have fairly clearly defined roles and role relationships, which can be redefined and adapted as the need arises.

The second concept of family organization, family cohesion, is the extent to which family members are connected to, or separate from the family. It is defined as, "the emotional bonding that family members have toward one another" (Olson et al., 1985, p. 4). Family cohesion, like family adaptability, can be placed along a continuum from low to high as represented in Figure 3.

Hill refers to families with little cohesion as disengaged. Individuals in these families have very little contact with one another. There is minimal communication among family members. In fact, they may know very little about one another. These families are clearly at risk following an injury to one of their members, since the stress associated with the injury may erode the family's already fragile sense of connectedness. Families with moderately low levels of cohesion are classified as separated. Family members have more contact but are still relatively isolated from one another, having relatively little interaction. Families with moderately high levels of cohesion are identified as connected. Family members retain their individuality, but they feel a bond between themselves and other family members. They are able to support one another and work toward common goals. Finally, families with extremely high levels of cohesion are labeled enmeshed. These families tolerate very little individuality. Each person is part of an undefined, amorphous, family

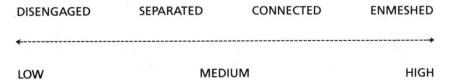

Figure 3. The continuum of family cohesion.

group. Family members find it very difficult to disagree and almost impossible to leave the family to go away to school or even marry. Because there is no sense of personal boundaries, one person's problems threaten everyone in the family. Such families are often very overprotective and stifle attempts by family members to assert their independence. As with adaptability, Hill maintains that families who maintain a balanced or moderate position along this continuum are best able to cope with stress. These are the families in which family members feel a bond with, and are able to support one another, while at the same time allowing the expression of each person's individuality.

There is research (Maitz, 1989) that supports the theoretical and clinical utility of this model in families in which a spouse has sustained a severe head injury. The author found that couples in the "head injury families" reported significantly less family cohesion ($p = .001$) than in the "non-injury families." In order to determine whether these two constructs had an impact upon the couples' marital relationships, the combined scores for couples in the "head injury families" on one set of variables (family adaptability, family cohesion, and time since injury) were compared with their scores on an instrument (Olson et al., 1985) that measures areas of marital conflict (EN-RICH). The results of the canonical correlation revealed a significant correlation between the two sets of variables ($p = .006$), thereby supporting the contribution of family cohesion and family adaptability to marital functioning in couples in which a spouse has sustained a severe head injury.

Variable C in the equation in Hill's model is the definition the family makes of the event. The family's definition of an event appears to reflect cultural norms and values. Within some social, cultural, and economic groups, a child's decision, for example, not to finish high school may be accepted or even supported by the family. In others, it may produce a family crisis. In the situation of a person with a head injury, some families may perceive the person as an embarrassment to be segregated from family functions. Others may make it a point to include the person in family functions.

The definition the family makes of the event may also be affected by the family's ascription of responsibility or blame. If the responsibility for the event is thought to be extra-familial, as in a fire or flood, the family system may be strengthened as the family rallies its resources in order to protect itself from the source of the perceived threat. If the responsibility for the event is thought to lie within the family, as in alcoholism or teenage parenthood, demoralization may occur. The ascription of blame is often subtle and is not always verbalized, which makes it difficult to resolve. After an accident or injury, family members may not openly discuss feelings of blame because they think their feelings are irrational or unfair. Nevertheless, the feelings persist and need to be addressed. In some cases, the person with the head injury may in fact be responsible for the accident. This becomes increasingly problematic if he or she was being reckless or using drugs or alcohol at the time of the accident. The blame, and associated guilt, may be intensified if other family members were also injured. If these issues remain unresolved, they can contribute to demoralization and the eventual dissolution of the family.

SUMMARY

It is critical that rehabilitation programs for individuals with head injuries involve the person's family throughout the rehabilitation and reintegration process. A head injury is not an isolated event. It has a profound impact on the family system and on individual family members. Helping the family adjust to the injury minimizes the impact of the injury on the family and strengthens the family system to which the person with an injury returns.

The intervention team should include someone who understands family systems, can help the family adjust, and can enlist the family's support in the rehabilitation process. It is imperative that the team maintain contact with the family after the person is discharged. Problems may not surface until after several months or even years, as the stress of caring for the person with the injury builds. It is also important to recognize that family adjustment is an ongoing process. It is not a linear progression that proceeds in stages and ends in acceptance. It is ongoing and cyclical and requires continued readjustment as the individual and the family mature. After a person has a brain injury, he or she is forever changed. Families mourn the person who was. The mourning occurs and reoccurs at significant times during the life cycle. The therapist may need to help families acknowledge that their grief is real and valid.

Most important, anyone who works with families should recognize that each family is unique and has its own culture, values, and personal history. Every family experiences, and responds to, stress in their own fashion. Only by assessing the scope of the event, the family's resources, and the family's definition of the event can the impact of the event be understood and appreciated. Because every family's history and resources are unique, so are their needs. A range of services should be available to families after careful assessment of each family. Not every family requires intensive family therapy. Families like Mr. M's, which have successfully coped with crises and have good crisis meeting resources, may require only support and/or brief family intervention. These families often benefit from an educational approach that helps family members understand the nature of the head injury and the changes in the family system. Other families benefit most from the emotional support that is available in family support groups. High-risk families include those who have not coped well with crises in the past, have experienced recent multiple stressful events, or have very limited crisis meeting resources. These families should be referred to a family therapist who is familiar with family systems theory and understands head injury.

The family systems model helps the person with a head injury relinquish behaviors associated with the role of patient and begin to redefine his or her place in the family system. Each step in this process has implications for family members, who must also redefine their roles in response to the reintegration of the person with the injury. If the family system is not considered in the design and implementation of the intervention plan, the plan may fail because it is inconsistent with the organization and/or operation of the family system. In this situation, staff and/or family members are often left feeling confused, angry, and resentful. When family members are involved in the intervention, the family system is strengthened, and the likelihood of successful outcome is increased.

REFERENCES

Brooks, D., Campsie, L., Symington, C., Beattie, A., & McKinlay, W. (1986). The five year outcome of severe blunt head injury: A relative's view. *Journal of Neurology, Neurosurgery and Psychiatry, 46*, 330–344.

Gurman, A., & Kniskern, D. (1981). Family therapy outcome research: Knowns and Unknowns. In A. Gurman & D. Kniskern (Eds.), *Handbook of family therapy* (pp. 742–776). New York: Brunner/Mazel.

Hill, R. (1958). Social stresses on the family. *Social Casework, 39*, 139–158.

Klonoff, P., & Prigatano, G. (1987). Reactions of family members and clinical intervention after traumatic brain injury. In M. Ylvisaker & E. Gobble (Eds.), *Community re-entry for head injured adults* (pp. 381–402). Boston: Little, Brown.

Lezak, M. (1976). Living with the characterologically altered brain injured patient. *Journal of Clinical Psychiatry, 39*, 592–598.

Livingston, M., & Brooks, D. (1988). The burden on families of the brain injured: A review. *Journal of Head Trauma Rehabilitation, 3*, 6–13.

Livingston, M., Brooks, D., & Bond, M. (1985). Three months after severe head injury: Psychiatric and social impact on relatives. *Journal of Neurology, Neurosurgery and Psychiatry, 48*, 870–875.

Maitz, E. (1990). *The psychosocial sequelae of a severe closed head injury and their impact upon family systems* (Doctoral dissertation, Temple University, Philadelphia). *Dissertation Abstracts International, 51*, 4.

Mauss-Clum, N., & Ryan, M. (1981). Brain injury and the family. *Journal Of Neurosurgical Nursing, 13*, 165–169.

McLaughlin, A., & Schaffer, V. (1985). Rehabilitate or remold: Family involvement in head trauma recovery. *Cognitive Rehabilitation, 3*, 14–17.

Olson, D., McCubbin, H., Barnes, H., Larsen, A., Muxen, M., & Wilson, M. (1985). *Family inventories*. Minneapolis: University of Minnesota.

Panting, A., & Merry, P. (1972). The long term rehabilitation of severe head injuries with particular reference to the need for social and medical support for the patient's family. *Rehabilitation, 38*, 33–37.

Rosenbaum, M., & Najenson, T. (1976). Changes in life patterns and symptoms of low mood as reported by wives of severely brain injured soldiers. *Journal of Consulting and Clinical Psychology, 44*, 881–888.

Rosenthal, M., & Geckler, C. (1986). Family therapy issues in neuropsychology. In D. Wedding, A. Hortan, & J. Webster (Eds.), *The neuropsychology handbook: Behavioral and clinical perspectives* (pp. 325–344). New York: Springer.

Sachs, P. (1985). Beyond support: Traumatic head injury as a growth experience for families. *Rehabilitation Nursing, January–February,* 21–23.

Turnbull, A.P., & Turnbull, H.R. (1990). Families, professsionals, and exceptionality: A special partnership. Columbus: Charles E. Merril.

Watzlawick, P., Beavin, J., & Jackson, D. (1967). *Pragmatics of human communication.* New York: W.W. Norton.

White, R. (1972). *The enterprise of living growth and organization in personality.* New York: Holt, Rinehart & Winston.

Williams, J. (1987). Families: The line between hope and reality. *Trends in Rehabilitation, 3,*14–18.

Zarski, J.J., Hall, D.E., & DePompei, R. (1987). Closed head injury patients: A family therapy approach to the rehabilitation process. *The American Journal of Family Therapy , 15,* 62–68.

ADDITIONAL READINGS

DePompei, R., Zarski, J., & Hall, D. (1987). A systems approach to understanding CHI family functioning. *Cognitive Rehabilitation, 5,* 6–10.

Olsen, D., Sprenkel, D., & Russell, C. (1979). Circumplex model of marital and family systems. *Family Process, 18,* 337–351.

Willer, B., Arrigali, M., & Liss, M. (1989). *Family adjustment to the long term effects of traumatic brain injury of husbands* (Report No. 89–2). Buffalo: University of Buffalo, The Rehabilitation Research and Training Center.

8

FAMILY REACTION
TO HEAD INJURY

JANET M. WILLIAMS

The presentation of how all families react to head injury is far too ambitious a goal for a single chapter. However, it is possible to review several existing paradigms of family reaction to disability and create a framework to understand the short- and long-term implications of head injury on the family system.

There are two distinctions to make when describing a family's reaction to head injury. First is the family's reaction to the event of head injury itself. The family experiences a profound loss, often realizing that the person is significantly different than before the head injury. This psychological reaction is intense at first and becomes episodic as time passes. Second is the family's reaction to the person's actual behaviors and characteristics as well as the ongoing events they encounter. The family must learn to react and cope with different behaviors and caretaking needs across the life cycle of the family. The reactions become more predictable, and families learn to draw on resources to develop or strengthen coping responses. Families deal with both reactions at the same time, constantly trying to anticipate the reaction to their new day-to-day life while dealing with the unpredictable loss reaction that may occur. In both instances, the loss reaction is episodic in that it comes and goes, lasts for different lengths of time, and is only sometimes predictable.

This chapter describes the traditional view of the experience of loss and family recovery after disability. The two distinctions of how families react to

The author expresses appreciation to Jane Dean, Beth O'Brien, Mary Pat Beals, and Ann P. Turnbull for their helpful comments.

head injury are then presented. The overlap of distinctions is presented in a new paradigm as a window through which to view how the family system regroups and deals with ongoing events they encounter. This paradigm will enhance the ability to elaborate on four areas of concern to families and professionals: 1) the immediate impact of head injury on the family system, 2) the interaction between the family system and other significant systems, 3) the long-term implications of head injury on the family system, and 4) ways to support families in understanding and dealing with their reactions. This new understanding can lead to more creative ways for families and professionals to support one another after a family member experiences a head injury.

LOSS AND TRADITIONAL FAMILY RECOVERY PARADIGMS

For most people, the ending of an episode of illness will be the result of cure, of remission, or of death (Mailick, 1979). In the case of cure or remission, families are thankful that the illness is gone, with some ongoing concern about its return. For the most part, they rely upon the advice of medical experts to predict their future, and family members are able to take on their former roles within the family. In short, the family resumes their interrupted existence (Murphy, Scheer, Murphy, & Mack, 1988). In the event of death, each family member goes through a defined process of mourning for all family members, with proper regard for the memory of the person who died. Roles and expectations among the remaining members are redefined, and new or altered relationships are established outside the family. In both instances, some sort of resolution is achieved by the family and they are able to move on with life.

For families of people who experience head injury, a different set of tasks is required. There is a loss reaction, but for the family there is no final resolution. The person, as they knew him or her before, is no longer there and they must get to know a new person. There is a paradox of coping with the horrors of head injury and at the same time being grateful that the person is alive (Corbin & Strauss, 1988). Roles and relationships change, often many times, and the entire family system must adapt. The family must deal with the loss of the person while taking on responsibility for the person who now has a new role in the family. In Chapter 2, JoAnn Kramer views her experience:

> I have vivid memories of Jenny receiving a basketball as a Christmas present the day before her accident. The agile, aggressive, little bubbly blond girl dribbled that ball all over our farm house and was so excited. Twenty four hours later she was lying in intensive care, eyes closed and decerebrate. This is where the new and different Jenny began. I cried every day for at least a year out of frustration, and at intermittent times later. It took me 5 years to truly accept the personality change and to totally convince myself that I could handle this new person in my mind. (JoAnn Kramer, parent)

To understand how families adjust to a family member with a head injury, it is useful to learn more about the adjustment of families of people with mental retardation. The adjustment model of the experience of parents of children with mental retardation has evolved over the years. In the late 1960s and early 1970s, the model of grief response to the death of a loved one, developed by Kubler-Ross, was applied to the reaction of families to disability (Kubler-Ross, 1969). Families worked through their grief over time and came to a final acceptance of the loss of the family member. This model was applied to families of people with a variety of disabilities, including people with mental retardation, mental illness, and chronic illness. Families heard of the "impairment," grieved in response to the loss, and followed a linear progression that led to full acceptance. The stages of anger, denial, anxiety, and fear were the predictable milestones that people reached at specific time intervals.

Over time, a different understanding of family reaction to the loss experienced after disability evolved. "Chronic sorrow," introduced by Olshansky (1962), described families of people with mental retardation as experiencing repeated sadness over time. In this framework the family never fully reconciles themselves to the loss, and continues on with life never fully coming to terms with the lost possibility of how good life could have been had the injury not occurred. Later, Wikler (1981) noted that the stages of adaptation did not have predictable linear progression. A family's reaction was based upon life cycle changes and other types of crises related to the disability (Wikler, Wasow, & Hartfield, 1981). Each family differed as did each child with a disability.

Viewing family recovery through these models has been a quite useful approach, but it also has certain drawbacks when applied to families of people with head injury. In the first framework, families are considered to be reaching for a specific destination of acceptance, in a linear fashion. To accept a situation without striving to meet new challenges is fatalistic. In everyday life people seek to overcome challenges. After head injury, the challenges may be far greater and seem overwhelming at times, but the family continues to draw upon needed resources to meet the challenges. To accept is to give up hope. To adjust is to realize what is, while continuing to strive for what could be. Additionally, the linear approach denies life cycle stresses that families encounter when they approach new stages and transitions.

In the second framework, families are seen to be in a constant state of sorrow about the person's current abilities. There are, however, families who believe that head injury is not necessarily the worst thing that has happened to their family (O'Brien, 1987); as traumatic as the situation may continue to be, not all families persist in chronic sorrow. They have episodes of sorrow, but they are able to balance the sorrow with the coping mechanisms that allow them to gain a sense of meaning in their lives. Both theories may be applied to a specific point in time in some families, but they do not address the constantly changing dynamics of family life.

Wikler's (1981) concept of stages of reaction based upon life cycle changes more closely represents a family's reaction to head injury. The process of recovery is a journey, not a destination (Power & Dell Orto, 1981). Grief for families is not time-bound, nor does it follow a predictable course. Grief changes over time as the life cycle of the family leads to changes and transitions. If it were time-bound, professionals would facilitate the family working through specific Kubler-Ross–like stages, discontinue these services at the conclusion of adjustment, and identify those families who did not go through these stages as dysfunctional. Given the great variation in family reaction and the ongoing nature of challenges faced by families, all families would be labeled dysfunctional.

Over time, families interact with many systems and strive to achieve a balance in their lives. The event of dealing with the disability of a member of the family can become one of many life circumstances with which families cope quite effectively. The loss reaction may be present in the family's life, but it does not have to create an overwhelming situation, preventing families from creating meaning in their lives. The very presence of the person may bring a new sensitivity to the importance of new life goals which were previously unrecognized. The presence of the person with a disability in the family is not denied, but his or her presence does not continue to be the focal point of the family. A balance is achieved in which all family members can have their needs met.

EPISODIC LOSS REACTION

The framework of the changing life cycle that all families experience points away from the notion of final acceptance and chronic sorrow to a different path. Families experience an episodic loss reaction over time associated with the event of head injury in the family. This framework for understanding the family's reaction combines the psychological reaction to the loss of the person the family knew, with the reaction to the stress created by the reality of daily living problems. It recognizes the family's need to grieve, as defined by Kubler-Ross, as well as the sorrow that families experience, as defined by Olshansky. In addition, it recognizes the family's need to deal with ongoing events and to adapt to the situation, regaining some balance. The framework is a dynamic one that is adaptable over time, recognizing the family's changing nature.

As shown in Figure 4, the episodic loss reaction is most often precipitated by an event. The event may be an unpredictable one, such as a memory of the person pre-injury, or a predictable event, such as a transition point or milestone that a person is not able to reach because of the head injury. The event may be a fleeting memory of a favorite movie that the person can no

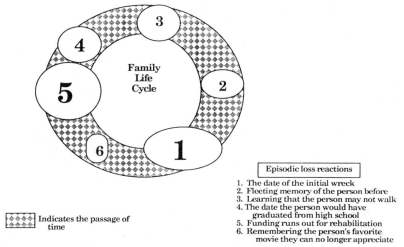

Episodic loss reactions

1. The date of the initial wreck
2. Fleeting memory of the person before
3. Learning that the person may not walk
4. The date the person would have
   graduated from high school
5. Funding runs out for rehabilitation
6. Remembering the person's favorite
   movie they can no longer appreciate

Indicates the passage of
time

Figure 4. Episodic loss reaction.

longer appreciate, or the milestone that marks the date of the injury. A transition point may be the time when the person is discharged from one treatment program to another. Families experience many such events in the life cycle, both developmental and nondevelopmental, as described in Chapter 6 by Turnbull and Turnbull. In the new framework, the event will lead to an episode of loss reaction that the family may or may not have anticipated.

Each episodic loss reaction triggers the emotions of a grief reaction. Each emotion is a feeling resulting directly from the type of event the family experiences. For example, a mother may feel great sadness and even depression when her daughter's friends are having children, while her daughter remains in a coma. Individual family members may experience different emotions as a result of the same event. For example, if for a short time a person with a head injury takes on a role within the family that he or she held before the injury, one family member may express joy at the future possibilities, while another family member may express sadness that the person could not maintain the role.

Often unexpected and intense, the psychological reaction can occur immediately after the injury or years later. Families may go through common reactions at the outset, but as time progresses family members will jump differently from grieving state to grieving state. The time between each reaction may lengthen as families begin to adjust to the situation. The more predictable loss reaction is the reaction to the daily events that the family encounters. The practical needs of the family member who was injured may bring on anger, denial, and frustration. The family must find the resources necessary to cope with the situation.

Families use existing coping strategies to develop new coping strategies to deal with the ongoing loss reactions. Existing strategies may be present as a result of dealing with a previous crisis. If the mother in a family had been ill in the past and family members had assumed new roles within the family, they may have developed the coping skills to better adjust to the injury of another member at a later time. Families may develop new coping strategies to deal with the reactions and may even learn to anticipate the reactions, allowing them to take measures to be sure that they receive the support they need at different times. For example, the mother of a youth with a head injury may realize that the graduation of her son's high school class may bring on an intense reaction, and she may choose to be out of town the weekend of graduation.

Ongoing Events and the Episodic Loss Reaction

As Viktor Frankl stated in his book, *Man's Search for Meaning,* "An abnormal reaction to an abnormal situation is normal behavior." Problems that families with a member with a head injury face are not inherent personal deficits (Dunst, Trivette, Gordon, & Pletcher, 1989), but natural reactions to unnatural events. Initially, the constant pressure on families to react to every situation prevents them from acquiring and using the competencies necessary to mobilize the resources to meet their needs. In being reminded of the loss over time, the family will continue to have reactions but will be able to predict more of the day-to-day situations and to acquire some of the competencies needed to move from situation to situation.

For some families, moving on after each event is not as smooth as it is for others. There is no clear definition of how families should react to each event. Each family differs in their adaptability, cohesion, and communication, thereby differing in their reaction. In addition, the event itself and family interaction with other systems create even greater disparity in how different families react to each event. Providing consistent support during the process of reaction allows professionals to understand how and why families react as they do to each event.

The ongoing nature of having to regroup after each situation helps the family learn from previous reactions and redefine roles within the family in a positive way. As a single mother, Beth O'Brien (1987) describes how she was able to deal with one situation:

> Helping John become a part of the teenage world had its notable moments, especially during outings and vacations. John's favorite activity has always been fishing. Despite the tremors, he has been able to relearn fishing, except for baiting the hook. Handling night crawlers is not exactly my line of work. On one fishing expedition there were no other fishermen to bait the hook, and I wasn't having an easy time of it. Finally, in frustration, I dumped all those worms on the dock and chased them with the hook until I got one. After that it was only shrimp and minnows for bait, but I did learn from a friendly fisherman how to bait a hook. John was very proud of me. (p. 426)

Understanding episodic loss reaction contributes to a framework for understanding the immediate impact of head injury on the family system, how families must interact with other systems, and how families deal with ongoing events they encounter. It is important to understand that the episodic loss reaction is present throughout the life cycle and has great bearing on how events are perceived by families.

THE IMMEDIATE IMPACT
OF HEAD INJURY ON THE FAMILY SYSTEM

There are many anecdotal reports by families about the experience of being informed about a family member's head injury (Bush, 1986). Often, the family receives a telephone call to come to the hospital immediately; there has been a tragedy. The family rushes to the hospital playing out all possible scenarios they may face upon arrival. They prepare themselves for the worst possible outcome. When they arrive, they find that the person has survived the injury, but the ongoing uncertainty of whether the person will live may last for days or weeks. The family maintains a vigil at the hospital. Perhaps having no previous experience with tragedy, the family hopes for survival; they just want the person to live.

The immediate crisis that a family experiences after learning of a loved one's injury has a profound and lasting effect. The immediate reaction is a combination of disbelief that the injury has occurred, shock that the situation is so critical, anger that this has happened to their loved one, with feelings of guilt and fear about the immediate future. After such intense emotions are set into play, families must continually react to events, having little opportunity to plan for future information that they receive. The intense web of pain and fear sets the stage for many future situations in which the family must make critical decisions in an effort to rally to support the member with a head injury.

While the family is experiencing the shock of head injury, perhaps for the first time, professionals deal with the event as one of many that have occurred, bringing their own set of values and experiences to the situation. Professionals often proceed with caution when informing family members about the medical condition of their relative. Some give the worst possible case scenario, believing that a report of any better future outcome will be perceived by the family as reason to rejoice. They may tell the family that the person will be a "vegetable" or would be "better off dead." While the family is praying for survival at any cost, the professionals are trying to deliver information about how high that cost may be. Some families are given concrete information without the doom and gloom predictions for the future. The information, while it may not be encouraging, is not presented as a yardstick to measure future outcome. This initial delivery of information by professionals, and how the family then translates that information into their own reality, has a lasting effect on families.

The delivery of this initial information by professionals is often the first in a long series of encounters the family will have with professionals. The family's perception of how professionals deliver this initial information may set the tone for future encounters. If the family is given negative information that is not born out, they may develop immediate disbelief in all subsequent information given by professionals. After all, they've proven the professional wrong once, why not again? For those who perceive that the bad news was delivered without predictions of dire outcome, a balance of guarded optimism for the future may develop.

Professionals need to be open and honest about the fact that they are having a hard time finding the right words to talk to the family (Poyadue, 1988). Also, it is important not to inject one's own negativism about the situation based upon previous situations. In addition, professionals should refrain from predictions for the future, especially negative ones, at such an emotional time.

For the family of a person with a head injury, the loss reaction is intense and often lasts for prolonged periods of time. The intensity is exacerbated by the fact that the family is anxious for the return of the previous person. Soon after survival is assured, the family assumes that the next logical step is cure, leading to full recovery. But the family must deal with a complex set of problems that are unique to head injury. Also the person will be in the acute care setting for weeks, maybe months, before becoming medically stable.

When survival is assured, the family focus must shift to the next set of tasks presented by the crisis, again in a reactive way. The continued reactive posture, over a long period of time, throws off the balance of the family system presented in the framework by Turnbull and Turnbull in Chapter 6. The family's life cycle, functions, resources, and interactions are altered to accommodate the needs of the person in jeopardy. Implications for such a profound effect on family homeostasis are enormous. The issues of such ongoing turmoil are covered in Chapter 7 by Maitz.

Once a person who experiences a head injury is medically stable, he or she may take different routes in rehabilitation. Which routes are taken may depend upon finances, availability of services, the person's level of disability, the family's decision, or a combination of all four. In many instances, a person leaves the acute care hospital after a head injury and enters a specialized rehabilitation program to address specific needs. If, after some time in rehabilitation, a person needs ongoing services and is fortunate enough to have the finances, he or she may have several options for where to live, including an extended care program or a supported community setting. Often, people with head injuries and their families are not able to gain access to any rehabilitation services or they are forced to cut the process short, due to financial constraints or lack of knowledge about options that exist.

During this acute period, families are in a continual state of loss reaction. Since the family focus has shifted completely to the person with the head injury and events are changing on a daily basis, the family is in a constant state of differing emotions. Each piece of news brings on a different reaction. It is at this time that families are the most vulnerable and may rely upon denial as a coping mechanism for extended periods of time (Romano, 1974). The family does not always recognize the enormity of the situation, which would allow them to mobilize their own emotional energy to face the future.

THE INTERACTION BETWEEN
THE FAMILY SYSTEM AND OTHER SIGNIFICANT SYSTEMS

The family is the single social unit in human society inextricably interwoven with all other systems (Anderson & Carter, 1978). Before a head injury occurs, a family has usually established relationships with other systems outside of the family that allow them to function as a unit. They become comfortable with their interaction with their church, school, work, and other systems. After a head injury, the family suddenly finds themselves immersed in a medical system they may never have needed before and interacting with professionals who seem to speak a different language. In addition, all of the relationships in which they were involved pre-injury must be renegotiated. They must turn to the church they formerly supported and ask for help, they must ask the school and employer to allow some flexibility so that family members can rally around the family member in need. If the person with the injury is in school or employed, the family must hope that the person's return will be accommodated. At times, the former ties must be severed and families must search out new systems for support.

After crisis, some families return to the old order, while others undergo major transformations (Reiss & Oliver, 1980). After a head injury, there is no clear-cut definition of when the crisis is over. Crisis becomes redefined by the anxiety of not knowing what will happen, the fantasies and fears about what might be wrong, the guilt, and the constant belief reinforced by society that when a person gets sick, he or she is cured and sent home. Furthermore, crisis affects the practical issues of family life. For Marty Beaver, in Chapter 3, crisis became the termination of her husband's program for behavior problems. And for Hope Hardgrove, in Chapter 4, crisis became each time her father hit 100 on the anger scale. The family is transformed to live in constant anticipation of a new crisis, and crisis becomes a way of life.

Family Interaction with the Medical System and Professionals

The initial shock and disbelief that a family experiences is compounded by their ongoing need to rely upon a rehabilitation system for the future quality of life of their family member. The interaction between a family system that is out of balance and a rehabilitation system that enters the family's life for a period of time, changes the functioning of the family system in subtle and more obvious ways. For example, as families interact with professionals, the professionals seem to speak a different language that families often find confusing and intimidating. Beth O'Brien (1987) describes her experience:

> The first formal meeting with the staff of the center was a nightmare. It was brutally demoralizing to face a set of professionals who had very important information and not be able even to understand their titles, much less their jargon. "Physical therapy" and "speech therapy" made some sense to me, but what did "occupational therapy" mean? Wasn't it a bit early to be thinking about occupations? And what was "cognitive rehabilitation therapy"? And Aphasia? Apraxia? Agnosia? When they first mentioned John's premorbid characteristics, I thought they might be predicting his death! These strange and bewildering words made me feel uneducated and uncomfortable and initially formed a barrier between me and the staff. (p. 424)

Many families begin to pick up the jargon and become as adept as professionals at speaking "the language." Not only is this common, it is necessary. Families are involved with professionals for a number of years after a head injury and must adapt to dealing with the medical system to receive the services and programs they need. It is probably unrealistic to think that the entire medical community will change their jargon to use words like "walk" instead of "ambulate" or "right arm" instead of "right upper extremity." Therefore, it is necessary to educate families early on to the fact that medical language is different, is intimidating at first, and that families will begin to learn the language over time. Families should be provided with a list of common medical terms and their meanings.

Family Interaction with Extended Family and Friends

Often relatives and friends do not know how to respond over time to the profound loss that families experience. Morton (1985) in *Parents Speak Out,* describes her thoughts on how others react to a family's grief:

> There is no established way of announcing the time for grief (in fact no real certainty that one is entitled to out-and-out grieving) since it takes a while before anyone can know how severe the disability is. One should not be gloomy and expect the worst. But there is certainly little reason to feel happy. Family and friends face the same ambivalence. Just what is their role? What words should they say? Should they extend their sympathy? None of the usual comforting gestures are appropriate, so most people, under such circumstances, do and say nothing. The absence of a response to an event of such enormous significance and impact on the lives of the parents simply compounds their loneliness. (p. 146)

For families of people with head injury, the reaction of friends to their loss is similar. When someone experiences a head injury and enters the hospital, families and friends, alike in their previous experience with the medical community, believe the person is "ill" and will be "all better" when he or she is ready to return home. As time goes on and progress slows, families are bombarded with information about head injury, and they begin to realize that the person may not fully recover. Extended family and friends are more removed from the situation without the benefit of information and contact with the person, and they continue to anticipate full recovery. The gap of understanding between friends and family widens. Families find that they are not able to explain the situation, and friends do not know what to ask or how to react.

In addition, as families take on the jargon of the medical community, they often begin to use it outside of the medical community. By doing so the family unknowingly alienates extended family and friends who are not directly involved in the situation. For example, there probably are not too many neighbors who understand how "an increase in range of motion can lead to feeding oneself or combing one's hair." Families should be sensitized to this possibility and remind one another to use the layperson's language.

When thinking about family interaction with other systems, we must reflect back upon the "Copernican Revolution" referred to by Turnbull and Turnbull in Chapter 6. For the family to truly be the center of the rehabilitation process, professionals must begin to recognize how they interact as a system themselves, and also how as a system, the family interacts with other systems. Presently, it is often necessary for families to change their functioning to adapt to other systems; in the future, other systems must recognize and adapt to the needs of families.

LONG-TERM IMPLICATIONS
OF HEAD INJURY ON THE FAMILY SYSTEM

Families may be involved in some type of rehabilitation for as long as 6 years after a head injury and have support from the medical community (Jacobs, 1988). Other families may not have access to any rehabilitation, which would force them to return home directly from acute care (Bush, 1988). In both situations, the families are largely on their own, intensifying their understanding of the permanence and irreversibility of head injury. Now, families must negotiate a new set of service delivery systems with little preparation and few mentors. They continue to face many challenges that bring on stress.

It is the stress of daily reality that brings on the second distinction in how families react to head injury. Some situations, repeated often enough, can be anticipated by families, and they can change their reaction to the situation accordingly. For example, a family may predict that there will be no services when their child needs respite care, but they may find that they react differently the third time they seek it. Instead of feeling helpless and forfeiting a planned trip, they become charged with energy to find the service and call countless agencies until they receive help. It is the constant stress of situations over the life cycle that drains the family's energy and resources.

Marcelissen, Winnubst, Bunk, and DeWolff (1988) define stress as those factors in the environment that are perceived by the individual as being problematic. Specifically, there are two kinds of stress that may threaten the family as they deal with the long-term implications of head injury: 1) the perceived imbalance between the resources that a family possesses and the demands of the environment on those resources, and 2) the family's needs exceeding the opportunities that the environment has to meet those needs. Both forms of stress threaten families after head injury. In the first, the environment becomes all of the systems that families are now forced to interact with in a new way. Demands come from the medical system, the insurance system, and the social system, all of which clearly tax the resources that a family possesses. Many families have never before dealt with many of the systems they find themselves using. For example, very few families have reason to apply for vocational rehabilitation services before a head injury occurs. In the second form of stress, the threat is most apparent to families who do not have access to rehabilitation services or to families who are forced to face a community that does not have the resources they need. For example, the family who cares for someone with a severe head injury at home may not live in an area where respite services are available. The environment does not possess the resources that the family needs.

Ongoing Events Families Encounter

The stress described by Marcelissen et al. can be exemplified by eight situations that commonly contribute to the ongoing stress families experience after head injury. These situations do not exist exclusively or in any specific hierarchical order. Often, the situations overlap, with one having a further impact upon another. The factors that cause the greatest stress for families over time include: cognitive and social problems of the individual, lack of information, lack of services, uncertainty of the future, finances, role changes, social isolation, and prolonged caretaking. Each stressor increases the frequency and intensity of episodic loss reactions.

Cognitive and Social Problems   Studies have indicated that cognitive and social problems of the individual cause more stress on families than physical problems (Lezak, 1986). Hope Hardgrove's experience concurs with the research:

> I would say over the past 10 years Dad has improved a lot. He has been in a behavioral modification program, which really benefited us all. Thanks to this, Daddy is usually very, very happy. He is constantly singing, humming, talking, etc. Although the change from being almost constantly angry to continually happy may seem better to you, the singing etc. gets very annoying. Have you ever had to stay in a house with someone who 90% of the time is singing, whistling, etc., while you are studying, reading, or talking on the telephone? I will admit, though, after 8 years of this it really gets very amusing sometimes, but it gets old fast too. (Hope Hardgrove, child)

Lack of Information   Families do not receive information they need to plan for the long-term future of their family. Clinical researchers have conducted studies over the past 10 years that document that families do not receive information about the long-term consequences of head trauma in the acute care setting (Bond, 1983). At the time of injury, families believe that the episode of hospital care and recovery will be minimal. Often families do not know that their loved one may have severe problems with attention, concentration, memory, and problem-solving (Boll, 1982), as well as changes in emotions, personality, and behavior (Bond, 1983) that are often the consequence of head injury. In addition, families do not realize that the entire family system will experience ongoing stress associated with financial, legal, psycho-social, and care issues resulting from the head injury (Panting & Merry, 1972). As a result, people with head injuries and their families are unaware of the short- and long-term problems that may occur and affect all family members, and they are not prepared to manage these problems.

In one study (Seligman & Darling, 1989) families indicated that the most important type of help they had received from professionals was information. Beth O'Brien (1987) recalls her experience:

> Like most people, I had some idea about heart attacks, but I had absolutely no frame of reference for head injury. . . . But I wanted information. The first hospital had taught me nothing about brain damage; and the books that I found in the local library were of little help. During those long months of acute care, when I wondered if John would ever wake up, I wanted to learn about head injury: What happened to my son's brain? What would he be like? What happens to families in this situation? How do they cope? (p. 143)

Lack of Services   Usually, information about options and choices is not available, which makes the planning even more complicated. Families of people with head injuries do not always have information about their options and choices, and services may be restricted because of geographical location or type of service needed. A wide range of services are needed but are not available in many areas (Jacobs, 1988). Marty Beaver relates her experience:

> We began our search for a specialized head injury rehab facility, but no center was found. I needed more family help and support so we moved closer to John's family. John was unable to handle a different environment, and due to his anxiety and agitation, he had to be admitted to a psychiatric facility. This was certainly not in John's best interest, but we had no other choice at the time. (Marty Beaver, spouse)

Uncertainty of the Future   The rapid progress an individual makes early on after the injury only heightens expectations for prolonged steady progress. Planning for the future becomes as uncertain as the person's progress thus far. Why plan for semi-independent living when, as the family may believe, there is certain to be full recovery? The family may find themselves on a roller coaster of expectations, with hopes for the future alternately raised and dashed as the person makes progress or falls back (Wadsworth & Wadsworth, 1971).

Furthermore, when someone experiences a head injury, the family's expectations are heightened by constant thoughts of how the person was before the head injury. Families are forced to live in two worlds, striving to balance present capacities with hope for improvement and return to previous functioning. Marty Beaver describes her family's experience:

> I had been told that John would reach his "full" recovery at 6 months. As this time line drew closer I became more and more anxious. I needed and wanted some answers. The "not knowing" what the immediate future would bring was hard for me to deal with. After all, I was a health care professional and my business was that of making people well. Why couldn't something be done for John? Those months at home were exhausting, as I aimed toward providing structure and therapy for John along with balancing my role as mother for two young children. (Marty Beaver, spouse)

As time goes on, the family may begin to realize the importance of future planning, yet have difficulty carrying out the many tasks this requires. Many parents worry about what will happen to their dependent child who has experienced head injury, after the parents die (Jacobs, 1988). However, families often express the need to live 1 day at a time, thereby making the planning process a series of stressful events (Turnbull, 1989).

Finances   In addition to the previously mentioned stress factors that affect families on an ongoing basis, short- and long-term financial issues are reported to be of major concern to most families (Jacobs, 1988). The financial factors include both direct costs, such as inpatient care, home modifications, and respite care, as well as indirect costs, such as lost income, interference with career advancement, and travel expenses to visit family members who may be receiving rehabilitation in another state.

Joseph Maurer relates how not having insurance that covers rehabilitation caused financial stress on his family:

> My parents, as is so often the case in other families with head injuries, became Ed's primary caregivers during those first few months that became years. My mother rented a house in Seattle for a time and brought my brother there after his 8-week stay in various hospitals. His HMO had determined that, since he was ambulatory, he was no longer in need of rehabilitation—just one of the many incongruous medical realities my family and brother have faced since this phase in our lives began. (Joseph Maurer, sibling)

Role Changes   The person with a head injury may have cognitive, emotional, and behavioral difficulties that affect perception of reality, adequate judgement, and flexibility in thinking. These difficulties affect adjustment, which in turn affects a person's role within the family system (Florian, Katz, & Lahav, 1989). The family may have found new ways to function while the person was in rehabilitation, and they may be reluctant to relinquish the new roles. In addition, the person with the head injury may only be able to function in new roles intermittently.

The literature is replete with examples of role changes within the family after a head injury. Rosenbaum, Lipsitz, and Abraham (1978) describe the change in roles of wives of men who experienced head injury in the Arab/Israeli war of Yom Kippur. Bond (1983) describes the role of a wife who cannot mourn the injury of her husband which has meant she has lost her partner, her affectional and sexual needs cannot be fulfilled, and her husband has a role in which he is childlike and dependent. Brown and McCormick (1988) report that sibling birth order dynamics may be altered. A younger sibling may reach developmental milestones toward independence as the sibling with a head injury moves into a functionally lower position in the family. Joseph Maurer describes his relationship with his twin brother:

> My relationship with Ed, too, is changing. We are, in many ways, more dependent on each other than before. It is a delicate transition which allows me to sometimes be "the older brother," and other times forces me to "know my place." There is much Ed does *not* need me for. And the dance, as his brother, I am learning, involves equal steps forward and back. (Joseph Maurer, sibling)

Social Isolation   In the early stages of recovery relatives may rally around the family, but as time passes and recovery slows, they may withdraw their support (Bond, 1983). Former friends begin to move on to new life experiences and do not know how to incorporate the person with a head injury into their lives. Beth O'Brien (1987) describes the social isolation and loneliness her son John experienced after a local football game:

> He was with people who knew him, who were patient with him and who accepted him most of the time. The crunch came after the games were over. John had to go home with his mother while the others partied or hung out downtown. It was not that I insisted that John go home with me; rather it was just too much for young people to include John in after game activities. . . . The most difficult part of John's injury for both of us has been his terrible loneliness. He yearns for the company of other young people, for activities that are important for anyone his age. (p. 428)

Often a person's social network increases in density over time, with a corresponding decrease in the size of the network (Kozloff, 1987). People with head injuries become more socially isolated, have fewer friends, and rely more heavily on remaining support systems for emotional and physical needs. Most single people spend more time with the family, partly because peers are apparently disinterested in maintaining previously established relationships. Married couples also have their own unique experiences, as related by Maureen Campbell-Korves:

> I thought I was doing great. I was working hard on my speech, but apparently not hard enough to put some of my friends at ease. One person literally bolted from my room not to be heard from again for years. Another person told people, "that it would be best not to call me because it was painful for me to speak." As a couple, if people dropped me, they also dropped Doug. There was also the

sense that since I was beginning to look physically all right, I must be all right. I was being made to feel that I was somehow letting the side down. (Maureen Campbell-Korves, person with a head injury)

Prolonged Caretaking   Many families are not able to gain relief or even a temporary respite from the daily needs of a loved one with a head injury. Between 70,000 and 90,000 people between the ages of 15 and 35 experience head injury each year severe enough to require ongoing care and supervision (NHIF, 1986), thus becoming dependent upon their families to meet their daily needs for the rest of their lives. These numbers, combined with the fact that these individuals have an average life expectancy, make it evident that a family may have 20–30 years of caretaking ahead of them. Some families, like JoAnn Kramer's, are able to come to an understanding of the best way for their family to support their loved one with a head injury:

> This summer Jenny applied for low-income housing in a town near our farm. Once there is an opening she would like to move back to Iowa to be closer to her family. We believe that we will be ready for that when the time comes if we have a third party to provide service coordination for her. She will always need some support, and we know that we would become burned out in a short time helping Jenny manage her daily living. We believe that it is important to her future for her to continue developing her self-advocacy skills. (JoAnn Kramer, parent)

The factors contributing to the ongoing stress imposed upon families after head injury do not exist distinctly. They are interrelated and often have an impact on one or more other factors. For example, continual lack of information contributes to the family's uncertainty about the future. If they have no prognostic factors to look to, they cannot plan, nor can they strive to surpass suggested goals. If role changes exist over an extended period of time in an unacceptable way, the family will be reminded of the person's previous abilities, which will prompt more frequent and intense reactions to the loss.

Therefore, alleviating one factor may alleviate other factors. For example, if a family has additional financial resources, they may be able to purchase respite services, which may alleviate prolonged caretaking. Additional information may teach families to enhance their social network and decrease social isolation.

WAYS TO SUPPORT FAMILIES
IN UNDERSTANDING AND DEALING WITH THEIR REACTIONS

Like earthquakes, head injury is viewed as something that "happens to other people." Those "other people" are actually entire networks of family and friends who must rely upon one another and many new systems to deal with the future. The psychological and daily stress reaction occurs for ordinary people as a result of extraordinary events.

Despite the shock and aftershocks (stressors) families face, they find the resources to rebuild, adapt, and cope. As exemplified in Section I in the accounts by Maureen Campbell-Korves, JoAnn Kramer, Marty Beaver, Hope Hardgrove, and Joseph Maurer, stressors become challenges that are overcome when families mobilize resources and take action.

Families should be given information about their natural reaction to head injury. It is natural to be angry, feel guilty, and use denial as well as other coping mechanisms in some situations after a head injury or when any other traumatic event happens to a family. Too often families experience years of difficulties that bring on emotional reaction before they realize the reaction is part of the coping process. If families are supported to express these emotions and use the coping mechanisms most available to them, they may deal with the day-to-day reality of head injury more effectively. With this support, fewer families will have to say, "If I only had known then what I know now."

Services should support, not supplant, the family's coping resources (Vincent & Salisbury, 1988). Professionals must reexamine the current intervention methods. Family-focused services should be directed to support the family as well as the person. Rather than "enlisting the family," as is the common approach in rehabilitation, families should "enlist the professionals" to truly bring about a Copernican Revolution. Families should be given enough information early on to understand options and choices.

Families have been consumers of many services for many years. In the care of a family member, they should take on the same consumer role. The many trappings of medical jargon and expert advice should be replaced with clear, concise information and support as a basis for making sensible decisions.

Rushing in to "fix" families may meet the family's short-term needs (Dunst, Trivette, Gordon, & Pletcher, 1989) but still leaves the family ill-equipped to face the many challenges, common yet unique, over the long-term future. Section V of this book presents specific techniques to be used to support families in different ways.

REFERENCES

Anderson, R.E., & Carter, I. (1978). *Human behavior in the social environment: A social systems approach.* New York: Aldine Publishing Company.

Boll, T. (1982). Behavioral sequelae of head injury. In P. Cooper (Ed.), *Head injury.* Baltimore: Williams & Wilkins.

Bond, M.R. (1983). Effects on the family system. In M. Rosenthal, E. Griffith, M. Bond, & J.D. Miller (Eds.), *Rehabilitation of the head injured adult* (pp. 209–217). Philadelphia: F.A. Davis.

Brooks, D.N., Campsie, L., Symington, C., Beattie, A., & McKinlay, W. (1986). The five year outcome of severe blunt head injury: A relative's view. *Journal of Neurology, Neurosurgery and Psychiatry, 49,* 764–770.

Brown, B.W., & McCormick, T. (1988). Family coping following traumatic head injury: An exploratory analysis with recommendations for treatment. *Family Relations, 37,* 12–16.

Bush, G. (1986, April). *Coma to community.* Paper presented at the Santa Clara Conference of Traumatic Head Injury. Available from Southboro, MA: National Head Injury Foundation, Inc.

Bush, G.W. (1988). The National Head Injury Foundation: Eight years of challenge and growth. *Journal of Head Trauma Rehabilitation, 3*(4), 73–77.

Corbin, J., & Strauss, A. (1988). *Unending work and care: Managing chronic illness at home.* San Francisco: Jossey-Bass Publishers.

Dunst, C.J., Trivette, C.M., Gordon, N.J., & Pletcher, L.L. (1989). Building and mobilizing informal family support networks. In G.H.S. Singer & L.K. Irvin (Eds.), *Support for caregiving families* (pp. 121–141). Baltimore: Paul H. Brookes Publishing Company.

Florian, V., Katz, S., & Lahav, V. (1989). Impact of traumatic brain damage on family dynamics and functioning: A review. *Brain Injury, 3*(3), 219–233.

Jacobs, H.E. (1988). The Los Angeles head injury survey: Procedures and initial findings. *Archives of Physical Medicine and Rehabilitation, 69,* 425–431.

Kozloff, R. (1987). Networks of social support and the outcome of severe head injury. *Journal of Head Trauma Rehabilitation. 2*(3), 14–23.

Kubler-Ross, E. (1969). *On death and dying.* New York: Macmillan.

Lezak, M.D. (1986). Psychological implications of traumatic brain damage for the patient's family. *Rehabilitation Psychology, 31*(4) 241–250.

Mailick, M. (1979). The impact of severe illness on the individual and family: An overview. *Social Work in Health Care, 5*(2), 117–128.

Marcelissen, F.H.G., Winnubst, J.A.M., Bunk, B., & DeWolff, C.J. (1988). Social support and occupational stress: A causal analysis. *Social Science and Medicine, 26* (3), 365–373.

Morton, K. (1985). Identifying the enemy: A parent's complaint. In H.R. Turnbull & A.P. Turnbull (Eds.), *Parents speak out: Then and now* (pp. 143–148). Columbus: Merrill.

Murphy, R.F., Scheer, J., Murphy, Y., & Mack, R. (1988). Physical disability and social liminality: A study in the rituals of adversity. *Social Science and Medicine, 26* (2), 235–242.

National Head Injury Foundation. (1986). *The silent epidemic.* Available from NHIF at 333 Turnpike Rd., Southboro, MA 01772.

O'Brien, B. (1987). A letter to professionals who work with head injured people. In M. Ylvisaker & E.M. Gobble (Eds.), *Community re-entry for head injured adults* (pp. 421–430). Boston: College-Hill.

Panting, A., & Merry, P.H. (1972). The longterm rehabilitation of severe head injuries with particular reference to the need for social and medical support for the patient's family. *Rehabilitation, 38,* 33–37.

Power, P.W., & Dell Orto, A.E. (1981). *Role of the family in rehabilitation of the physically disabled.* Baltimore: University Park Press.

Poyadue, F.S. (1988). In my opinion. . . Parents as teachers of healthcare professionals, *Children's Health Care, 17*(2), 82–84.

Reiss, D., & Oliver, M.E. (1980). Family paradigm and family coping: A proposal for linking the family's intrinsic adaptive capacities to its response to stress. *Family Relations, 29,* 431–444.

Romano, M.D. (1974). Family response to traumatic head injury. *Scandinavian Rehabilitation Medicine, 6,* 1–4.

Rosenbaum, M., Lipsitz, N., Abraham, J. (1978). A description of an intensive treatment project for the rehabilitation of severely brain injured soldiers. *Scandanavian Journal of Medicine, 10,* 1–6.

Seligman, M., & Darling, R.B. (1989). *Ordinary families, special children: A systems approach to childhood disability.* New York: The Guilford Press.

Turnbull, H.R., Turnbull, A.P., Bronicki, G.J., Summers, J.A., & Roeder-Gordon, C. (1989). *Disability and the family: A guide to decisions for adulthood.* Baltimore: Paul H. Brookes Publishing Co.

Vincent, L., & Salisbury, C.L. (1988). Changing economic and social influences on family involvement. *TECSE, 8*(1), 48–59.

Wadsworth, H.G., & Wadsworth, J.B. (1971). A problem of involvement with parents of mildly retarded children. *The Family Coordinator, 28,* 141–147.

Wikler, L. (1981). Chronic stresses of families of mentally retarded children. *Family Relations, 33,* 281–288.

Wikler, L., Wasow, M., & Hartfield, E. (1981). Chronic sorrow revisited: Parents' vs. professionals' depiction of the adjustment of parents of mentally retarded children. *American Journal of Orthopsychiatry, 50*(1), 63–70.

9

ASSESSMENT
OF THE FAMILY

ROBERTA DEPOMPEI

JOHN J. ZARSKI

Various authors (Brooks, 1984; Brooks, Campsie, Symington, Beattie, & McKinley, 1986; Brooks, Campsie, Symington, Beattie, & McKinaly, 1987; DePompei & Zarski, 1989; Eames & Wood, 1985; Klonoff & Prigatano, 1987; McKinaly, Brooks, Bond, Martinage, & Marshall, 1981) indicate that the family is an increasingly important factor in the rehabilitation of its member with a head injury. Family members' participation in assessment, rehabilitation, and compensation activities is important if the person with a head injury is to experience intervention that is functional and that will return him or her to the real world. The family is an essential part of that return. Depending on family interactions, the family can contribute in several ways. It can interact positively to aid in successful reintegration, or it can contribute to problems in the reintegration process. Therefore, assessment of the family and its capacity to develop and change contributes an important facet to the reintegration of the person with a head injury.

The family, as noted in previous chapters, is a living, changing system that relates and reacts to all that happens to its individual members. The head injury of a member imposes major stressors on the family's interactions. While the impact of such an injury is a primary contributor to family unbalancing, it should be viewed as only one factor that challenges the family's

The authors wish to thank Amy Frankel-Smith for her helpful comments in the preparation of this chapter.

total functioning. The family's work in adjusting to the head injury progresses over time, just as the rehabilitation of the member with a head injury occurs over time. If the family is thought of as a changing, developing entity, a one time "diagnostic assessment" of the family may not be the most realistic means of understanding its functioning.

Assessment might be better viewed as an ongoing interactive process. Assessment of family interactions and how the family unit is functioning at any given time is a challenging and difficult task. The severity of the head injury does not necessarily dictate the extent to which the family will have difficulty adapting. Some families with a member who has received a minor head injury appear to have more difficulty with denial and family functioning around the injury than some families with a member with a severe injury. The problems families experience in dealing with the head injury appear not to be directly related to the severity issue alone, but appear to be more a function of overall coping, support, and family system issues (McCubbin & Patterson, 1982).

This chapter attempts to familiarize professionals who work with people with head injuries and their families with a variety of methods and techniques that may be employed to better assess how family members are thinking, feeling, and behaving. By better understanding the family's position, the professional may encourage more support and healing within that family.

Assessment of the family focuses on a three-pronged approach:

1. Presentation of empirical (objective) assessment methodologies for determining family functioning
2. Outline of clinical observation techniques (subjective) that contribute to understanding family functioning
3. Suggestion of methods to include the person with a head injury in the family assessment process

This assessment approach balances the need for employing selected standardized measures that supply data on families in general, with observational protocols that supply functional and unique information about an individual, specific family system. This combination of assessment methods is useful when determining whether families will be involved in psycho-educational sessions and counseling, referred for specific family therapy intervention by a family therapist, or involved in some combination of counseling approaches.

FORMALIZED METHODS OF ASSESSMENT OF THE FAMILY

Rationale

Obtaining formalized empirical data on family functioning is beneficial in understanding family interactions and is one way of informing third party payors and medical personnel of methods taken to assess and provide intervention for the family. With increasing demands for efficacy of intervention, formalized methodologies appear to be an excellent means of documenting how counseling can contribute to progress and change.

While a variety of measures have been developed for family therapy assessment in general, few have been used with people with head injuries. Bishop and Miller (1989) indicate that objective methods of quantifying family functioning in head injury are increasingly important, and continuation of documentation in their use is essential.

There are several benefits to evaluating the family on standardized forms:

1. Data is consistent from family to family.
2. Families are familiar, and therefore comfortable with this type of approach.
3. Information is quantifiable and tests can be repeated and compared.
4. Results of studies that are increasingly demanded can be compared across families for efficacy.
5. Generalization of data may help professionals to better understand all the facets of family functioning where head injury is concerned.

Bishop and Miller (1989) indicate that there are four methodologies for obtaining family assessments: self report, interview, observation, and laboratory. Table 2 is a list of the tests that are available for use with families. Test information in Table 2 is based on the work by Bishop and Miller (1989) and Brown and McCormack (1988). It should be noted that few tests have been routinely used with families of people with head injuries, and none to date have been normed on these families.

Suggestions for Use of Formalized Tests

Formalized tests should be used with the following considerations:

1. The family should be assessed after its member with a head injury is medically stable. Formal assessments in acute care facilities may be premature and, if they are administered, the results should be carefully interpreted in view of the family's emotional state.
2. As many members of the household as possible should be asked to complete the forms. The more input from family members, the better the chance to elicit a clear picture of the family system's perceptions. Many of the tests suggest lower age limits that are appropriate for participation. In most cases, children's ages and ability to read should be taken into consideration prior to their being asked to participate in formal surveys.
3. The family should understand the scope of the test they are asked to take and should have results explained.

Table 2. Measures of family functioning

I. SELF REPORT: Questionnaires that request information about an individual's perception of the family's functioning in a predetermined aspect, such as adaptation to illness

Tests	Documented with TBI	References
1. Family Environment Scale (FES)—A set of 90 true/false questions that look at family cohesiveness, independence, organization, control, and orientation issues	Not frequently	1. Moos, R. (1974). *Family Environment Scale: Manual.* Palo Alto: Consulting Psychologists Press.
2. Family Adaptability and Cohesion Evaluation Scales (FACES III)—A 20-question scale that assesses the family's real and ideal views of family functioning on the dimensions of cohesion and adaptability	Yes	2. Olson, D., Portner, J., & Lavee, Y. (1985). *FACES III. Family Social Science.* Minneapolis: University of Minnesota.
3. Family Assessment Device (FAD)—A series of 60 questions that assesses seven dimensions, including problem-solving, communication, role dimension, affective responsiveness, affective involvement, behavior control, and general functioning	Yes	3. Epstein N., Baldwin, L., & Bishop, D. (1983). The McMaster Family Assessment Device. *Journal of Marital Family Therapy, 9,* 171–180.
4. Strain Questionnaire—A set of 40 questions that the person with injury answers about physical, emotional, and cognitive functioning	Not frequently, but is in use	4. Lefebvre, R. C., & Sanford, S. L. (1985). A multi-model questionnaire for stress. *Journal of Human Stress, 11,* 69–75.
5. Family Inventory of Life Events and Changes (FILE)—An inventory that assesses the pileup of life events experienced by the family	Yes	5. McCubbin, H. I., Patterson, J. M., & Wilson, L. (1980). *Family Inventory of Life Events and Changes (FILE).* St. Paul: University of Minnesota.

Tests	Documented with TBI	References
6. Family Crisis Oriented Personal Evaluation Scales (F-COPES)—Assessment of effective problem-solving and behavioral strategies used by families in response to stressful situations	Yes	6. McCubbin, H. I., Larsen, A., & Olson, D. H. (1981). *Family Crisis Oriented Personal Evaluation Scales (F-COPES)*. St. Paul: University of Minnesota.
7. Coping Health Inventory for Parents (CHIP)—Measurement of family resources; Modified by Brown and McCormack (1988) for use with all family members dealing with head injury	Yes	7. McCubbin, H. I., McCubbin, M., Caubel, A., & Nevin, R. (1979). *Coping Health Inventory for Parents (CHIP)*. St. Paul: University of Minnesota.

II. INTERVIEW: Assessment of family functioning, which is completed by a trained therapist asking questions

Tests	Documented with TBI	References
8. Camberwell Family Interview—A semistructured interview that assesses a key family member's response to a psychiatric illness in the family	No	8. Vaughn, C., & Leff, J. (1976). The influence of family and social factors on the course of psychiatric illness; a comparison of schizophrenic and depressed neurotic patients. *British Journal of Psychiatry, 129*, 125–137.
9. McMasters Clinical Rating Scale—A seven-item rating scale designed to be used in conjunction with the FAD.	No, but demonstrates potential for use.	9. Kabacroff, R., Miller, I., & Bishop, D. (1982). *The McMasters Clinical Rating Scale*. Providence: Buttler-Brown Research Group.
10. McMasters Structured Interview for Families—A series of structured interview questions that aid in gathering information related to the seven areas of the FAD	No, but demonstrates potential for use.	10. Bishop, D., & Miller, I. (1988). Empirical family assessment techniques. *Journal of Head Trauma Rehabilitation, 3*(4), 16–30.

(continued)

Table 2. (continued)

Tests	Documented with TBI	References

III. OBSERVATION: An evaluator observes the family in its home in real life situations and rates its behaviors

Tests	Documented with TBI	References
11. Family Interaction Coding System—No	Reported in the literature of marital interaction; not documented with persons with TBI	11. Reis, J. (1978). *A social learning approach to family intervention (Vol. 2). Observation in home settings.* Eugene: Castalla Publishing Co.
12. Home Observation Assessment Method—No	No	12. Steinglass, P. (1979). The Home Observation Assessment Method (HOAM): Real time naturalistic observation of families in their homes. *Family Process, 18,* 337–354.

IV. LABORATORY MEASURES: Two or more family members complete standardized laboratory tasks and their behaviors are assumed to assess more general family functioning

Tests	Documented with TBI	References
13. The Card Sort Procedure	Has been employed with multiple family groups for persons with disabilities and may have some application for persons with TBI	13. Reis, D. (1981). *The family's construction of reality.* Cambridge, MA: Harvard University Press.
14. Beavers Timberlawn Family Evaluation Scale	No	14. Green, R., & Kolevzon, M. (1985). The Beavers-Timberlawn Model of family competence and the circumplex model of family adaptability and cohesion: Separate but equal? *Family Process, 24,* 385–408.
15. Family Task Interview	No	15. Kinston, W., & Loader, P. (1988). The family task interview: A tool for clinical research in family interaction. *Journal of Marital Family Therapy, 14,* 67–87.

4. Results should be interpreted for the family with caution, as little normative data exists for these families.
5. Tests should be considered as indicators of present family functioning and not as predictive of future behaviors.
6. The process of the family taking the test may be as informative as the formalized scores obtained. Note interactions, resistance, and spontaneous remarks, as the family proceeds. In one instance, the authors noted that a mother insisted on telling her teenage son what answers to mark on FACES III (see Table 2). This resulted in the son marking the same number on the entire score sheet and refusing to complete additional tests. This informal information contributed insight into the mother-son dyad that was as pertinent as the test results might have been.

CLINICAL OBSERVATIONS OF FAMILIES

Each family that experiences the trauma of head injury has a unique response pattern. The gathering of information about each particular family contributes to overall understanding of the family's functioning around the head injury. Clinical observation includes: 1) the gathering of data about the family member who sustained a head injury, 2) the assessment of family capabilities, and 3) the determination of other pertinent life-cycle issues. Benefits of clinical observation include:

1. Individual differences in families are not overlooked.
2. Specific issues for a given family can be explored.
3. Collaborative efforts with the therapist may improve intervention, as by contributing to better understanding and focus for the family and professionals.
4. Data that is gathered contributes to an overall understanding of the family system.

Following are suggestions for clinical observation methods:

A. Gather Data on the Physical and Cognitive Status of the Person with a Head Injury (Medical Status)

Rationale Families will attempt to understand the degree of involvement or severity of the head injury. The physical involvement usually can be seen and dealt with first; the cognitive communication impairments and the social and behavioral changes that often accompany the physical problems are experienced over a longer period and are not as well understood (DePompei & Zarski, 1989).

Some families will respond to the injury by becoming educated about the injury and by trying to accommodate the changed family member by changing roles, rules, and boundaries. They will perceive the situation as manageable and attempt to adapt.

Other families will perceive the situation as unmanageable and not adapt. They may focus on the medical problem (head injury) as a major crisis in their lives and organize their system around the injury. Muir, Rosenthal, and Diehl (1990) point out that the more severe the physical and cognitive problems, the greater the chance for the family to have difficulty in coping and adjusting.

Considerations and Methods for Gathering Data on the Person's Medical Status   Signed release of information forms should be obtained, and the medical information should be sent for. Considerations for obtaining medical information from the family are:

1. The family should be asked to review, in chronological order, the series of events that lead to the present.

    - Families who are in denial often cannot recount various aspects of the rehabilitation process.
    - Families who are having difficulty with blame may focus on portions of the rehabilitation process and be unable to retell the entire account in chronological order.
    - Families who lack appropriate education about the injury or who received the educational information before they were ready to hear it may not be able to recall pertinent events.
    - Families in depression may not recall time frames well.

2. Each medical recommendation should be reviewed to determine if it was carried out and why or why not.

    - Often families are frustrated by their lack of funds to complete the recommendations medical personnel have made. Financial difficulty can become a major stressor in their attempts to cope.
    - Denial may be a factor that is interfering with the family's ability to follow through.
    - Confusion and lack of education about the reasons for which a recommendation was made may be a factor in the family not cooperating.
    - Families who provide overly detailed accounts and chronologies of the process may be manipulative.
    - Enmeshed families may offer more complete chronologies than disengaged family systems.
    - Families with a belief system that focuses on the injury as a "matter of chance" may minimize the importance of their relationship to the injury and not see the importance of follow-through.
    - Families who have received conflicting medical recommendations may have been unable to proceed due to confusion.
    - Families may respond differently to recommendations, based on cultural background.

3. The family should be asked for a description of the communication patterns within their system prior to the injury and how they have communicated about or with the person with a head injury since the injury.

   • Individual family members may have different pieces of information and expectations about the recovery process.
   • Families who keep secrets may not be capable of sharing accurate information about the rehabilitation process of their loved one.
   • Families with a strong leader may not feel the need for everyone to have all the information.
   • Families who communicate feelings and actions well may demonstrate better overall coping skills.

4. Whether or not the injury was drug- or alcohol-related should be established. Rumbaugh and Fang (1980) indicate that substance usage is a factor in many families with a member with a head injury both pre- and post-injury. Obtaining this information in assessment allows the direction and focus of intervention to be altered to address substance abuse, if necessary.

   • Be aware that more injuries are substance abuse-related than previously believed (Substance Abuse Task Force, NHIF, 1988).
   • Determine whether there is alcohol or drug abuse with other members of the family, and be prepared to use this information for appropriate interventions and referrals for the family.
   • Understand that drug and alcohol use may begin for the person with head injury after the injury (Falonere & Tercilla, 1985), so pertinent questions about present substance usage, including prescription drug usage, should not be overlooked.

B. Assess the Family's Capabilities

Rationale   The degree of crisis or incapacitation of the family system is dependent on the family's ability to respond to multiple changes and demands (defined as stressor pileup by Lavee, McCubbin, & Patterson, 1985; McCubbin & Patterson, 1982) that occur during their adjustment to the head injury. McCubbin and Patterson (1982) and McCubbin and McCubbin (1987) developed a Family Adjustment and Adaptation Response (FAAR) framework in family medicine research that indicates that families adjust and adapt in a variety of ways that are helpful or nonhelpful. They suggest that families' perceptions, resources, and coping may be grouped under a general heading of family capabilities and that these capabilities indicate how the family will respond to the head injury. How the family copes with the head injury depends on its perception of the injury and on resources available to them.

Considerations and Methods for Assessing Family Capabilities   Perception is described as the assessment made by individual family members or collectively by the family unit in regard to how they view the injury, as well as their perceived ability to manage the total situation. McCollum (1975) suggests that some individuals will respond with helplessness, which may lower self-esteem. Coping with the situation becomes a monumental and impossible task for this family member and this feeling may be transferred to the entire unit. Other families offer consistent encouragement, and each small step of successfully meeting small crises along the way gives courage to face the next (DePompei, Zarski, & Hall, 1988).

Assessment of family perceptions may be best accomplished with several of the standardized methods described previously. (See Table 2 and the case study later in this chapter.) In addition, asking the family to explain verbally and in writing how they understand the impact of the injury on all members (not just the person with head injury) is beneficial. A further assessment might be conducted by asking family members to relate how they feel this injury compares with other family illnesses and how they were handled.

Family resources encompass two aspects: 1) strengths of individual family members that can be used to meet the challenge of the "changed" family member, and 2) the family's ability to use existing support systems such as house of worship and friends, as well as to take advantage of new systems such as support groups and educational facilities (Zarski, DePompei, West, & Hall, 1988).

Assessment of family resources may include the use of the ecomap (Atteneave, 1976; Hartmen, 1979; Sherman & Fredman, 1986) or the genogram (Bowen, 1978; McGoldrick & Gerson, 1985; Sherman & Fredman, 1986). An ecomap is a graphic depiction of a family's support from other families, institutions, and organizations. It enables others to see "where bonds, tensions, supports and a host of other relationship issues" (Sherman & Fredman, 1986, p. 96) are present in a family system.

A genogram shows a multi-generational relationship system that indicates how vertical patterns in the family may be influencing present day functioning. Penn (1983) suggests that a genogram that focuses on generational patterns of chronic illness and how family members coped with past illnesses, especially those that were sudden and unexpected, may be particularly useful.

Positive coping patterns include: 1) maintaining an optimistic definition of the situation, 2) developing social support, and 3) understanding the medical situation (McCubbin & McCubbin, 1987). The family that is unable to cope creates resistance to medical recommendations and increases family conflict. Increases in unacceptable behaviors of the person with head injury may also be seen (Burish & Bradley, 1983; Friedrich & Copeland, 1983). For example, a mother overcompensates for her son who sustained a head injury by dressing him when he can complete this task by himself with effort. The son eventually stops trying to accomplish this task on his own and becomes more dependent on his mother, wanting her to feed him as well. She reacts with dismay and states that she resents his dependency on her. He reacts with temper tantrums when she resists helping him.

Coping strategies employed by the family might be understood by employing the FAD (see Table 2). Family coping patterns can be observed in behaviors of denial, blame, overcompensation, too much tolerance, and so forth (DePompei, Zarski, & Hall, 1988). These behaviors are readily observable within the family's interactions. Following is a series of questions that might be asked of each family member to ascertain information on such behaviors:

1. What is the explanation of how this injury occurred? (Look for issues of blame of a particular family member and family mythology, which can include punishment for prior deeds, bad luck, or negligence by a family member.)

2. Who is the best person to direct the care of the member with a head injury? (If the family has a strong internal locus of control, members may feel they have an individual who can direct the remediation and believe, "He will do better if we can just bring him home." If the family has a strong external locus of control, members may feel the medical team should always be in charge. They may feel abandoned when recommendations are made for the family member with head injury to go home, and responsibility for further decisions is given to the family (Rolland, 1988b).

3. What ethnic and or religious background may influence beliefs about the rehabilitation process? McGoldrick, Pearce, and Giordano (1982) indicate that families tend to have different cultural identities that may dictate who will be responsible for care of the person, what the role of extended family will be, and how the medical team will be involved in the planning process. "Deference to distinctions between professionals' cultural beliefs and those of the patient and his or her family may forge a working alliance that is basic to the treatment of a long term illness. Disregard of these issues can lead families to wall themselves off from health care providers and available community resources—a major cause of non-compliance and treatment failure" (Rolland, 1988b, p. 47)

C. Determination of Other Family Life Cycle Issues

Rationale While the head injury becomes of paramount importance to the family, the therapist must remain cognizant that the family continues to move within other normal life cycle patterns that may have an equal effect on family behaviors, but are unrecognized by the family (Carter & McGoldrick, 1988; Rolland, 1988a). By determining what other life-cycle issues might be pertinent for a particular family, the therapist can better integrate information about the person with head injury and where he or she fits into the family's ongoing life cycle. Dodson (1977) indicates that there are a number of normal life crises that each family system experiences. These include marriage, birth, first and last child attending school, graduation from high school, leaving home, last child leaving home, and retirement. If other life cycle issues are arising in the family simultaneously with the head injury, family stress may be inadvertently increased. The head injury may be cited as the focus of family stress while other factors are equally affecting family functioning.

Assessment Considerations   Determining what other life cycle issues are present in the family, in addition to the issues surrounding the person with head injury, may be helpful. For example, if the person is the last child at home and was a senior in high school, parents may have been anticipating beginning a new phase of their relationship. One parent may be resentful that the parent's own plans to attend college will have to be placed on hold, perhaps permanently, because of the demands of caring for the child. The other parent may be concerned over finances and the extra burden of working instead of beginning to plan for retirement. Siblings may be resentful of the person's need for the parents' time and money and the potential sibling commitment to caring for the person at the time when they are leaving the parents' home themselves to live independently, begin careers, begin marriages, or become parents.

Families that are already stretched by a variety of life cycle issues may find the addition of the head injury to be the stressor that causes the family unit to believe that they are unable to continue to cope. Determining other significant and co-existing life cycle issues and helping the family to place them into perspective may aid in supporting the family and its interaction with the member with head injury.

Assessment can be aided with an information sheet such as Lifeline (1982), which includes questions about family life cycle issues. Rolland (1988a) and Combrinck-Graham (1985) provide additional information about life cycle issues and their implications in assessment of chronic illness. They suggest that assessment include determining centripetal (moving together) versus centrifugal (moving away) family styles and life cycle phases. Knowing whether families are in centripetal or centrifugal periods will be helpful in establishing relationship patterns. Any information about other members of the household and where they are in the life cycle should be documented when it is provided.

INCLUSION OF THE FAMILY MEMBER
WITH A HEAD INJURY IN THE ASSESSMENT PROCESS

Often, the family member with a head injury is established as the "identified patient" within the family system (Wachtel & Wachtel, 1986). As a result, many intervention decisions are made and counseling is completed without this family member present. In some cases, where the injury is severe and the cognitive-communicative impairment profound, it is impossible to involve this very important family member. However, in other cases, it seems the family member with a head injury is inadvertently omitted as a participating member of the family unit. It is strongly suggested that this family member be included whenever possible so that his or her perceptions of family functioning can be employed in the overall assessment of the family system.

It could be argued that the cognitive-communicative impairments of the individual will interfere with accurate perceptions of his or her position within the family unit. However, it might be stated that regardless of the accuracy of the perception, assessment results give a picture of where the family member with a head injury *believes* himself or herself to be within the family system. Additional information from the family member with a head injury is, therefore, pertinent to understanding the family system's functioning. The following suggestions are made for involving this family member in the assessment process:

1. Determine the physical problems that may interfere with completing a formal assessment, and accommodate wherever possible. For example, if there will be problems in holding a pencil, special adaptations to the pencil may be made. Other special accommodations can be made by an occupational therapist so that any physical problems will be minimized in the testing.

2. Establish the cognitive-communicative competencies of the person. Ability to understand a question and process an answer should be documented by the speech/language pathologist. Even highly verbal individuals with head injury should be evaluated for cognitive-communicative functioning, and this assessment used as a basis for interpreting test results.

3. Modify test administration if necessary. For example, print may need to be enlarged, questions may have to be presented orally, answers may have to be circled by the therapist rather than the person with head injury, and the test may have to be given in short segments.

4. Redirect attention if needed in order to complete the testing.

5. Use Strain Questionnaire and FACES III (see Table 2) if formalized assessment is desired.

6. To obtain a personal perception of family structure, roles, and rules, ask the person to tell about his or her role in the family and how it has changed.

7. Observe interactions among family members when the member with the head injury is included. This observation will provide clues about the self-perception of the person with head injury, as well as family unit perceptions of this individual member.

8. Ask the person to share his or her ideas about who (self, parent, spouse, medical personnel) is in charge of decisions regarding rehabilitation.

9. Determine how well the person believes he or she is communicating with the family.
10. See Chapter 19 (Table 3) for additional suggestions that may be helpful when including the family member with a head injury in discussions.

CASE STUDY: GERALD AND VIRGINIA

Gerald, age 32, was injured when a truck ran a red light and hit his car. He was hospitalized for 7 months and participated in intensive cognitive-communicative therapy for memory, organizational skill development, problem-solving, and reasoning. He has no physical problems except for some motor coordination problems with his left hand and arm. Prior to the accident, Gerald was a manager for a computer programming company. Gerald is married to Virginia, age 29, who is a registered nurse. She has always worked part time, but since the accident has taken a full-time position. They have two children, Mary, age 6 and Jeffrey, age 4.

Gerald continues to have difficulty with organization; for example, he has problems remembering to shave both sides of his face, how to care for the children (e.g., preparing meals, getting them ready for school), telling time when it is essential to be somewhere, and doing the laundry. He spends much of his time in his woodworking shop where he completes bookshelves and small cabinets. He has learned to follow a step-by-step outline when completing his woodworking activities.

Virginia expresses concern that she has been forced to take a full-time position and guilt that she cannot spend time with her children. She is also worried that her parents must "babysit" for her husband while she is at work. Additionally, the situation is such that her children "tattle" on their father, and she feels compelled to discipline her husband for not completing the laundry or for forgetting to prepare lunch for the children.

They have been referred for family therapy because they are having difficulty adjusting to his staying home and her working full time. Virginia states, "I want my sweet little life back."

Empirical Assessment

1. FACES III, couples version, was administered with the following results:

Gerald and Virginia are dissatisfied with the current family system. Virginia is more dissatisfied with Gerald, as indicated by the greater discrepancy between her score for how she sees the family now compared with her score for how she would like her family to be. While Virginia wants the family to be more flexible, Gerald wants more rigidity. Virginia sees the family as rigidly enmeshed. The couple perceives their relationship at extremes of the adaptability/cohesion continuums and tends to endorse negative communication skills such as nonsupportive statements, incongruent messages, and lack of empathy.

2.   FAD results indicate the following:

FAD results suggest poor problem-solving skills, with particular emphasis on difficulty identifying problems and formulating approaches. On the communication dimension, the couple scores high on the masked and indirect style, which indicates conflict between nonverbal and verbal messages. Affective results indicate there is constant overprotection of emotion and lack of personal privacy within the dyad. Behavior control data indicate the couple has reasonable standards, but a lack of effective follow-through. General functioning results suggest that the couple have difficulty expressing feelings to each other, are unable to be supportive of each other, and are not able to confide in each other.

3.   The Strain Questionnaire administered to Gerald indicated the following information:

A.   Physical: Gerald reports few problems with physical symptoms and does not use alcohol or drugs. No problems with headaches or muscle aches other than those related to his left hand or arm were reported.

B.   Behavioral: Gerald indicates no problems other than being accident prone and feeling some irritability.

C.   Cognitive: Gerald has a high number of responses indicating that thinking about himself is causing stress. He feels he is no good, has nightmares, believes the world is against him, and experiences feelings of unreality. He has these experiences on a daily basis.

Clinical Observations of Family Capabilities (See Figure 5)

Both Gerald and Virginia have support systems that they employ. Gerald is obtaining support from his family, although they are too far away to make

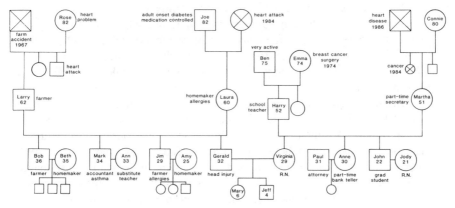

Figure 5. Ecomap of Gerald and Virginia's support system.

regular visits. He also receives support from his health care therapists and his church. He does not, however, indicate that the support is two-way. That is, he is always the recipient and never the provider of the support. He enjoys woodworking and includes his children in this activity. It is a major area of strength for him. He has tenuous relationships with his old friends and feels they do not respond to him as they did before his injury. He has stressful relationships with his in-laws (they report a previously good relationship) and with his ex-colleagues from work.

The ecomap indicates that there is outside support for Virginia, which includes her family, friends, church, and nurses' organization. Virginia has support at work. Because she feels guilty about full-time employment, work provides a tenuous support relationship. While Virginia's parents are supportive of her and care for the children, Gerald believes that they are also caring for him. Therefore, this family support relationship is deteriorating. Gerald's parents and family are reacting to Virginia by demanding their son have more responsibility. Therefore, while Gerald indicates support from his family, Virginia believes her relationship with her in-laws is deteriorating.

2.   A four generational genogram (Figure 6) indicates that both individuals are from extremely stable family systems. Gerald comes from a large farm family. His grandparents, parents, and three brothers have traditional roles, with husbands as major income providers and wives as primarily homemakers. There is some history of chronic illnesses such as diabetes, allergies, and asthma in Gerald's mother's family. Gerald reports that no major complications arose from any of the illnesses. He states the family handled any illness by working together to get the ill member "back on his feet" and by relying on good medical care. There were no major hospitalizations for long periods of time until Gerald's accident. He is the first male in three generations to be unable to provide the primary income for his family due to an injury or illness.

Virginia also comes from a traditional family where no members have been divorced, and there have been no major, ongoing illnesses. Virginia reports that she has been the only family member involved with chronic illness. The family allows her to provide the medical "fixing" because she is a nurse. The husbands provide the income, as with Gerald's family; wives work part time.

Because Gerald and Virginia come from such traditional male-female work ethics, the role of full-time income provider may be an especially difficult one for Virginia, as no other females in either family have assumed that role. While Gerald hopes to return to full-time employment so that Virginia can become employed part time again, it remains questionable whether he can achieve this goal. Information obtained from the ecomap and genogram indicates that rules and roles related to who should be the primary income provider may be a source of considerable stress for this couple. In

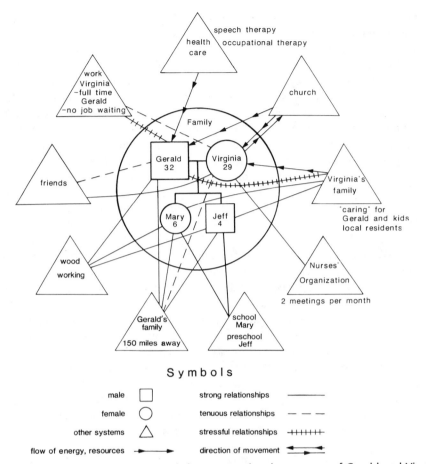

Symbols

male	☐	strong relationships	——————
female	○	tenuous relationships	– – –
other systems	△	stressful relationships	++++++
flow of energy, resources	——▶	direction of movement	◀══▶

Figure 6. Chronic illness oriented, four generational genogram of Gerald and Virginia.

addition, historical information about chronic illness in both families indicates that they have little experience to draw from, and both families prefer to let the medical people "take care of it." Because head injury does not follow traditional medical models of treatment, Gerald's injury is especially difficult for both families to assimilate into their systems' functioning.

3.   Lifeline information about this couple indicates that they have minor financial worries for the next year. They have begun socializing with old friends, but Gerald is less comfortable than Virginia in these situations.

Virginia describes her husband as childlike and feels it is necessary to help him with learning adult behaviors. She does not notice when her children tattle on their father that she disciplines him as she would one of them.

Virginia's paragraph about her husband prior to his injury reveals her picture of him as a well-organized professional who ran most household business. He was responsible for the check book and for decisions about major purchases. He was a "fun father" who played with the children. She was the disciplinarian. She indicates that he is the only love in her life. No problems in the sexual relationship were reported.

4.   Family life cycle issues include the fact that their daughter began school while Virginia was working and that Gerald has assumed responsibilities that Virginia would like to have in regard to preparing their child for school, contacting the school, and so forth. In addition, Virginia's youngest brother has married and her parents now have no children living with them. Virginia's mother recently retired from her part-time job and was looking forward to taking interior decorating classes. She has placed these plans on hold to care for her grandchildren.

5.   An extremely positive consideration is both individuals' sense of humor. They are able to laugh at situations and find humor where others may find frustration and stress. This use of humor is a major strength in coping.

By assessing the unique relationships and stressors that Gerald and Virginia were experiencing, the rehabilitation team devised an intervention program that addressed the needs of the family system while taking into consideration the effects of the head injury. Rehabilitation was directed toward developing functional skills that were deemed important within the family system. Because the family system was assessed, and continued to be assessed as they participated in a variety of rehabilitation programs, their energies were channeled in a positive manner to aid the family reintegration process. Formal and informal assessment and ongoing rechecks are essential to aiding the family in developing the capacity to change and adapt. The professional who works with the person with head injury should consider assessment a vital contribution to the overall rehabilitation plan.

REFERENCES

Atteneave, C. (1976). Social networks as the unit of intervention. In P.J. Guerin (Ed.), *Family therapy theory and practice*. New York: Gardner Press.

Bishop, D.S., & Miller, I. (1989). Traumatic brain injury: Empirical family assessment techniques. *The Journal of Head Trauma Rehabilitation: Families of the Brain Injured, 3*(4), 16–30.

Bowen, M. (1978). *Family therapy in clinical practice*. New York: Jason Aronson.

Brooks, D.N. (1984). *Closed head injury: Psychological, social and family consequences*. Oxford, England: Oxford University Press.

Brooks, D.N., Campsie, L., Symington, C., Beattie, A., McKinlay, W. (1986). The five year outcome of severe blunt head injury: A relative's view. *Journal of Neurology, Neurosurgery and Psychiatry, 49*, 764–770.

Brooks, D. N., Campsie, L., Symington, C., Beattie, A., & McKinlay, W. (1987). The effects of head injury on patient and relative within seven years of injury. *Journal of Head Trauma Rehabilitation, 2*(3), 1–13.

Brown, B., & McCormack, T. (1988, May). *Successful family coping in response to head injury: Preliminary results*. Paper presented at New York State Head Injury Association, Sixth Annual Conference, Rochester.

Burish, T.G., & Bradley, L.A. (1983). *Coping with chronic disease*. New York: Academic Press.

Carter, B., & McGoldrick. (1988). *The changing family life cycle: A framework for family therapy* (2nd ed.). New York: Gardner Press.

Combrinck-Graham, L. (1985). A developmental model for family systems. *Family Process, 24*(2), 139–150.

DePompei, R., & Zarski, J.J. (1989). Families, head injury, and cognitive-communicative impairments: Issues for family counseling. *Topics in Language Disorders, 9*(2), 78–89.

DePompei, R., Zarski, J.J., & Hall, D.E. (1988). Cognitive-communication impairments: A family-focused viewpoint. *Journal of Head Trauma Rehabilitation, 3*(2), 13–22.

Dodson, L.S. (1977). *Family counseling: A systems approach*. Muncie, IN: Accelerated Development, Inc.

Eames, P., & Wood, R. (1985). Rehabilitation after severe brain injury: A follow up study of a behaviour modification approach. *Journal of Neurology, Neurosurgery Psychiatry, 48*, 613–619.

Falonere, J. & Tercilla, E. (1985). *Chemical abuse and head injury*. Tigland, OR: Rehabilitation Psychology Associates.

Friedrich, W. N., & Copeland, D. R. (1983). Brief family-focused intervention on the pediatric cancer unit. *Journal of Marital Therapy, 9*, 293–298.

Frieson, J.D. (1985). *Structural-strategic marriage and family therapy*. New York: Gardner Press.

Hartman, A. (1979). *Finding families an ecological approach to family assessment in adoption*. Beverley Hills: Sage.

Klonoff, P., & Prigatano, G. (1987). Reactions of family members and clinical intervention after traumatic brain injury. In M. Ylvisaker & E.M. Gobble (Eds.), *Community re-entry for head injured adults* (pp. 381–402). Boston: College-Hill.

Lavee, Y., McCubbin, H.I., & Patterson, J.M. (1985). The double ABCX model of family stress and adaptation: An empirical test by analysis of structural equations with latent variables. *Journal of Marriage and the Family, 47*, 811–826.

Lifeline. (1982). Akron: Department of Communicative Disorders, Akron City Hospital.

McCollum, A.T. (1975). *The chronically ill child: A guide for parents and professionals*. London: Yale University Press.

McCubbin, H.I., & Patterson, J.M. (1982). *Family stress, coping and social support*. Springfield, IL: Charles C Thomas.

McCubbin, M.A., & McCubbin, H.I. (1987). Family stress theory and assessment: The t-double ABCX model of family adjustment and adaptation. In H.I. McCubbin & A.I. Thompson (Eds.), *Family assessment inventories for research and practice* (pp. 3–34). Madison: University of Wisconsin Press.

McGoldrick, M., & Gerson, R. (1985). *Genograms in family assessment*. New York: Norton Press.

McGoldrick, M., Pearce, J.K., & Giordano, J. (1982). *Ethnicity and family therapy*. New York: Guilford Press.

McKinlay, W.W., Brooks, D.N., Bond, M.R., Martinage, D.P., & Mashall, M.M. (1981). The short term outcome of severe blunt head injury as reported by relatives of the injured persons. *Journal of Neurology, Neurosurgery & Psychiatry, 44*, 527–533.

Minuchin, S., & Fishman, H.C. (1981). *Family therapy techniques*. Cambridge, MA: Harvard University Press.

Muir, C., Rosenthal, M., & Diehl, L. (1989). Methods of family integration. In M. Rosenthal, E. Griffeth, M. Bond, & J.D. Miller (Eds.), *Rehabilitation of the adult and child with traumatic brain injury* (2nd ed.). Philadelphia: F.A. Davis.

Muir, C., Rosenthal, M., & Diehl, L. (1990). Methods of family intervention. In M. Rosenthal, E. R. Griffith, M. Bond, & J. D. Miller (Eds.), *Rehabilitation of the adult and child with traumatic brain injury* (2nd ed.). Philadelphia: F.A. Davis.

Penn, P. (1983). Coalitions and binding interactions in families with chronic illness. *Community Mental Health Journal, 1,* 339–345.

Rolland, J. (1988a). Chronic illness and the family life cycle. In B. Carter & M. McGoldrick (Eds.), *The changing family life cycle: A framework for family therapy* (pp. 3–28). New York: Gardner Press.

Rolland, J. (1988b). A conceptual model of chronic and life-threatening illness and its impact on the family. In C. Chilman, E. Nunnally, & F. Cox. *Chronic illness and disability* (pp. 17–68). Newberry Park, CA: Sage Publications.

Rosenthal, M., Griffith, E., Bond, M., & Miller, J. (1983). *Rehabilitation of the head injured adult*. Philadelphia: F.A. Davis.

Rumbaugh, C.L., & Fang, H.E.H. (1980). The effects of drug abuse on the brain. *Medical Times, March,* 37–52.

Sherman, R., & Fredman, N. (1986). *Handbook of structured techniques in marriage and family therapy*. New York: Brunner/Mazel Inc.

Substance Abuse Task Force, National Head Injury Foundation. (1988). *White paper*. Southborough, MA: National Head Injury Foundation.

Umbarger, C.C. (1983). *Structural family therapy*. New York: Grune & Stratton.

Wachtel, E., & Wachtel, P. (1986). *Family dynamics in individual psychotherapy: A guide to clinical strategies*. New York: The Guilford Press.

Ylvisaker, M., Szekeres, S.R., Henry, K., Sullivan, D., & Wheeler, P. (1987). Topics in cognitive rehabilitation therapy. In M. Ylvisaker & E.M. Gobbel (Eds.), *Community re-entry for head injured adults*. Boston: College-Hill.

Zarski, J.J., DePompei, R., & Zook, A. (1989). Traumatic head injury: Dimensions of family responsivity. *The Journal of Head Trauma Rehabilitation: Families of the Brain Injured, 3*(4), 31–41.

Zarski, J.J., DePompeii, R., West, J., & Hall, D.G. (1988). Chronic illness: Stressors, the adjustment process and family focused interventions. *Journal of Mental Health Counseling, 10*(2), 145–158.

Zarski, J.J., Hall, D.E., & DePompei, R. (1987). Closed head injury patients: A family therapy approach to the rehabilitation process. *The American Journal of Family Therapy, 15,* 62–68.

10

EVOLUTIONS

RESEARCH AND CLINICAL PERSPECTIVES ON FAMILIES

THOMAS KAY

MARIE M. CAVALLO

INTRODUCTION: AN EVOLUTIONARY PERSPECTIVE

Traumatic brain injury (TBI) is a catastrophic life event that permanently changes a person and the family system in which he or she exists. Since 1983, the authors' study of recovery from head injury has revealed a complex and variable process of evolution that families go through after an injury to one of their members. Families are as different as individuals, and each family's struggle to "recover" after head injury is as *unique* (because of the enormous differences among families) and as fraught with themes *common* (because of the common realities of traumatic brain injury) to the "recovery" of the individual person. Just as with the person with TBI, "recovery" remains qualified: neither the person nor the family system will ever be exactly as it was. Professionals step in and out of the picture at various points along the rehabilitation continuum, but both the individual with TBI and the family system have lives of their own and will evolve in their own particular ways. Professionals only help adjust the course here and there in a swiftly flowing current strewn with obstacles, seen and unseen, and send families on their way.

It has become clear that families do not march through a series of stages, reaching a final stage of "acceptance" (so that those who fail to "accept" are somehow "stuck" and in need of our help). Rather, families, and their members with TBI, evolve. Evolution, by definition, does not end; it is an ongoing process of adaptation to current realities. As realities change, as they inevitably do over the course of a family's life cycle, the family must adapt and change again and again. Of course, the history of evolution is replete with species that have branched off and pursued a dead end path; families do get stuck, do fail to adapt, and there is a legitimate role for professionals in the family's evolutionary struggle to survive.

From a different vantage point, the field of rehabilitation has evolved in the way it views, provides intervention for, and documents the family's role in recovery from traumatic brain injury. The explosion of interest in traumatic brain injury began in the 1970s. In less than 20 years the professional literature has evolved away from being interested in families primarily for what they could reveal about changes in the person with head injury, through an incidental interest in the effects of the injury on family members, to focusing on the determinants of stress and burden on individual family members, and most recently has shifted to studying the impact of head injury on the family system as a social unit.

This chapter is about these evolutions. First, the change that has taken place over time in how families have been dealt with in the professional literature on traumatic brain injury, in both formal research studies and clinical descriptions, is selectively examined. (In this examination, the authors briefly describe their own work with families at New York University Medical Center, specifically the development of an instrument to track changes in families.) The second part of the chapter takes a more clinical perspective, and traces parallels in the process of changing self-perception and self-identity in persons with head injury, in individual family members, in the family as a system, and even at the level of national organizations. The unifying theme is evolutions: the gradual, continuous process of change whose goal is adaptation to present realities and future needs.

EVOLUTION OF THE PROFESSIONAL LITERATURE

Literature Reviews

Because of this chapter's focus on the evolutionary aspect of the professional literature, a formal and comprehensive review of all the literature on head injury and the family has not been undertaken. This chapter attempts to include most significant contributions to the literature; however, a number of other reviews, each with its own particular point of view, have been published in the late 1980s. The interested reader is referred to the following sources:

In both editions of his excellent book on head injury, Mitchell Rosenthal has included chapters that focus on reviewing the current literature on families. Bond (1983) and Livingston (1990) blend reviews of relevant literature with clinical perspectives on families after TBI.

Livingston and Brooks (1988) specifically reviewed the literature (largely their own) on the burden family members experience after TBI. The review by Florian, Katz, and Lahav (1989) contrasts head injury and spinal cord injury family studies, to make stronger observations on the specific impact of brain damage on family systems. Romano's (1989) review is particularly striking for its integration of research with clinical perspectives on both situational (community) and interactional (within the family system) issues faced by families after head injury. Bishop and Miller (1988) present an overview of the family assessment approaches and tools available to the family researcher, and summarize the studies to date utilizing empirical family assessment techniques after head injury. Finally, it should be noted that the December 1988 issue of the *Journal of Head Trauma Rehabilitation* (Volume 3, Number 4) was devoted to "Families of the Brain Injured" (the Livingston & Brooks, and Bishop & Miller reviews appear in this issue).

Research Literature

The specific focus on the impact of TBI on the family system is a relatively new development in the history of head injury research. Four stages in this evolution can be identified; while each stage came into prominence in temporal succession, no stage entirely disappeared, with the result that the current literature spans a range of approaches. These four stages are considered in order below.

Family Members as Windows on the Person with Head Injury   The earliest studies, primarily concerned with the nature of TBI and its outcomes, tended to use family members as windows onto the changes and deficits in persons with head injury. Hpay's (1970) study is typical: "Each case was interviewed, along with one or more close relatives or friends from whom information was obtained about changes in personality characteristics which are not generally available from the patient himself" (pp. 110–111). Bond (1976), part of the Glasgow group, which made such rich contributions to understanding family burden, began his research with a study interviewing family members about their observations of the person with head injury. The driving force behind these early studies was the fact that persons with head injury are often poor self-observers; the utilization of the perceptions of family members was a natural adjunct when the goal was to objectively evaluate the impact of TBI on the person with the injury. One result of this literature was documentation of the range of physical, cognitive, and behavioral changes that persist after head injury (e.g., Oddy, Coughlan, Tyerman, & Jenkins, 1985). This line of research is a valid one, and continues today (e.g., Klonoff,

Costa, & Snow, 1986). It does not, however, directly bear on the impact of head injury on the family system, and is not considered further here.

Incidental Impact on the Family   The second line of TBI family research focused, as did the first, primarily on the person with head injury as the object of study, but *incidentally* took note of the impact of the injury on the family, usually on individual family members. These studies predominated in the 1970s and early 1980s.

Panting and Merry (1972), in studying long-term rehabilitation after severe head injury, noted that TBI was more difficult for wives than for parents (a clinical observation brought into question by later empirical studies by the Glasgow group); that 61% of wives and mothers required medication to help them cope with relatives with TBI; and that more than half of all relatives felt that supportive services had not been adequate. This study is important as one of the earliest studies of persons with TBI that paid significant attention to family issues.

Also in 1972, Walker noted the personal sacrifices (social, economic, and sexual) that wives made in adapting to living with husbands with TBI, and speculated that wives who stayed with husbands with TBI possessed devoted, maternal types of personality.

The Danish studies of Thomsen are significant both for long-term follow-up, and for their clinical detail about individual cases of severe head injury. In her earlier study, Thomsen (1974) reported that burden on families came primarily from personality changes, then cognitive deficits, and least from physical disabilities (these clinical observations were empirically verified years later by the Glasgow group). These studies reiterated Panting and Merry's observation that wives coped less well than parents. In her later study, Thomsen (1984) emphasized that 10–15 years post-injury, two thirds of the subjects continued to have personality changes that were stressful for their families; that families became isolated from their communities; and that family relations, in particular father-son relations, were prone to deterioration.

Many of the reports in which incidental observations of families contributed to the understanding of the impact of TBI on families came from Oddy and colleagues in a series of studies done in London and published in the late 1970s and early 1980s. Oddy, Humphrey, and Uttley (1978b) studied subjective impairment and social recovery after TBI. They noted that single persons tended to be more dependent on parents when their injury was more severe. They also found that there was no change in marital or sexual relationships, and no increase in family friction, at 6 months post-injury. (In part this may reflect an initial "honeymoon" stage, which dissipates with time.) In 1980, Oddy and Humphrey extended their 6-month study to 1 year. They found that dependency of single persons had decreased, but that friction had increased between the person with TBI and siblings (although not between parents and the persons with TBI). At 1 year, poorer family relationships were associated with personality changes in the person with head injury, *but only when a sibling was present*. (This provocative finding, to our knowledge, has not been followed up.) By 1 year, the authors claimed that the person with TBI interacted as well with their families as did a control group of persons with limb fractures.

Also in 1980, Weddell, Oddy, and Jenkins studied a group of persons with more severe TBI (PTA [Post Traumatic Amnesia] of more than 7 days, compared to 24 hours for the Oddy et al. [1978b] study), and found that persons with personality changes were more dependent on their families than patients without personality changes. They postulated that the friction in families resulted not from personality changes in general, but from the presence of irritability in particular in the person with TBI.

From an evolutionary point of view, these studies went beyond using family members as windows on persons with TBI; while continuing to focus on the person with the head injury, they began to incidentally report changes in family members or changes in family relationships.

Focus on Individual Family Members   The next development in the evolution of family studies was a series of studies, beginning in the late 1970s, but peaking in the mid to late 1980s, that focused not on the person with TBI as the subject of study, but on individual family members, and the impact of the head injury on their lives. Ironically, this line of research tended to use the person with the head injury as the window on the stressed family member. Measures of cognitive and behavior changes in the person with TBI were interesting not in and of themselves, but to the extent that they helped illuminate burden in the family system.

One of the early studies of the Oddy group was typical of this trend. Oddy, Humphrey, and Uttley (1978a) focused specifically on the stresses upon relatives of persons with TBI. They administered the Katz Adjustment Scale (Katz & Lyerly, 1963) to relatives to rate changes in the person, and the Wakefield Depression Scale (Snaith, Ahmed, Mehta, & Hamilton, 1971) to measure depression in the relatives. They found that depression in family members at 6 and 12 months correlated with the extent of the most common cognitive symptoms; depression correlated not with neurological variables (e.g., coma, PTA), but with the neuropsychological consequences of brain injury. At 12 months post-injury, relatives were more depressed when the person with TBI took longer to go back to work, and had fewer social contacts. The more symptoms the relatives rated the persons as having at both 6 and 12 months, the greater the relatives' depression.

The epitome of this line of research is the studies on burden conducted by the Glasgow group. Throughout the 1980s, Brooks, Livingston, McKinlay and colleagues published a series of studies attempting to elucidate when and why family members experience subjective burden after TBI. This literature has been reviewed in depth by Livingston and Brooks (1988) and Livingston (1990), and only the highlights are summarized here.

McKinlay, Brooks, Bond, Martinage, and Marshall (1981) introduced the 7-point subjective burden rating scale, a global scale on which a family member was asked to rate how stressful (from "no strain" to "severe strain") it was living with the family member with a head injury. (See the section on the NYU Head Injury Family Interview later in this chapter for an extension of this approach.) Two significant findings emerged from this study. First, the relationship between neurological indices (e.g., post-traumatic amnesia) and subjective burden decreased with time; in the long run, severity of the injury itself had less to do with stress in the family. Second, mental and behavioral changes were much more related to burden in family members than were physical or speech/language changes. This theme remains constant throughout the literature on family burden: neurological severity of injury affects family burden only to the extent that it is translated into behavioral change on the part of the person with TBI. Changed emotions, personality, and behavior are what make life difficult for family members, much more than physical or even cognitive changes, regardless of severity of injury.

Brooks and McKinlay (1983) extended these findings. They found that reports of personality change increased from 49% to 60% between 6 and 12 months post-injury. More important, the relationship between the person's personality change and the relative's burden *increased* over time. Over the course of the first year, changes in personality became more linked to higher levels of burden in the family. This helps in understanding the Oddy et al. (1978b) study; the burden of coping with changed personality emerges gradually over the course of the first year. An additional important contribution of this report was the observation that while all relatives who experienced high burden reported personality changes in the person with TBI, not all relatives reporting personality changes experienced high burden. When burden is high, it is attributable to personality changes in the person with TBI; however, there are significant (unspecified) individual differences among relatives which determine who will experience how much burden as a result of personality changes in the person with TBI.

McKinlay and Brooks (1984) found that relatives and persons with TBI tended to agree closely when rating physical problems, agree moderately when rating cognitive problems, and agree poorly when rating emotional and behavioral problems; disagreement on emotional/behavioral problems occurred because ratings of relatives were higher than ratings of persons with TBI. Relatives who rated emotional/behavioral problems as high also had higher neuroticism scores on the Eysenck Personality Scale (Eysenck & Eysenck, 1975), which itself correlated with the amount of stress they reported feeling. The authors point out that little attention was paid (nor has it been paid since) to the personality characteristics that enable relatives to cope.

Livingston, Brooks, and Bond (1985b) and Livingston (1986) focused on relatives' adjustment after *severe* (PTA greater than 48 hours, Glasgow Coma Scale [GCS] less than 8 on admission) versus *mild* (concussion with discharge after 48 hours) head injury. They found that relatives of the persons with severe TBI had more psychiatric disturbance and more subjective burden than relatives of persons with mild injuries. Within the severe group, wives and mothers showed no differences, but mothers of persons with severe TBI had higher Leeds anxiety scores (Snaith, Bridge, & Hamilton, 1976) than mothers of the mild group. (These results should not be misinterpreted as minimizing the potential impact of minor head injury on the family system. Individual cases become lost in group data. While minor head injuries *as a group* cause less stress than severe injuries, any given minor head injury has the potential to disrupt family functioning significantly.)

Livingston, Brooks, and Bond (1985a) reiterated the fact than no statistically significant differences were found between wives' and mothers' scores on the General Health Questionnaire (Goldberg, 1978), the Leeds scales for anxiety and depression (Snaith, Bridge, & Hamilton, 1976), the Social Adjustment Schedule (Weissman, Prusoff, & Thompson, 1978), or the perceived burden rating scale, at 3, 6, or 12 months post-injury. When psycho-social functioning of wives and mothers were combined, it was found that the best predictor of adjustment was the level of subjective complaint voiced by the person with TBI. The more complaints the person made, the more stress on the family member.

Sobering conclusions about family adjustment emerged from a study by Brooks, Campsie, Symington, Beattie, and McKinlay, reported in 1986. Studying changes in subjective burden in relatives over a 5-year period, the authors found that perceived burden actually increased over time. While 76% of relatives reported low/medium burden at 1 year (with 24% reporting high burden), at 5 years only 43% reported low/medium burden (with 56% reporting high burden). This fits in with clinical observations that families only really come to grips with the realities of dealing long-term with family members with TBI years after injury. The implications for rehabilitation are clear: from the family's point of view, it may be 5 years or more before they require—and are ready for—significant psycho-social interventions.

Brooks, Campsie, Symington, Beattie, and McKinlay (1987) provided the most in-depth look at the burden issues. They reiterated that persons with TBI tend to underreport problems compared with relatives' complaints. They found that, with the exception of physical problems, increasing deficit in the person (as rated by the relative) was associated with increasing burden on the relative; this was particularly true of emotional and behavioral problems. Lower levels of burden were associated with lower levels of deficit; however, high levels of burden might or might not be associated with higher levels of deficit (except in behavioral areas, where high burden was associated with greater personality change).

More neurologically severe injuries (as measured by post-traumatic amnesia) were associated with higher levels of relative burden. Less severe injuries, however, could be associated with low, medium, or high burden. With milder head injuries, apparently a wider range of intervening variables determine the level of family stress; in more severe injuries, the neurological impairments are more likely to be translated into neuropsychological problems that lead directly to family burden. Finally, counter to earlier clinical observations, burden scores of parents did not differ from those of spouses; when mothers and wives were directly compared, mothers were found to have higher burden scores.

Another piece of the family burden puzzle was put in place by Livingston (1987), who addressed the clinically important but difficult-to-document issue of premorbid family functioning as a variable in family coping post-injury. Livingston (1985) had documented that the level of subjective complaints of the person with TBI was the best predictor of relatives' stress. He now adds that previous psychiatric and health problems *of the relative* accounted for more than 30% of the variance in relatives' ratings of subjective burden. Livingston (1987) correctly emphasizes the premorbid adjustment of relatives as a factor in their ability to cope after a family member's head injury.

What has not been adequately addressed in the literature is this potential for interaction between the family member's coping and the patient's subjective complaints. It is usually assumed that neuropsychological deficit determines the patient's subjective complaints, which determine the relative's subjective burden. It may also be, as Livingston's data suggest (and as would be predicted from a family systems perspective), that premorbidly determined difficulties in coping for relatives could serve to magnify the person's subjective complaints, above and beyond neuropsychological factors, which would then feed back into relatives' subjective burden. This could, in part, account for family crisis in which both the person with TBI and family members seem engaged in a mutual intensification of the symptom-stress synergy that escalates out of control, far beyond what would be expected from the neurological severity of the injury. This maladaptive synergy has been observed to be particularly common in families of persons with minor head injury.

Focus on Family Systems   So far, the studies reviewed in this chapter have used family members as windows on persons with TBI, have incidentally commented on impact on the family while focusing primarily on the person with TBI, or have focused primarily on the impact of head injury on individual family members, using the members with TBI as windows on the other family members. The current line of research focuses on the family system as a unit and attempts to document the impact of head injury not on individual family members, but on the family system or situation as a whole. While the roots of this research reach back into the late 1970s and early 1980s, virtually all of the important work has been done since 1988. In the authors' opinion, the significant advances will be made along this line of research in the 1990s in the area of the effect of traumatic brain injury on the family.

The precursor to this literature was the work of Rosenbaum and Najenson (1976). They compared two small groups of wives of men with TBI and men with paraplegia from spinal cord injuries, and measured family interaction outcomes. They found that compared to the wives of the men with spinal cord injuries, wives of men with TBI reported more changes in their family lives and being more disturbed by them, especially in the area of family activities. Wives of men with TBI reported more interpersonal and social disruption in their lives; also, they ascribed less importance to their role as sexual partners and found themselves handling family matters outside the home to a greater degree than they would have liked. Wives of men with TBI were also more depressed than wives of men with paraplegia. This early work was unique at the time in documenting the interpersonal and role changes in families of persons with head injuries.

Mauss-Clum and Ryan (1981) studied wives of 40 men with TBI; their study was important for its documentation of the type of help wives felt they needed (explanation, discussion, support, financial counseling); who provided support (relatives, friends, and physicians, much more than mental health professionals); and what coping mechanisms they used and were helpful.

A study by Kozloff (1987) marked an important step in the evolution of the family TBI literature by applying social network analysis of families after head injury:

> Network analysis focuses on the interactional and structural properties of social and personal networks and provides a means of understanding the process by which the head-injured person and his or her significant others seek and receive support from their relationships. (p. 15)

Independent of its specific results, this study represents a radical departure from the language—and the conceptual basis—of the work earlier reviewed in this chapter. From this point on, research attempts to conceptualize the family system as the unit of study; this represents the most advanced stage of the evolution of research on the family after head injury.

In fact, the results of this study confirmed clinical experience, but were not startling (the early family systems research yielded findings that only begin to approximate the richness of family systems revealed clinically). As time post-injury increases, the person's social network decreases in size and increases in density (the product of length of time and degree of commitment in a relationship). The number of multiplex relationships increase (family members serve more and more functions, as nonrelatives drop out of the picture). Persons with higher socioeconomic status are more likely to maintain existing relationships, which then serve multiple functions. Kozloff's discussion of these and other findings correctly points to the individual differences in familial patterns of responding to head injury, based in large part on culturally determined beliefs and values related to conflict resolution.

A number of other studies have focused specifically on the family system as the unit of observation. Zarski, DePompei, and Zook (1988) applied existing empirical family assessment tools to families after head injury, with results that focused more on methodological measurement issues than substantive outcome (although family satisfaction was found to be higher in families rated as functioning at a higher level).

Maitz (1989) compared 43 couples in whom one member had a head injury, to 18 couples in whom neither member had a head injury, but where one member had a sibling with TBI or a sibling married to a person with head injury. He used two measures of family functioning, the FACES III (measuring dimensions of adaptability and cohesion) and ENRICH (measuring marital conflict). He found no group differences in adaptability, but less, and more variable, cohesiveness in the TBI group, and less satisfaction within the TBI group with the personality traits of spouses with TBI. In addition, there was more variability in conflict resolution within the TBI group (suggesting unexplored variables in familial conflict resolution independent of the presence or absence of head injury), and (not surprisingly) marital conflict was associated with less family cohesion. Within the TBI group, there was no evidence that cohesion or adaptability improved with time post-injury.

Peters, Stambrook, Moore, and Esses (1990) attempted to predict dyadic adjustment in groups of wives of men with mild, moderate, or severe brain injury. Dyadic consensus, affectional expression, and overall dyadic adjustment were generally worse in the group with the most severe injuries. While a diversity of variables predicted outcome in these three areas, three variables overall were most strongly related to *good* dyadic adjustment: less financial strain, low spousal ratings of patient psychopathology, and less severe injuries (as measured by Glasgow Coma Scores).

In addition to these studies of family systems, a number of studies have reported on the impact of TBI on various aspects of family life (as opposed to the system as a unit). In a major survey in the Los Angeles area, Jacobs (1988) documented the financial and role stress on the family after TBI. Families played the role of providing the major source of support, socialization, and assistance to persons with TBI, and two thirds of the families experienced financial adversity. The financial devastation of TBI on the family was further documented by McMordie and Barker (1988), who examined changes in who works, loss of income, loss of personal possessions, and debt among family members. Finally, Willer, Arrigali, and Liss (1989) utilized a creative group technique to identify problems and solutions among men with TBI and their wives. Among the family systems problems identified (by the husbands with

TBI) were being included in family decisions, and understanding the concerns of other family members, and (by the wives) reduction in financial resources, loss of emotional support, and feeling unable to meet children's needs.

Of note is the fact that to date no studies have been made of women with head injury and their spouses; all studies reviewed have been of men with TBI, or men and women together. This is presumably because of the much higher incidence of head injury in men than women (Kalsbeek, McLauren, Harris, & Miller, 1980). If the researcher is unable to obtain a sex-balanced sample, groups of men are much more readily accessible. There is a danger, however, in generalizing about the impact of TBI on the family by only studying men with head injury. Studies are needed that look at the family impact when women are injured, and that compare changes in family functioning with situations in which the husband is injured.

Summary—Research Literature   Since 1970 four distinct but overlapping lines of research have evolved in quasi-sequential fashion, which focus on the family after traumatic brain injury. First, initial studies (early 1970s) utilized family members as windows to view recovery of persons with head injury, with no focus on the family members themselves. The second line of research (1970s and early 1980s) focused primarily on the recovery of individuals with head injury, but incidentally reported on the impact on individual family members. Third, a later line of research (1980s) focused primarily on the subjective burden incurred by relatives of persons with TBI and used data on patients as windows through which to view relatives. Fourth, the current stage in the evolution of family TBI research (late 1980s and into the 1990s) focuses on the family itself: either the system as a unit of study, or various aspects of family life after TBI. The evolutionary trend is toward broadening the unit of study toward the network of individuals surrounding the person; each line of research, however, retains its specific advantages and should survive as a viable method of learning.

The NYU Head Injury Family Interview

Overview of the Instrument   The Head Injury Family Interview (HI-FI) was developed by the authors, along with Dr. Ora Ezrachi (Kay, Cavallo, & Ezrachi, 1988) within the New York University Medical Center's Research and Training Center on Head Trauma and Stroke (funded by the National Institute of Disability and Rehabilitation Research). The HI-FI evolved over a 5-year period out of our need to study the natural course of recovery after head injury. We found that no existing instrument met our need to document the demographic and premorbid situation of the person with head injury; the facts of the episode of injury, medical procedures, neurological variables, and the information given to families; the utilization of community and government resources, medical and social; attempts to return to work, school, and home-making, and the related qualitative problems encountered; changes in physical, cognitive, social, and behavioral functioning, as perceived by both the person with TBI and a family member; changes in activities of daily living and socialization patterns; and impact on the family system as a whole, including intrapersonal and role changes in parents, spouses, siblings, and children. All of these areas are covered within the HI-FI.

In its current version (1.2), the HI-FI is a structured interview comprising five parts: 1) Demographic and Pre-Injury Form, 2) Follow Up Interview, 3) Survivor Interview, 4) Significant Other Interview, and 5) Impact on the Family Interview. The interview consists of three levels of questions, which are always presented in the following order: First, open-ended questions elicit unguided, spontaneous perceptions (e.g., What changes have you noticed since the accident?). Second, structured questions ask for information in specific domains revealed by the open-ended questions (e.g., Have you noticed any changes in your thinking ability?). Third, specific checklists and rating scales are presented to document particular problems along uniform dimensions, which can be translated into statistically analyzable data (e.g., Do you have problems with concentration? If so, is this a change from before the injury? If yes, rate this problem on a scale of 1–7 indicating how much of a problem it is for you.).

The interview can be administered as a structured interview (which is preferable because of the opportunity to probe and follow up answers), or given to the family to fill out and return (particularly useful in preparation for a formal evaluation). A triaging system is built into the interview so that family members only answer those questions that are relevant to them. The interview takes about 1–2 hours to complete, depending on how many family members are involved, how much return to functioning the person with TBI has attempted, and the extent to which the examiner follows up questions. Families report enjoying the interview process, especially early on after injury, when the interview is often the first time the entire range of their experience has been explored. Clinicians, once they become practiced in administration, value the comprehensiveness of the format. We believe the HI-FI is particularly useful for less-experienced clinicians, who benefit from a structured framework for gathering information in a systematic way. The interview has proved useful for both clinical and research purposes. Clinically, it is most useful as an intake instrument for outpatients being evaluated for intervention. Research applications include tracking both individual and family changes over time, and changes in functioning and self-perception as an outcome of intervention.

Currently the HI-FI is being field tested in a multi-center study. Following completion of this study, the instrument will be revised based on clinical feedback, a database will be developed, and then the interview will be made available for use throughout the field.

Research Applications of the Problem Checklist   With the partial exception of studies such as Livingston (1987) and Peters et al. (1990), which attempted to predict family functioning from a variety of variables, the entire body of family TBI literature reviewed in this chapter asks the question: How does a head injury affect the family? Our particular research approach since 1985 at NYU has been to ask the question: How do individual persons and families differ in their responses to TBI, and what variables influence those different responses? Within our family studies, this philosophy has led us to examine the differences among families, and to work toward a taxonomy of families related to outcome, and potentially to differential rehabilitation approaches.

One small piece of the HI-FI that is amenable to this process and affords comparison with other studies is the Problem Checklist (PCL). The PCL consists of 34 items that describe common problems after head injury in physical, cognitive, emotional, and behavioral domains. Both the person with head injury and a significant other indicate (yes/no) whether the person with TBI *experiences* that symptom. If the answer is yes, the person with TBI is asked to rate at what level of severity that symptom presents a problem (on a scale of 1–7). The significant other is asked to indicate whether this is a change from the situation pre-injury (to control for pre-existing problems), and if so, to rate on a scale of 1–7 not only the severity of the problem for the person with TBI as an individual, but also how much of a burden this problem presents for the person as a family member.

This approach clearly builds on the research on burden by Brooks and colleagues in Glasgow. It differs, however, in a number of ways. First, rather than employing a single global burden scale, we ask relatives to rate the differential burden associated with different problems in the person with head injury. Second, by asking the same questions of the person with TBI and a relative, we can group families by how well they agree in their perceptions. Rather than attempting to characterize all families, we are interested in identifying different subgroups of families with different characteristics.

Very few studies have taken this approach. Fordyce and Roueche (1986) used a similar Competency Rating Scale, filled out by persons with TBI, relatives, and staff, to subgroup families in an intensive intervention program. Three groups emerged: 1) persons with TBI, staff, and families having similar ratings pre- and post-program; 2) persons with TBI underestimating their impairment pre-program compared with staff, but congruent with staff estimations post-program, with family ratings intermediate pre-program; and 3) persons with TBI underestimating their impairment pre-program (this difference between self and staff ratings increased post-program), with families intermediate but still overestimating patient competency. There were no differences among the groups in etiology of injury, age, education, chronicity, or in Katz adjustment scores. While the three groups did not show statistically significant differences in vocational outcome, there were trends toward complex differences in emotional distress, awareness, and neuropsychological capacity over the course of rehabilitation.

Hendryx (1989) asked persons with TBI and family members to rate physical, cognitive, and emotional changes in the person with the head injury. Both groups agreed on the extent of physical changes. Persons with TBI rated cognitive changes as greater than emotional changes, and family members rated emotions as more changed than did the persons with head injury. Hendryx did not attempt to group families by response patterns.

Our own work has looked at how families differ when asked to rate the person's problems. A number of interesting findings have come out of these studies (Cavallo & Kay, 1988). Thirty-one of the 34 families in our original sample could be categorized into one of three groups, using 75% endorsement rate as the criterion for patient-family agreement. Group I consisted of 12 High Agreement families, with both patients and family members agreeing on at least 75% of the items (problem vs. no problem). Twenty-two families by this criterion were High Disagreement families and were divided into the following groups: Group II consisted of high disagreement families where the person endorsed at least twice as many items as the significant other (8 families). Group III consisted of high disagreement families where the family member endorsed at least twice as many items as the person with the head injury (11 families). Only three families did not fit one of these patterns.

The groups did not differ on age, sex, education, duration of coma, time since injury, or relationship of the family member to the person. They did differ, however, on employment outcome. To our surprise, Groups I (high agreement) and III (high disagreement, family member rate higher) had employment rates of about 50%, whereas all but one person with TBI in Group II (high disagreement, person with TBI rate higher) were employed. Rating one's own difficulties as higher in severity than the perception of others was associated with a higher rate of return to work. Perhaps being in a work situation brought out a recognition of problems, or perhaps a greater awareness of deficits enabled persons to compensate better and therefore be more successful at returning to work.

When we compared the two high disagreement groups, the Group II (problems rated higher by person with TBI, higher rate of return to work) items that accounted for the disagreement were mainly cognitive in nature. In contrast, when we looked at the items that Group III disagreed on (problems rated higher by family, lower rate of return to work), they were largely emotional and behavioral in nature. Persons who returned to work were more aware of their cognitive difficulties and did not have unrecognized personality changes, whereas persons rated by their families as having emotional and behavioral changes were less likely to recognize them and were less likely to go back to work.

When we looked at what items caused most burden for family members, we found that affective and behavioral items were associated with the most burden, and physical and cognitive items were associated with less burden.

Our approach to studying burden *directly* asks the family member to rate the degree of stress associated with each particular problem; the work of the Glasgow group (cited above) asks for a global rating of burden, then *indirectly* infers the relationship of burden to problem by correlating problem ratings with global burden scores across families. While the results of our direct approach are consistent with the indirect approach of other researchers, the item-by-item approach has a number of advantages. For example, we were able to document the fact that certain personality changes, while they might not occur often, imposed enormous burden when present. Mood swings, physical violence, temper outbursts, and high sexual drive fell into this category.

A further surprise occurred when we looked at burden scores within our three groups. Exactly the opposite of our expectations, Group I (high agreement group) family members had higher burden scores than Group II or III, who disagreed in their perceptions, despite the fact that the most common problems were similarly rated across the three groups. Although Group I did not show more severe neurological ratings, it may be that the persons with head injury in this group in fact had more severe symptomatology, to the extent that it could not be ignored on either side, and caused a severe burden on the family. The intuition that families in which persons with TBI consistently rated their problems lower than did relatives would carry more family burden was not borne out.

While these preliminary observations raise more questions than they answer, they do suggest a methodology for analyzing family data in terms of individual differences among families, the variables that predict such differences, the outcomes attached to various subgroups, and ultimately, differing rehabilitation approaches for different families.

Descriptive Literature

In addition to the research literature on families and head injury, there is a broad and qualitatively variable descriptive literature that treats family issues after head injury from a clinical perspective. The following section samples some of the more significant publications in this area, but makes no attempt to document every comment in the literature on families of persons with head injury.

Denial and Stages of "Recovery"   Within this volume, different authors have taken different approaches to conceptualizing stages families go through after head injury. These models are neither right nor wrong; rather they should be judged by their utility in making sense of clinical experiences with families.

A seminal article in observing the reactions of families to TBI was Romano's 1974 observations on family denial. Observing a small group of families of persons with TBI in a rehabilitation unit, Romano was struck by the extent to which the families focused their lives around the person, decreased contact with the outside world, denied (despite counseling) the extent of deficits, and how friction developed between family members who could and could not acknowledge long-term problems.

With time these dynamics came to be seen as one stage in the family's experience early on in the rehabilitation process. A number of authors (e.g., Groveman & Brown, 1985; Henry, Knippa, & Golden, 1985) have applied the Kubler-Ross model of emotional responses to death and dying to stages families go through after head injury. Under this model, denial and isolation, anger, bargaining, depression, and acceptance follow upon each other in succession, with the final stage, acceptance, being a steady state in which families remain. Under such a model, the denial seen as pathological by Romano becomes transformed into a necessary stage. Ridley (1989) has reassessed the entire concept of denial after head injury, and interprets it as an adaptive, hope-oriented coping strategy in the early stages of adjustment. Denial is seen as negative only if it interferes with problem-solving, not if it is an emotional response in the service of new meaning. Stern, Sazbon, Becker, and Costeff (1988) have addressed the particular problems faced by families of patients who remain in prolonged coma; they interpret the hostility acted out toward staff in terms of an understandable process of anger, frustration, disconfirmed expectations, and inability to mourn.

Our own response to the Kubler-Ross model is that while the various emotional reactions defined as stages can certainly be helpful in understanding some families at certain points in time, the stages as presented oversimplify and make uniform the complex and variable processes that real families go through. We are particularly concerned about implicitly expecting families to "accept" the injury in the sense that is often meant. It is impossible to mourn (and accept the disappearance of) someone who has not died, especially one who may be behaviorally disruptive, especially in the context of a family life cycle where developmental crises re-precipitate the cycle of despair and adjustment all over again.

Other authors have gone beyond a simplistic application of the Kubler-Ross model, to define a series of stages specific to traumatic brain injury. Lezak (1986) has outlined a six-stage process that unfolds over at least a 2-year period of time, and linked the stages to time since injury, the family perception of the person with TBI, the family's expectations, and the family's reaction to the person. Words like denial, anger, and acceptance are not used. The family's perceptions are seen as progressing from "a little difficult," through "not cooperating" and "irresponsible," to "a different, difficult, childlike person." Expectations evolve from "full recovery," through "independence if we know how to help him," to "little or no change." The family reactions, which sound most like the Kubler-Ross model, proceed from "happy," through "bewildered," "discouraged," and "depressed," to "mourning" and finally "reorganization" (Lezak, 1986, p. 244). Two advantages of this model over the Kubler-Ross model are that it casts the family response in more of a systems framework, and does not decree that a steady state of "acceptance" is the ideal and healthy long-term outcome.

Finally, McLaughlin and Schaffer (1985) have taken the approach of conceptualizing the family's reactions as "remolding," and drawn parallels with a child's developmental stages.

Family Systems and Dynamics   A second group of descriptive papers can be characterized as not taking a stage approach, but describing the impact of living with a person with TBI, either on the individual or on the family system, at a particular point in time.

The classical article in this area was written by Lezak (1978), and vividly described "Living with the Characterologically Altered Brain Injured Patient." The tone of this article is clearly sympathetic with the plight of the significant other, and does not attempt to view the family system from the point of view of the person with a head injury. In a later article Lezak (1988) redefines the situation more from a systems point of view: "Brain Damage is a Family Affair." Specific family relationships are explored in terms of their susceptibility after brain injury.

A few articles are beginning to unite the rehabilitation and family systems literature. DePompei, Zarski, and Hall (1987) outlined the basics of family systems functioning for a rehabilitation audience, while Henry et al. (1985) outlined the cognitive and behavioral realities of brain injury for a family systems audience, before putting the impact of TBI on the family into a family systems context.

Reflecting on the overall trend within this descriptive literature, one can see an evolution from viewing family reactions as pathological maladaptations, and reactions of family members to the changes in individuals with TBI, toward an attempt to understand the process that families go through in an attempt to integrate and adapt to the changes that are taking place within their system.

Interventions with Families   In both editions of his book on traumatic brain injury, Rosenthal has included chapters surveying intervention approaches with families (Muir, Rosenthal, & Diehl, 1990; Rosenthal & Muir, 1983). Their approach has been to define levels of intervention for families (e.g., education, counseling, therapy), as well as to identify the factors that put families at risk for system breakdown. The latter chapter in particular places family interventions squarely at the intersection of family and rehabilitations systems, and provides case examples of intervention. Chapter 18 in this volume summarizes much of this previous work.

A number of authors have discussed interventions with families at various levels of the rehabilitation process. Brown and McCormick (1988) link a survey of families to recommendations for social and medical system interventions.

At the level of inpatient rehabilitation, the best family intervention is often a formal plan for family involvement. Johnson and Higgins (1987) describe a highly structured inpatient rehabilitation family program emphasizing: 1) a primary contact and resource person, 2) family support group, 3) orientation to the unit, 4) formal discussion of goals, 5) shared educational objectives, 6) scheduled teaching sessions, 7) family input into the care plan, 8) shared discharge planning, and 9) standardized documentation of each component of this plan.

In contrast, Klonoff and Prigatano (1987) present a plan of family involvement for an outpatient head injury program for post-acute clients. They emphasize the heterogeneity of families, and the dependence of family adjustment on a number of factors including the coping style of the family, the pre-injury personality and role of the person with TBI, and the effects of brain injury on behavior. They also emphasize the need for a strong alliance with families if successful community reintegration is to occur. Dysfunctional families are defined as those that fail to cope and adjust, and a number of dysfunctional family characteristics are identified. A major contribution of this article is the parallel drawn between the "awareness and acceptance" of the person with TBI of his or her acquired deficits and altered capacities, and the "awareness and acceptance" of the family of the person's changes, capacities, and new family role. This is not "acceptance" in the sense of emotional passivism, but acceptance in the active sense of awareness of change and a willingness to make decisions on the basis of revised goals. They define a number of programmatic interventions within their particular setting, including participation in an intake interview; feedback after evaluation; orientation to the program; and weekly family groups, which provide a framework for both understanding and concrete ways of coping.

A final area of intervention with families involves the controversial use of families as therapists. McKinlay and Hickox (1988) see family members as a "cost-effective and highly motivated adjunct to trained staff" (p. 65), specifically in the areas of memory retraining and anger management. Quine, Pierce, and Lyle (1988) reported on a study asking family members to spend up to 8 hours a day providing therapeutic stimulation to severely impaired hospitalized persons. They found family involvement decreased with time as motivation and hope for improvement waned.

Our own perspective on the use of family members as therapists is a cautious one. We are concerned about the implications for the family system when family members are called therapists—and what limitations that may cause for the healthy reintegration of the family system. We have seen families burn out, and be filled with guilt and resentment when they felt the burden of making the person with TBI "better"—which is the role of the therapist.

We suggest it is preferable to help family members find a level of involvement with the person that both is appropriate to the stage of recovery and makes sense in terms of smooth family functioning and needs, but *not* to call this therapy. Every family must learn how to manage behavior, provide structure, and so forth, but this should be seen as a family matter in the service of system homeostasis, rather than intervention for a patient by surrogate therapists.

Only one article to date has directly applied family therapy techniques to the problems of families after head injury. Zarski, Hall, and DePompei (1987) in the *American Journal of Family Therapy* outline the changes families face after brain damage, define a structural family therapy approach, and present a case example. While a number of rehabilitation experts have privately expressed doubt about the appropriateness of family therapy after brain damage, we believe that an exploration of how the family therapy model can be most appropriately adapted to the needs and limitations of families with a member with TBI will be a later stage in the evolution of interventions with families after head trauma.

CLINICAL EVOLUTIONS AFTER HEAD INJURY

There are evolutions also after each individual head injury. There is a process of continual, and only partially predictable, change during acute care hospitalization, formal rehabilitation, community reentry, and lifelong adaptation. A large part of this process involves evolving a new sense of self—a reorganization of self-perceptions, expectations, and goals.

The authors have been struck by certain parallels in the evolutionary process of self-definition. Not only the person with TBI, but each individual family member, and the family system as a unit, seem to move through evolutionary processes that bear striking similarities to each other. Currently, there are very similar changes in self-definition at the organizational level, within the National Head Injury Foundation. The remainder of this chapter attempts to sketch some of these clinical evolutions after head injury.

The Person with Head Injury

Issues of awareness and acceptance play a prominent role in successful rehabilitation programs. Following traumatic brain injury, one of the most devastating neuropsychological impairments is often organically-based lack of self-awareness: the inability to recognize the changes and new limitations in oneself. Very different from (although sometimes coincident with) psychologically-based denial, lack of awareness is rooted in damage to the frontal lobes, which impairs executive functions: the ability to anticipate, plan and organize, develop a strategy, self-monitor and self-correct, and judge the appropriateness of one's own behavior. After traumatic brain injury, most persons are initially unaware of changes in their own capacity. They operate as if they were their pre-injury selves. The unrealistic goals of many persons with head injury, and their resistance to attempts to work toward new, reduced goals, are due to this phenomenon, and are perhaps the single greatest obstacle to the ultimate rehabilitation goal of successful community reintegration and achievement of an optimal level of productivity and social relatedness.

In working with clients both programmatically and in private practice settings, we have been struck by a gradual evolutionary process that unfolds over time. At some point in their rehabilitation, all persons with head injury must struggle actively with the issue of self-redefinition. In its broadest outlines, this process involves moving from a state of relative unawareness of the new self, through identification of self as a "head injured person," to a final stage of identifying oneself as a person—who happens to have a head injury.

The transition from the old sense of self to identification as a "head injured person" is the most tumultuous one. It involves often bitter confrontation with failure, and honest but supportive feedback from professionals and family. (The extent to which the family is able and ready to participate in this process will ultimately block or facilitate the transition in the individual.) Clients must actually go through a process of learning what head injury is, and identifying their own behavior and problems as in large part due to their injury. Persons who fail to go through this process will never successfully reintegrate into the community because they will always fall prey to their own unrealistic expectations of themselves. They must learn that they cannot trust their memory and must write things down. Clients must also learn that they lack control over their anger and to identify the early warning signs of building rage. Clients must learn that they make unrecognized errors and must check and recheck their work at every step.

This learning process is complicated by the very fact that necessitates it: impaired executive functioning, which keeps a person from being aware of what he or she is not aware of. We have found that in order to make the transition to awareness of the changed self, clients need to rely on a benevolent but directive other who can help shape new self-perceptions. This is a major role of professional staff in a well-organized head trauma program. The personality of the person with the head injury will play a major role in determining whether this transition can take place. Some persons have the interpersonal relatedness and flexibility to allow themselves to trust another for guidance toward a new sense of self (what Dr. Yehuda Ben-Yishay, Director of the NYU Head Trauma Program, calls "malleability"). Other clients do not; they rigidly resist the efforts of others to help shape a new sense of self. These are the persons who often remain stuck, battling bitterly their whole lives to be who they were before the injury.

Closely tied to awareness is acceptance of one's new limitations. This is not acceptance in the sense of being pleased or happy with one's changed self and no longer troubled by it, but acceptance in the sense of a willingness to acknowledge that these changes have actually occurred, that they cannot be undone, and rather than continuing to struggle toward something impossible, one accepts the necessity of making decisions and setting goals based on the new self. It is the difference between angry, desperate attempts to be the old self, and the calm resignation (again Dr. Ben-Yishay's words) to the limitations and rewards of accepting a new person with new goals.

In the process of evolving from the old self to awareness of one's new self, we have watched clients take on the identity of being a "head injured person." As they begin to realize the reality of their changed self, they begin to understand themselves in terms of their brain injury. This is very freeing: it is what allows them to be aware of, and therefore to begin to compensate for, the deficits that have been holding them back.

This is not the final stage, however. We have seen persons become stuck at the stage of identifying themselves as "head injured persons." At its worst, this can become an abdication of responsibility, a message to the world that they are not responsible or capable because of their head injury. (Families who for their own reasons need to center on the person with the head injury, and thrive on their dependency, are often potent forces in keeping persons with head injury stuck at this stage.) This is partial learning, incomplete evolution. The final transition involves shedding the "head injury" identity that one has struggled to obtain, ceasing to identify one's injury as the dimensions of self-definition, and beginning to think of oneself as a person first—whose head injury imposes certain restrictions within which he or she must operate.

It is during this final stage of evolution that persons with head injury begin to pursue realistic goals with conviction. They seek meaningful jobs, pursue relationships, and struggle to live realistically with their disability. It can be an exciting time for the person, the family, and professionals. In a sense this final stage never ends. Many persons with head injury, because of their memory and executive deficits, lose the mental set of this new identity quite easily (this phenomenon is instructive in the role that memory and intact conceptualization play in establishing a stable identity in the course of normal development). These persons will always be dependent to some extent on others to help them hold onto the reality and rationale of the changed self.

The Family Member

Just as the person with the head injury evolves from lack of awareness, through identification with "being head injured," to a new identity as a person with a head injury, so too do individual family members move through a series of parallel evolutions to a new sense of self. We have been struck by how often changes in their current family rekindle unresolved issues in their own family of origin, and how this precipitates a crisis within the self. How this crisis is resolved will determine whether the family member becomes stuck and dysfunctional, or moves on to a new identity.

One family member, Emma, was 27 years old and had been engaged 6 months when her fiance Dave sustained a severe head injury in a fall at work. Along with his parents and brother, she threw herself into all aspects of his rehabilitation: daily visits to the acute care hospital (despite her evening job in a print shop), regular trips to an out-of-town inpatient head injury program, and regular participation in a local outpatient head injury program. She spent hours supporting and talking with him, attended family meetings, advocated for him with staff, and generally reorganized her own life around his care.

As her fiance improved, however, Emma's life did not. Her exhaustion, anger, confused feelings, and sense of losing herself intensified, rather than abating. Six months after Dave's injury, she sought therapy with the senior author. Initially therapy centered on head injury issues: each new development, decisions about discharge and programs, struggles with other family members, and so forth. Gradually, however, it became apparent that Emma's decision to seek help was based on issues that ran deeper than her coping with Dave's injury.

Figure 7 is a reproduction of a picture Emma drew in reaction to the logo of the National Head Injury Foundation (NHIF). (The original was done in heavy blacks and blood reds.) Three faceless, uninjured adults surround and contain six grimacing, screaming, contorted faces of head-injured persons. Blood runs from one who appears unconscious. Emma's reaction to the NHIF logo, which pictures a line drawn across a person's head, was powerful and clear. The line across the injured person's head touched off all her rage against the invalidation of the person, which she saw occurring during the medical and rehabilitation process. She reacted powerfully to limits, demands, and forced routines—and especially the tendency of staff to treat Dave and other persons with head injury as "brain damaged patients," rather than as individuals struggling to assert and express themselves.

As we talked about the strong sense of invalidation she felt at the sight of that line across the person's head in the logo, Emma's associations drifted more and more to a sense of invalidation in her own childhood. Her father had been an alcoholic—and ironically sustained a head injury in a motor vehicle accident, and even had the same name as her fiance. Beyond these ironic surface similarities, being thrown into Dave's rehabilitation recreated for Emma a prison from her own childhood. While she was growing up, Emma's entire life was dedicated to preserving the family's fragile stability by taking care of her father, aggressively ignoring his drinking and the chaos it wrought in the family, and systematically stamping out her own identity and needs, submerging them in the needs of others, especially her family. Emma grew up deeply ambivalent about, and distrustful of men. Her young adulthood, once she moved far from home, was spent attempting to discover and establish her own sense of self.

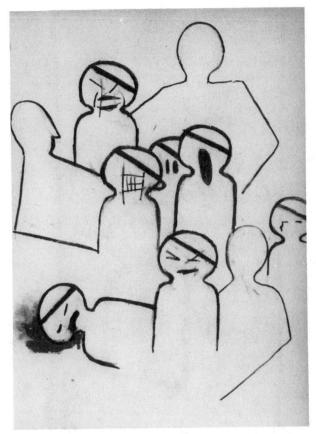

Figure 7. Emma's drawing in response to the NHIF logo.

Her fiance's accident undid all this and threw her back into the very situation she was struggling to escape. Once again her sense of self disappeared as she threw herself into taking care of the needs of others. Figure 8 is a reproduction of another drawing Emma did. Here the mouth with a silent scream of one of the persons in Figure 7 is enlarged and becomes the central identity of a small, single invalidated figure, who exists at the foot of a looming, faceless adult. In the therapy process it became clear that while on the surface the suffering person in Figure 8 was Dave or any other person with a head injury, on a deeper level the figure represented Emma herself. Therapy began to change; we talked less and less about Dave, and more and more about Emma. Not just about what she was going to do with her relationship with Dave, but Emma and her family (especially her father), who Emma was, what she wanted, her struggle to form and live out her own identity.

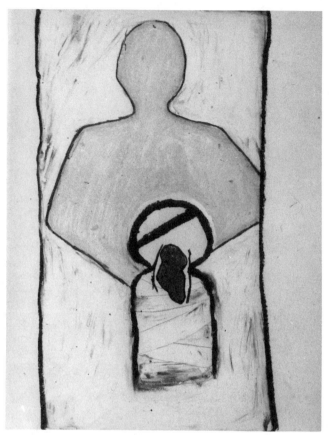

Figure 8. Emma's representation of her feelings about her position in her family.

How Emma resolved her relationship with Dave is less important than the evolution she went through as a result of Dave's injury. There was often the sense in therapy that Emma's family (parents and two sisters) were moving silently in and out of the room, watching, whispering to her. She often wanted to run out, and she glared mistrustfully at her therapist. The forming of a therapeutic alliance, with all the transference that entailed, was a deep and difficult struggle that went far beyond coping with Dave's injury. Emma was revisiting her own family and confronting for the first time the conflicts that were limiting her own life. In the process of resolving these conflicts, Emma was evolving a new sense of herself. This process would eventually allow her to emerge as a new person with a clearer and stronger identity.

The Family System

When one of its members has a head injury, the homeostasis of the family system is instantly destroyed. In all but the most dysfunctional families, there is an instant reorganization around the needs of the person with the injury. (This process is well documented in Chapter 8 of this volume.) As time progresses, the family as a system undergoes an evolution parallel in some ways to that of the person with TBI. The utility of various stage models of recovery has already been discussed earlier in this chapter. Regardless of what framework one adopts, certain broad outlines of the family's evolution are clear and strikingly parallel to the individual's. After hospitalization is no longer necessary and the person with the head injury returns home, the family begins the process of redefining itself as a workable system. Lezak's (1988) model suggests an early stage in which the family is on a "honeymoon": glad to have the person alive and back home, willing to overlook idiosyncrasies as temporary remnants of the injury, and hopeful of full recovery—explicitly of the individual, and implicitly of their family as a whole. This corresponds to early stages of unawareness of self for the person with the head injury. The family cannot yet know or appreciate what permanent changes will exist within the system itself.

As time goes on, the reality begins to sink into the family not only of the permanence of some of the changes in the person, *but the permanence of changes in the family system as well.* This is where vulnerable families are at risk for crisis or dissolution. As new roles and limitations in relationships, finances, or allocation of time, energy, and resources begin to take shape in a permanent way, cracks in the system may begin to widen. Latent parental schisms may emerge. Children may act out. Depression may overtake a young spouse. Divorces—legal and emotional—are common.

This is also the time during which healthy, coping families take on the identity of being "head injured families." Routines, vacations, financial planning, job decisions, social and recreational patterns, are all determined by the needs of the person with TBI within the family system. The extent to which this new identity is possible differs from family to family; how much conflict it creates depends on individual family members, and the flexibility and cohesiveness within the family system.

However, just as the individual must take on, but then shed, the identity of being a "head injured person," so too a system that has learned to be a "head injured family" (i.e., whose routines, roles, and relationships are centered on the person with TBI) must unlearn the identity. Often families, like individuals, become stuck at this middle stage, perpetually organizing themselves around the needs of the person with TBI. In the long run, this is destructive to all members of the family, and often to the system itself. As individual family members develop and face their own transitions, and as the family cycle evolves, change in family functioning and organization is essential. The system stuck in the "head injured family" identity will not be able to respond to such needs, and individuals will suffer. Gradually, most families find a way to gently disengage from the central needs of the person with the head injury. Routines remain to meet the needs of the member with TBI, but the energy focus of the system begins to diffuse again to meet the needs of all members.

Sometimes the evolutions of the person with TBI and the family system are out of sync, and problems occur. Often the person with TBI is ready to regain more independence and autonomy before the family is able to accommodate this. Conversely, the family system may push to decentralize its focus on the person with the head injury while he or she still solidly holds the identity of "being head injured," with the consequent needs of being cared for. Professionals can be helpful at these times, as long as they are not working with the person with head injury in isolation. The biggest practical mistake therapists make, especially at the community reentry stage, is to try to "treat" the "patient" without working within the context of the family system. Almost always these efforts are doomed to failure because guiding the evolution of the person with TBI requires a corresponding change within the evolution of the family system.

A National Organization

The National Head Injury Foundation is the national advocacy organization for persons with head injury and their families. This year it is celebrating its 10th anniversary. Events within the organization provide striking parallels with the process of evolution that affects individuals and families after head injury.

In the early years of its existence, persons with head injury played a rather passive and quiet role within this organization. Founded by family members and professionals, the organization had focused its energies on improving the lives of persons with head injury, and supporting and advocating for their families. Thought of as a system much like a large family, the organization was very centered on taking care of the member with TBI (actually the group of members).

A change began in the mid-1980s when persons with head injury became more vocal and involved in the organization. Support groups began to include persons with head injury. Wanting more of a voice in the organization, persons with head injury began to organize and formed survivor councils to make their voices heard. This both was welcomed and caused uneasiness, just as it does within a family when a person with a head injury starts to reclaim some power and control. This was clearly an evolution within the organization: persons with TBI, no longer content to remain the passive objects of beneficence of families and professionals, took on a new identity within the organization: survivor.

That label, which identified its bearers as persons with TBI, was worn proudly—until the late 1980s. The latest stage in the evolution is away from both the logo of the organization—which identifies the person with TBI with the invalidating slash across the head—and the survivor label. The label of survivor is being rejected precisely because it identifies its bearers by their injury. From a systems point of view, this is similar to an individual rejecting the identity of being "head injured," and instead wanting to be seen as a person with a head injury. And just as the family becomes uneasy when the previously dependent person wishes to assume new responsibility, not just for himself or herself, but also within the family, so too NHIF is now struggling to reorganize its own inner relations and find a new homeostasis.

SUMMARY

The evolutions continue at all levels because they are part of the dynamics of human systems. The struggles of the individual with head injury to take on a new identity are mirrored in the struggles of each family member, the family system itself, and even at the national organizational level. As professionals, we are undergoing our own evolutions in how we view and interact with families. One can never tell where evolution will go; what is certain is that we cannot go back. We have learned too much to try to "rehabilitate" the "head injured patient" to our goals, in isolation from the family and social context in which he or she exists. The next stage of our own evolution is to open our own eyes to the necessity of thinking in family systems perspectives as we go about our work in rehabilitation.

REFERENCES

Bishop, S.D., & Miller, I.W. (1988). Traumatic brain injury: Empirical family assessment techniques. *Journal of Head Trauma Rehabilitation, 3*(4), 31–41.

Bond, M.R. (1976). Assessment of psychosocial outcome of severe head injury. *Acta Neurochirurgica, 34,* 57–70.

Bond, M.R. (1983). Effects on the family system. In M. Rosenthal, E. Griffith, M. Bond, & J.D. Miller (Eds.), *Rehabilitation of the head injured adult* (pp. 209–217). Philadelphia: F.A. Davis.

Brooks, N., Campsie, L., Symington, C., Beattie, A., & McKinlay, W. (1986). The five year outcome of severe blunt head injury: A relative's review. *Journal of Neurology, Neurosurgery and Psychiatry, 49,* 764–770.

Brooks, N., Campsie, L., Symington, C., Beattie, A., & McKinlay, W. (1987). The effects of severe head injury upon patient and relative within several years of injury. *Journal of Head Trauma Rehabilitation, 2,* 1–13.

Brooks, D.N., & McKinlay, W. (1983). Personality and behavioural change after severe blunt head injury—A relative's review. *Journal of Neurology, Neurosurgery, and Psychiatry, 46,* 336–344.

Brown, B.W., & McCormick, T. (1988). Family coping following traumatic head injury: An exploratory analysis with recommendations for treatment. *Family Relations, 37,* 12–16.

Cavallo, M., & Kay, T. (1988). *Head injury and the family system: The N.Y.U. Head Injury Family Interview revisited.* Workshop presented at the Seventh Annual Professional Symposium of the National Head Injury Foundation, Atlanta.

DePompei, R., Zarski, J.J., & Hall, D.E. (1987). A systems approach to understanding CHI family functioning. *Cognitive Rehabilitation, March/April,* 6–10.

Eysenck, H.J., & Eysenck, S.B.G. (1975). *Eysenck personality questionnaire.* London: Hodder and Stoughton.

Florian, V., Katz, S., & Lahav, V. (1989). Impact of traumatic brain damage on family dynamics and functioning: A review. *Brain Injury, 3*(3), 219–233.

Fordyce, D.J., & Roueche, J.R. (1986). Changes in perspectives of disability among patients, staff, and relatives during rehabilitation of brain injury. *Rehabilitation Psychology, 31,* 217–229.

Goldberg, D. (1978). *Manual of the general health questionnaire.* Windsor: NFER Publishing Co.

Groveman, A.M., & Brown, E.W. (1985). Family therapy with closed head injured patients: Utilizing Kubler-Ross' model. *Family Systems Medicine, 3,* 440–446.

Hendryx, P.M. (1989). Psychosocial changes perceived by closed-head-injured adults and their families. *Archives of Physical Medicine and Rehabilitation, 70,* 526–530.

Henry, P., Knippa, J., & Golden, C.J. (1985). A systems model for therapy with brain-injured adults and their families. *Family Systems Medicine, 3,* 427–439.

Hpay, H. (1970). Psycho-social effects of severe head injury. In *International Symposium on Head Injuries. Edinburgh and Madrid, 1970* (pp. 110–119). New York: Churchill Livingstone.

Jacobs, H.E. (1988). The Los Angeles head injury survey: Procedures and initial findings. *Archives of Physical Medicine and Rehabilitation, 69,* 425–431.

Johnson, J.R., & Higgins, L. (1987). Integration of family dynamics into the rehabilitation of the brain-injured patient. *Rehabilitation Nursing, 12,* 320–322.

Kalsbeek, W.D., McLauren, R.L., Harris, B.S.H., & Miller, J.D. (1980). *Journal of Neurosurgery, 53,* S19–S31.

Katz, M.M., & Lyerly, S.B. (1963). Methods of measuring adjustment and social behaviour in the community: Rationale, description, discriminative validity and scale development. *Psychological Reports, 13,* 503–535.

Kay, T., Cavallo, M., & Ezrachi, O. (1988). *Administration Manual, N.Y.U. Head Injury Family Interview (Version 1.2).* New York: N.Y.U. Medical Center Research and Training Center on Head Trauma and Stroke.

Klonoff, P.S., Costa, L.D., & Snow, W.G. (1986). Predictors and indicators of quality of life in patients with closed-head injury. *Journal of Clinical and Experimental Neuropsychology, 8,* 469–485.

Klonoff, P., & Prigatano, G.P. (1987). Reactions of family members and clinical intervention after traumatic brain injury. In M. Ylvisaker & E.M.R. Gobble (Eds.), *Community re-entry for head injured adults* (pp. 381–402). Boston: College-Hill.

Kozloff, R. (1987). Networks of social support and the outcome from severe head injury. *Journal of Head Trauma Rehabilitation, 2,* 14–23.

Lezak, M.D. (1978). Living with the characterologically altered brain injured patient. *Journal of Clinical Psychiatry, 39,* 592–598.

Lezak, M.D. (1986). Psychological implications of traumatic brain damage for the patient's family. *Rehabilitation Psychology, 31,* 241–250.

Lezak, M.D. (1988). Brain damage is a family affair. *Journal of Clinical and Experimental Neuropsychology, 10,* 111–123.

Livingston, M.G. (1986). Assessment of need for coordinated approach in families with victims of head injury. *British Medical Journal, 293,* 742–744.

Livingston, M.G. (1987). Head injury: The relative's response. *Brain Injury, 1,* 33–39.

Livingston, M.G. (1990). Effects on the family system. In M. Rosenthal, E.R. Griffith, M.R. Bond, & J.D. Miller (Eds.), *Rehabilitation of the adult and child with traumatic brain injury* (pp. 225–235). Philadelphia: F.A. Davis.

Livingston, M.G., & Brooks, D.N. (1988). The burden on families of the brain injured: A review. *Journal of Head Trauma Rehabilitation, 4,* 6–15.

Livingston, M.G., Brooks, D.N., & Bond, M.R. (1985a). Patient outcome in the year following severe head injury and relatives' psychiatric and social functioning. *Journal of Neurology, Neurosurgery and Psychiatry, 48,* 876–881.

Livingston, M.G., Brooks, D.N., & Bond, M.R. (1985b). Three months after severe head injury: Psychiatric and social impact on relatives. *Journal of Neurology, Neurosurgery and Psychiatry, 48,* 870–875.

Maitz, E.A. (1989). *The psychological sequelae of a severe closed head injury and their impact upon family systems.* Unpublished doctoral dissertation, Temple University, Philadelphia.

Mauss-Clum, N., & Ryan, M. (1981). Brain injury and the family. *Journal of Neurosurgical Nursing, 13,* 165–169.

McKinlay, W.W., & Brooks, D.N. (1984). Methodological problems in assessing psychosocial recovery following severe head injury. *Journal of Clinical Neuropsychology, 6,* 87–99.

McKinlay, W.W., Brooks, D.N., Bond, M.R., Martinage, D.P., & Marshall, M.M. (1981). The short-term outcome of severe blunt head injury as reported by relatives of the injured person. *Journal of Neurology, Neurosurgery and Psychiatry, 44,* 527–533.

McKinlay, W.W., & Hickox, A. (1988). How can families help in the rehabilitation of the head injured? *Journal of Head Trauma Rehabilitation, 3,* 64–72.

McLaughlin, A.M., & Schaffer, V. (1985). Rehabilitate or remold? Family involvement in head injury. *Cognitive Rehabilitation, January/February,* 14–17.

McMordie, W.R., & Barker, S. (1988). The financial trauma of head injury. *Brain Injury, 2,* 357–364.

Muir, C.A., Rosenthal, M., & Diehl, L.N. (1990). Methods of family intervention. In M. Rosenthal, E.R. Griffith, M.R. Bond, & J.D. Miller (Eds.), *Rehabilitation of the adult and child with traumatic brain injury* (pp. 433–448). Philadelphia: F.A. Davis.

Oddy, M., Coughlan, T., Tyerman, A., & Jenkins, D. (1985). Social adjustment after closed head injury: A further follow-up seven years after injury. *Journal of Neurology, Neurosurgery, and Psychiatry, 48,* 564–568.

Oddy, M., & Humphrey, M. (1980). Social recovery during the year following severe head injury. *Journal of Neurology, Neurosurgery and Psychiatry, 43,* 798–802.

Oddy, M., Humphrey, M., & Uttley, D. (1978a). Stresses upon the relatives of head-injured patients. *British Journal of Psychiatry, 133,* 507–513.

Oddy, M., Humphrey, M., & Uttley, D. (1978b). Subjective impairment and social recovery after closed head injury. *Journal of Neurology, Neurosurgery and Psychiatry, 41,* 611–616.

Panting, A., & Merry, P.H. (1972). The long term rehabilitation of severe head injuries with particular reference to the need for social and medical support for the patient's family. *Rehabilitation, 38,* 33–37.

Peters, L.C., Stambrook, M., Moore, A.D., & Esses, L. (1990). Psychosocial sequelae of closed head injury: Effects on the marital relationship. *Brain Injury, 4,* 39–47.

Quine, S., Pierce, J.P., & Lyle, D.M. (1988). Relatives as lay-therapists for the severely head-injured. *Brain Injury, 2,* 139–149.

Ridley, B. (1989). Family response in head injury: Denial . . . or hope for the future? *Social Science and Medicine, 29,* 555–561.

Romano, M.D. (1974). Family response to traumatic head injury. *Scandinavian Journal of Rehabilitation Medicine, 6,* 1–4.

Romano, M.D. (1989). Family issues in head trauma. *Physical Medicine and Rehabilitation: State of the Art Reviews, 3*(1), 157–167.

Rosenbaum, M., & Najenson, T. (1976). Changes in life patterns and symptoms of low mood as reported by wives of severely brain-injured soldiers. *Journal of Consulting and Clinical Psychology, 44,* 831–888.

Rosenthal, M., & Muir, C.A. (1983). Methods of family intervention. In M. Rosenthal, E. Griffith, M. Bond, & J.D. Miller (Eds.), *Rehabilitation of the head injured adult* (pp. 407–419) Philadelphia: F.A. Davis.

Snaith, R.P., Ahmed, S.N., Mehta, S., & Hamilton, M. (1971). Assessment of the severity of primary depressive illness. *Psychological Medicine, 1,* 143–149.

Snaith, R.P., Bridge, G.W.K., & Hamilton, M. (1976). The Leeds Scale for the self assessment of anxiety and depression. *British Journal of Psychiatry, 128,* 156–165.

Stern, J.M., Sazbon, L., Becker, E., & Costeff, H. (1988). Severe behavioural disturbance in families of patients with prolonged coma. *Brain Injury, 2,* 259–262.

Thomsen, I.V. (1974). The patient with severe head injury and his family. *Scandinavian Journal of Rehabilitation Medicine, 6,* 180–183.

Thomsen, I.V. (1984). Late outcome of very severe blunt head trauma: A 10–15 year second follow-up. *Journal of Neurology, Neurosurgery and Psychiatry, 47,* 260–268.

Walker, A.E. (1972). Long-term evaluation of the social and family adjustment of head injuries. *Scandinavian Journal of Rehabilitation Medicine, 4,* 5–8.

Weddell, R., Oddy, M., & Jenkins, D. (1980). Social adjustment after rehabilitation: A two year follow-up of patients with severe head injury. *Psychological Medicine, 10,* 257–263.

Weissman, M.M., Prusoff, B.A., Thompson, W.D., Harding, P.S., & Myers, J.K. (1978). Social adjustment by self report in a community sample and in psychiatric outpatients. *Journal of Nervous and Mental Diseases, 166,* 317–326.

Willer, B., Arrigali, M., & Liss, M. (1989). *Family adjustment to the long term effects of traumatic brain injury of husbands* (Tech. Rep. No. 89-2). Buffalo: University of Buffalo RRTC.

Zarski, J.J., DePompei, R., & Zook, A. (1988). Traumatic head injury: Dimensions of family responsivity. *Journal of Head Trauma Rehabilitation, 3,* 31–41.

Zarski, J.J., Hall, D.E., & DePompei, R. (1987). Closed head injury patients: A family therapy approach to the rehabilitation process. *The American Journal of Family Therapy, 15,* 62–68.

III

FAMILIES AND THE
ARRAY OF SERVICES

Section III addresses the family and their interaction with the various aspects of service delivery. Rather than presenting service delivery as a continuum through which a person logically progresses, this section presents an array of services. This distinction reinforces the notion that a service delivery system must respond to each individual and family rather than forcing the individual and family to respond to a given system. This important distinction is yet another paradigm that challenges the current reality in many programs concerned with service delivery.

11

THE FAMILY SYSTEM IN ACUTE CARE AND ACUTE REHABILITATION

LYNN GRAHAME

Professionals who have been involved in the care of people who have had a head injury know that what is most certain about head injury is the uncertainty of its prognosis for any individual. How the injury will manifest itself, how it will affect the way a person is able to think, to learn, and to do will be almost infinitely variable. What we have come to know over the years of experience is that the quality of life after a head injury may have more to do with the quality and stability of the injured person's network of family and friends than with any organic aspect of the injury itself.

Obviously, this is not to say that medical and clinical interventions are unnecessary. It does mean that unless the injured person is to live permanently in our institution or program, he or she will go back to living within another system. The needs and rules of that system, therefore, must be the major concern if the rehabilitation program is to be relevant. Those needs and rules must determine the goals and will determine the outcome.

THE FAMILY SYSTEM IN ACUTE CARE

The possibility that "out of the blue" something could happen to me that could permanently change my ability to make decisions, to control the way I move, to do my work, or to fulfill other functions that are part of living in my world is disturbing. Likewise, the possibility that I might have to take over the decision-making "rights" of my spouse or one of my children on an indefinite basis is very threatening. As a social worker in a brain injury program, I know all too well the magnitude of demands that a family care system may suddenly have to face—demands that none of us ever is really prepared to take on as part of our busy lives.

That is what head injury is all about. The person who has been injured will be permanently different, in small and subtle ways or in a substantial way. Most likely, he or she will require help or supervision in some or all areas of decision-making and/or physical functioning. Possibly, this need will go on for the rest of the person's life.

Where will the bulk of assistance that a person with head injury requires over time come from? The answer, as we know, is that for the majority of persons affected by any sort of injury to the brain, the family or other close psycho-social system will be the primary, long-term resource for physical, emotional, and managerial support. It is only in the minority of cases that professional care is required indefinitely for medical or clinical needs. It is also true that funding resources for professional care are increasingly limited. Rarely can funding be counted on for indefinite assistance.

Given the need that any of us might have of our family system in the event of catastrophic injury, it is fortunate that relatively few of us are truly alone in the world. However, there is great variability in the extent to which people are entwined with others. Linkages of expectations and responsibilities are subtle, and people generally live and work in many overlapping systems without much thought as to how they operate and "who" is to "whom" and for "what." An enlightening exercise might be to identify the persons who might "be there" for us and for what responsibilities.

Crisis alerts the primary system, usually the family, and the person with severe illness or injury is visited at the acute care hospital by those who see themselves as most involved. Family members may show up even though there have been years of separation or alienation. However, though many may show care and concern, it will be commitment that counts over the long run. The first psycho-social task for social workers and nurses in acute care is the identification of those who are "primary" within the family or other social network, that is, those who seem to have potential for meaningful helping involvement.

Observations about who visits, the visitors' questions, how they seem to be interacting with the patient, and how they appear to be coping provide valuable information about the strength or potential of possible caregivers. However, observations and inferences made by inexperienced staff may lead to incorrect conclusions. How people behave in a time of crisis is related to many variables: their state of health or level of fatigue, the pressure they feel from daily responsibilities, finances, and their access to support from others within the system are among the variables that may influence the way they appear or behave. Strategies for coping in crisis are learned out of past experiences. These strategies may have been similar but not necessarily positive. When there are no relevant experiences to draw from, people make up strategies out of raw material that comes from values and a sense of what is expected. Comfort with and access to information about the situation at hand is vital.

Three of the most important psycho-social interventions for promotion of coping skills in potential long-term care providers are:

1. Access to accurate information about head injury
2. A supportive climate for learning and adjustment
3. The opportunity for family members and/or other close support persons to physically interact with the person who has been injured

Information

Access to information means access to a way to understand head injury in addition to protection from confusion as a result of inaccurate or misleading information. All people ask questions in one way or another and if denied answers, may simply "make something up." A problem for professionals in acute care is that a family's questions can take up a good deal of time and schedules may be hectic. In addition, the knowledge and understanding that we as professionals have gained through experience and training may commonly lead us to use terminology or utilize concepts to which the family has had no prior exposure. We know what we mean; they often do not. Without enough of a knowledge base they may interpret our words inaccurately.

When family members or other potential caregivers ask questions about brain injury, they need information provided as concretely as possible, at a level that facilitates understanding. Information needs to emphasize the key facts as we know them.

Brain cells can be injured or "damaged" in many different ways. A medical event such as a stroke or aneurysm (ruptured blood vessel) may result in bleeding or loss of oxygen, which injures or kills cells. In a traumatic event such as a fall, motor vehicle accident, or an assault, there may be impact that results in contusions (bruising). Especially in motor vehicle accidents, there may be the effect of stretching or shearing of brain tissue as a result of the rapid movement of the brain within the skull at the time of forceful impact. In both kinds of trauma there may be additional injury to cells from bleeding or swelling. Surgery, which frequently is necessary to save a life, will also inflict further damage. Seizures or infection may occur and take their toll as well.

Family members need to be introduced at the acute care stage to the concept of permanency of impairment, to learn that brain tissue, as we currently understand it, is not able to regenerate or to "fix itself." It is also important that they learn that the technology they are hearing so much about can only show relatively large areas of problem, and much of the injury to the brain may actually be at a microscopic level, which cannot be seen. Helping families avoid or limit unrealistic expectations must include informing them that the technology cannot predict exactly how the person with the injury eventually will be able to think, talk, move, learn—to be and to do. The family will have to learn these things about the person over a period of time.

Learning whom to ask for information is also important, and it is essential that staff understand and respect their own limitations as information providers. Many people are unintentionally misled by "helpers" who feel they must answer a question but do not really have the correct answer themselves. It is also common that families may seem to pick the most inconvenient times to want information, such as on weekends or night shifts when the doctor or social worker is not available and the nurse on duty just came in that morning and knows very little about the case. Having access to literature about head injury that is written in language a lay person can understand can be invaluable to the family in the acute care hospital. This is also a mechanism for providing information about head injury resources, including the National Head Injury Foundation (NHIF) and its state chapters, as well as local support groups.

Regardless of the effort expended to provide accurate information, there are bound to be misconceptions. People in crisis simply are not good receivers of information, especially when the information is painful to hear. They may seem to take in only a fraction of what is provided. Also, the professional may be perceived as threatening, and often it seems that the anxious person goes to the most unlikely informant for a comforting word.

Support

Access to support during this difficult time is essential. People feel alone and out of control when they are powerless to help an important person in their world who is in grave danger. Information is itself supportive because when people find help to understand a situation, they feel more able to cope with it. Acute care staff who convey the message that they are there to help answer questions and that information sharing is an appropriate use of their time help families in crisis to feel less alone.

Support also means giving information in a climate of hope. We know that, more than ever, people are surviving the injuries that commonly resulted in death only a decade ago. Although the process of rehabilitation may be painful and lengthy, many more people with severe injury are eventually able to resume much of the responsibilities of their lives. Although for most people, significant adjustments may be required in life plans and goals, there can still be some quality to life.

Psycho-social and nursing staff also provide valuable support when, in privacy, they provide family and friends the opportunity to vent feelings of grief or anger or loss. These obviously human and normal feelings consume energy needed for other coping activities. Some situations, especially where the person with severe injury is the victim of a violent act, may require special attention for psycho-social intervention. The normal desire for retribution can escalate, especially when a peer group comes from a social setting where violence is not uncommon and getting back at a perpetrator may be expected.

As medical stability is achieved and the time comes to make decisions about the next step, the potential caregivers need support and assurance in order to be open and honest about the very real limitations that they may have for long-term involvement. Not all members of the system will have the hours and availability required. Those who do not, may need help not to feel guilty and may be able to find smaller but not unimportant ways to be helpful later in the care plan.

Interaction

The opportunity for physical interaction with the person who has been injured is obviously available to anyone who simply comes into the room. However, there are no clear rules for how people can or should behave in this interaction. Ordinary sickroom conversation generally is out of the question, at least initially. It can be devastating to look at a loved one's changed appearance. Tubes and tracheostomies look dangerous or painful. Smells and sounds may be unpleasant or embarrassing. It is especially hard to be in the room with a loved one and not know what to do or to say. Someone who is uncertain about what is safe or appropriate in this situation may find it difficult to want to show affection.

Assisting in reacquaintance with an injured loved one through touch and personal care may be one of the most important ways that acute care nursing staff can help re-establish relationships between the person and his or her care system. Time for training and supervision in such activities may be in short supply for acute care nursing staff but this investment can pay off in many ways in the future. Such simple acts as providing skin care or mouth care or grooming someone's hair will help the "helper" to feel useful and will promote comfort for the injured person where counseling alone would be limited.

Such physical interaction helps potential caregivers to become more comfortable with the person and enables the caregiver to develop a sense of competency that will be invaluable as decisions are made about eventual caretaking roles. Also, through this interaction, members of the care system can be prepared for the kinds of involvement that will be necessary and expected when the patient is ready to move on to acute rehabilitation and the real "training process" for going on with life.

The task of acute care is to achieve medical stability and to provide the involved psycho-social system, usually the family, with information, support, and preparation so that an informed decision can be made about what they should do next to meet their loved one's needs.

Formal rehabilitation in an inpatient setting obviously is not necessary in every circumstance. Some head injuries may be sufficiently mild so that the patient is able to recapture competency in basic skill areas while in the acute care hospital. There may be no readily apparent need for any further inpatient hospitalization, or there may seem to be only limited need for outpatient therapies. However, there may be areas of severe deficit that are not apparent as problems until the individual returns to the real-life expectations of home. It is extremely important that health care providers warn these seemingly unaffected individuals that problems may occur and that help can be available where necessary.

For other persons, especially those with extremely severe head injuries, the fact of medical stability does not necessarily mean that the person is ready for rehabilitation or, in fact, can derive any benefit from it. The family is likely to feel very anxious or even angry about this situation; they may almost feel that the loved one has somehow "failed." They may conclude that the recommendation against rehabilitation is a matter of lack of insurance coverage, that if financial resources were better there would be no problem. There may also be the fear that if the opportunity for rehabilitation is not seized immediately, the person will somehow be lost in the system and forgotten.

The family may also feel that they themselves have in some way failed. Perhaps a different choice of physician or a different hospital would have made a difference. Guilt feelings about the circumstances of the injury, even where obviously inappropriate, may surface. Reiteration of the facts about head injury and the differences in individual "readiness" for rehabilitation can help the family support system to feel much more comfortable about a nursing home or sub-acute placement. Identification of the kinds of indicators of "readiness" and explanation of how the family can be part of a program of observation and recording are also important in helping the family cope with an injured loved one's slower course.

THE FAMILY SYSTEM IN ACUTE REHABILITATION

Decisions about referral to formal rehabilitation should always address the question: "Rehabilitation to what, for what?" When a person has achieved medical stability but continues to display severe impairments in cognitive and/or physical functioning, it is obvious that we cannot assume that "good rehabilitation" will effect the return of all of the person's previous abilities. However, what is obvious to us as professionals is not necessarily obvious to the person's family. "To life as before; to work as before," is the answer to the question about rehabilitation that families generally would prefer to give, and sometimes do give. Those who have had an opportunity for education about head injury in the acute care setting will be more likely to conceptualize a post-rehabilitation destination plan with some reasonable elements.

The initial task of the psycho-social team in acute rehabilitation is to tease out the options for where the person will be able to go and what the person will have to be able to do to stay there. These questions are at once the simplest and the most complex that the acute head injury rehabilitation team will have to answer. From it will come the development of the initial Destination and Activity Pattern Plan for after the injured person leaves the institution: Where and with whom will the person live, and what will the person do with her or his time? (The concept of Destination Stability and Activity Pattern as essential to favorable TBI outcome was developed by Dr. Nathaniel Mayer and the rehabilitation team at Drucker Brain Injury Center, Moss Rehabilitation Hospital, Philadelphia, Pennsylvania.)

This plan for living and doing must be ecologically relevant. Ecology means the interaction between an organism and its environment. There is ecological stability when the organism and the environment meet each other's needs in an adaptive and nonstressful way. After head injury, the real product of rehabilitation is not only enhanced physical or cognitive functioning, but also the relevance of this functioning to both the needs of the individual and the needs of the system to which he or she returns.

A healthy ecological system is flexible and able to adapt to changes from internal and external forces over time. Likewise, a stable Destination and Activity Plan is one that is adaptable to changing needs and deals effectively with stresses.

Identifying what is realistic and acceptable to a family system is a tall order for the head injury rehabilitation team. In most cases families do not come into this stage of the process with the complete and accurate information that the first part of this chapter advocated providing. They do not come in with a full acceptance of the changes that have occurred in their loved one, and they are not necessarily as "committed" to potentially indefinite care as they might have indicated on the admission application.

Rather, most families come into the inpatient rehabilitation setting still in a state of crisis. Generally they are anxious. Often, they have come to feel mistrustful of or even angry towards care staff because of previous medical or other care problems or miscommunications. They may be resentful of requests for financial or insurance information that they believe they have already given to too many people, too many times. Because of missed work time, they may be fearful for their own economic future.

They may feel increasingly guilty about home chores left undone or the needs of other family members left unmet. Siblings may feel angry and resentful about disruption of family life and the attention being given to the member with an injury. They may actually be physically uncomfortable during much of visit time, having missed meals or having made do with snacks or fast foods for too long. Even the opportunity to handle basic personal needs in privacy may be limited in the hospital setting.

Consequently, the family system coming into the rehabilitation setting generally is not ideally prepared for realistic, productive planning. The rehabilitation team, however, may feel pressure to move quickly when it appears that the length of stay may be brief and there is much to accomplish. What help, then, does the family need to become sufficiently comfortable with the team and the setting so that, together, they can tackle the work ahead?

Attention to the Comforts of the Setting

In the rehabilitation setting, just as everywhere else in life, it is often the "little amenities" that mean the most for establishing comfort. Being able to feel safe and comfortable in a setting is often one of the most important elements that families look for in the process of choosing among rehabilitation options. Once they have made their choice, those comforts may be major factors in the relationships they form with the professionals with whom they will work.

Important comforts include introduction to the team members and identification of their various responsibilities. Knowing the appropriate team member to contact for information and knowing the patient's daily schedule can help reduce overly vigilant attitudes that may have developed out of insecurity in the previous setting. If the psycho-social team is able to provide evening or weekend times for information sharing, caregivers may be freed for resumption of daily routines without sacrificing the opportunity to stay closely informed. The physical attractiveness of the facility and its grounds may be very important initially, but it will be the quality and comfort of the relationships that are built between the family system and the rehabilitation system that will make the difference in how they work together.

Evaluating the Family System

The development of an ecologically relevant Destination and Activity Plan requires that the family or other potential care system disclose enough information about how that system operates for the rehabilitation team to have an accurate sense of strengths and needs and potential problem areas. Learning about the physical layout of a home is not difficult. People generally are quick to identify the steepness of staircases, where bathrooms are located, and who is present and at what times. However, the more important information for destination planning is information about the family system's emotional health, values, and coping strengths. This information is less readily shared and less easily gathered.

The art of psycho-social counseling is that process of teasing out the family stories and making the observations that give the information about how these particular people live. It is in this way that we learn what is valuable, as well as what is unimportant, what is expected, and what may be tolerated.

A real danger in the exploration process is that if we professionals are unable to tease out the relevant material, we may make up our own impressions of what must be needed or wanted by the family system. Even though there are enough good goal options in rehabilitation, needs of little relevance to the real world of the patient may be given an inordinate amount of time. A complicated program of communication strategies may be technically correct, but if the family members find it impractical or already have a way of understanding each other that is adequate, our time is wasted. At the same time, it may be the patient's bad table manners or demanding behavior that is driving the family crazy. Attention to those concerns will be far more valuable to the family system's coping ability.

In addition to drawing out needs, the psycho-social team must often delve into areas that are potentially threatening or embarrassing. Drugs and alcohol very often are factors in the circumstances that resulted in the patient's present condition. Attention must be given to how the family understands and expects to deal with this issue in the future. It is important for the psycho-social team to be nonjudgmental in their presentation of how to deal with drug or alcohol abuse and that the family and friends involved reach a consensus on what rules will be followed around the family. Even where usage is a highly infrequent part of a family system's activity pattern, the information about the risks of drug and alcohol use is crucial. Bringing in members of a peer group may be especially important if we are to protect a person with head injury from being inadvertently harmed by socializing with friends who do not know the dangers.

Often, drug or alcohol abuse is more of a problem than can be handled through family counseling and education. Referral to a more extensive drug or alcohol program may be needed as part of the total rehabilitation process. This is a step that may not be acceptable to the person with head injury or to the family care system. In many cases, the fact that drug or alcohol abuse has led to such a devastating situation is enough that everyone concerned is sure that there will be no more of this behavior. It is important to emphasize that something positive must be developed in the person's life to replace the substance abuse. Otherwise, it may return.

Sexuality is also an area that may be difficult for the family to discuss. From the sexually inappropriate behavior that is common when a patient is agitated and not yet attending to the expectations of the environment, to changes in affect or personality, there are many reasons to be concerned about how to be sexually intimate with someone again. Sexual partners may need explicit discussion about changes in sexual functioning. A change in contraceptive method may also be indicated for any number of reasons but most commonly because of the need for antiseizure medication, which may dilute the effectiveness of an oral contraceptive.

How a partner may feel about just being in a situation of potential intimacy is often a relevant question as plans are made for living at home. Especially where there is incontinence or some other sort of management problem, the significant other may need to talk out the options with a rehabilitation team member who is comfortable with the issue and has the correct information.

Sexuality is also an issue of concern, realistic or not, for a patient's vulnerability because of inappropriate behavior or poor judgment after head injury. Families may be very uncomfortable about a patient's uninhibited use of vulgarity or inattention to whether or not he or she is fully clothed. There may be concern that the person could be taken advantage of sexually because of this behavior, or that he or she might become sexually aggressive toward someone else. Indeed, the family may be hearing that other persons with head injuries or families at the rehabilitation center are upset or fearful about what the person is doing. Information about how head injury relates to behavior change is important in helping the family to understand. The family also needs training in how most effectively to respond to inappropriate behaviors. Just plain support and concern for what they are experiencing are also important.

The Education Process

The process of providing education about head injury must proceed concurrently with the process of drawing out information from the family about their issues and concerns. The education process, including actual training in the strategies that are useful, is most important in empowering the members of the family system for the roles that they must eventually take. Although ideally the education process should begin in the acute care facility, it is often incomplete there, or the family is not ready during the time spent there to absorb it.

The education process needs to include both general information about head injury and information on the specifics of the particular case. The most effective method may be a combination of education/counseling sessions with the psycho-social team, integrated with training sessions for practice in specific strategies. Training sessions at home as part of a therapeutic leave of absence from the hospital are another opportunity for the family to practice and internalize what they have learned.

The family's receptivity to education and their ability to use what is taught is facilitated with attention to their specific learning style. Knowing something about the family system's educational level and previous educational experience may help to predict abilities, but it is generally through trial and error that the team best learns how to help the system internalize the information they need. When they are not "getting it," it is often because we are somehow not "giving it" in the most understandable way. We must sometimes deliberately analyze whether words, pictures, or hands-on experience are most useful to meet the caregiver's learning needs. The most beautifully written and packaged set of discharge instructions will be useless for the family system that does not read or cannot make sense of our written instructions. Others may feel comfortable only when every detail is written down so that they may refer to their instructions and confirm that what they are doing is right.

The aim of the education and training process is for the team and family care system together to establish the living plan that is most reasonable for both the person with head injury and the members of the care system. A plan has potential for stability only when all involved in it know what they are getting into and what needs will have to be met. The material resources of the patient and/or family system will also have to be considered for obvious reasons. Additionally, the assigned managers, or major decision makers, in the family system will need special attention from the team for education around maximizing the accompanying benefits and entitlements that they may need to make use of.

Developing an Ecologically Valid Plan

A Destination Plan is empty if it does not include a plan for what the person who has been injured will do with his or her day. This Activity Plan must also realistically consider the person's strengths and limitations as well as what is available from others for supervision and assistance. As with the overall Destination Plan, it must also be ecologically relevant so that it considers and reflects the activities that are normal and acceptable components of the day in the setting where the person will be living.

Thinking about and planning for what the changed person can do with his or her time may be more difficult for the care system than thinking about and planning for how to provide care. Family members may more easily decide how to entertain someone, but understanding how the person's new roles and responsibilities might be developed is more complicated.

For most adults, competitive work and/or home management responsibilities make up the bulk of the activity of the day. For someone unable to manage these activities it may be difficult to discover what else is available within the person's specific world that feels useful. Also, professionals must be concerned that the Activity Plan provide continued opportunity for problem-solving and further skill development.

Again, it is through learning about what activities are acceptable to the care system and by practice of specific activities that this plan can be developed. Families may need help accepting the fact that the person's new activities will be different from the person's activities pre-injury, especially if the new activities will be substantially different. Washing dishes or folding laundry may seem to be very reasonable activities for a person with a severe impairment from the staff's point of view, but if the notion of "macho Dad" doing housework is too foreign (or perhaps painful) for a family, these activities will not be practiced at home. Other possibilities that seem more comfortable should be explored. Additionally, the caregiver's needs, limits, and general emotional comfort must be respected. If a wife states that she will do anything for her injured spouse except "allow" him to work in her kitchen, then so be it.

A stable Destination and Activity Plan is enhanced by identification of how more peripheral members of the family or other support persons can remain involved over time. For example, a cousin who was identified during acute care as having only limited availability may still be willing to give some of that limited time. If this person has only a few hours for card games or walking in the park every other Saturday, this is still a useful and valuable option for respite. Those few hours could make a considerable difference in how more involved care system members feel about their responsibilities and are able to continue coping.

Just as a workable environment is able to adapt to needs and issues, the workability of the Destination and Activity Plans also is affected by how caretakers or managers are able to permit and encourage more complicated roles and responsibilities as there is improvement. The family system that is really educated and empowered will be more likely to be able to adjust and expand, as well as to know when additional assistance from professionals is required to solve problems or plan new directions.

The intensity of involvement that develops between the rehabilitation team, the person with head injury, and the family commonly leads to considerable team anxiety at the time of discharge from the rehabilitation hospital. Even when we know that we have put together a good plan, the needs may be so many and the care plan so complicated that we fear the individual and her or his support systems will be lost without our constant assistance. Often, to our amazement, they are able to go on with their daily lives with very little of the difficulty we anticipated. These are truly the most successful situations, that is, those in which the person with a head injury is able to continue rehabilitation through daily life itself.

12

FAMILY AND COMMUNITY REENTRY

SALLY KNEIPP

Since its inception, the National Head Injury Foundation (NHIF) has proclaimed that "life after head injury is never the same." Clearly this is true for the family members of a person who has experienced a head injury, as well as the person with the head injury. The full impact is rarely realized until the person begins the process of community reentry. At the time of discharge from the rehabilitation hospital, family members and people with head injuries often believe that the hardest part is over. This is understandable considering that such major events as emergence from coma, or learning to walk or talk again occur there. Family members frequently anticipate, especially when their loved one has exceeded the treatment team's prognosis, that progress will continue at essentially the same rate, to full recovery. Moreover, because of the focus on physical functioning during the early stages of rehabilitation, people with head injuries and family members tend to underestimate the extent of cognitive, psycho-social, and emotional dysfunction. Family members report that the person's personality changes are a major source of long-term stress and are more difficult to handle than the physical changes.

Family members often comment that they were not prepared for the problems in the later stages post-injury. In investigating the stress felt by relatives of patients who experienced head injury, Oddy, Humphrey, and Uttley (1978) found that the "most common dissatisfaction expressed [by relatives] was with the level of communication between medical staff and themselves" (p. 511). Panting and Merry (1972) and Thomsen (1984) also found that relatives believed they had received insufficient information, es-

165

pecially regarding prognosis and anticipated difficulties. Lezak (1978) has suggested that, when the family is reunited following a head injury of one of its members, information and guidance are needed but may not be accepted.

Underlying the issue of whether the family can assimilate the information is whether the family and the person with a head injury are ready to hear it at all. Having weathered the intensity of emergency treatment, acute care, and comprehensive medical rehabilitation, family members and people with head injuries may need, psychologically, to believe that reintegration into the community will be straightforward. The demands on their personal resources have already been enormous. They need to feel optimistic about future recovery in order to maintain energy and momentum for the next and final stage of rehabilitation after head trauma.

During acute rehabilitation, professionals evaluate and treat the person clinically and, on the basis of their observations, make predictions as to his or her level of functioning during community reentry. However, once the individual is discharged, the change in setting and structure can lead to a very different clinical picture. Individuals who did quite well in a hospital setting may exhibit extreme difficulties in the community. They may respond negatively to the reduced structure and the additional stimulation of family life and community living. For example, they may find it particularly difficult to plan meaningful activity to fill their days or to initiate household chores.

The proliferation of head trauma programs has included a significant increase in the number of programs labeled "community reentry." Many of these programs are residential and/or transitional and aim to increase one's ability to function independently in the community. However, these programs are not necessarily located in the person's community. For the purposes of this chapter, the focus is on the salient issues for families with a member with head injury returning to the home community following acute rehabilitation, transitional living, or other post-acute residential program.

This focus is not intended to minimize the fact that there are complex family issues involved when the person with a head injury is placed outside the home following acute rehabilitation or when the family ultimately recognizes that they cannot provide a beneficial environment for the person at home. When family members decide that placement outside the home is necessary, they frequently feel enormously guilty, as if they have abandoned their member with a head injury. They may need reassurance that alternative placement is a viable option and frequently indicated, particularly if family dysfunction is contributing to regression or impeding additional progress for the person. The purpose of narrowing the focus of this chapter is to avoid trying to cover all community reentry issues, with inevitably unsuccessful results. The magnitude of the problem demands some delimitation.

SCOPE OF THE PROBLEM

In fundamental ways a head injury interrupts the normal developmental stages and transitions in family life cycles. Roles and functions of family members are often altered dramatically and permanently. While anyone is vulnerable to having a head injury, head injuries are most often sustained by persons 18–30 years of age. After having fulfilled the major parenting responsibility of raising their children to the point of independence, it is devastating for parents to have to reverse the psychological process and accept the possibility of their offspring's head injury causing lifelong dependence on them. Likewise, for the young adult with a head injury, the acceptance of dependence, following the maturational struggle for independence, is a very difficult psychological shift.

There are many other scenarios as well, which demand that the spouses, parents, and siblings of persons with head injuries change their familiar roles as they are thrust into new ways of interacting with their family members. A husband, for example, must learn to assume roles previously held by his wife with a head injury. The role changes invariably affect each family member and the way each member relates to every other member. As a result, family functions are affected.

The changes are felt much more acutely by families at the point of community reentry. Until that time, the attention of the family is focused on milestones for recovery. Although the tension is felt, there are goals (for example, emergence from coma) that are reasonably clear and that become the focal point of communication among family members. In a sense, these goals help to bind the family. At the time of community reentry, life is presumed to be returning to some semblance of normalcy; family members redirect their attention to their own personal goals. There is often lack of consensus regarding the goals of the person who has experienced a head injury; conflict among family members may surface. Conflicts over intervention for the person can escalate into legal battles for conservatorship, guardianship, and so forth. Individual personality style determines the responses and behavior of family members at this stage. There are frequent reports of guilt, anger, resentment, hostility, anxiety, depression, and despair.

When divorce occurs in couples after a partner has experienced a head injury, the guilt of the partner choosing to separate (usually the noninjured partner) can be tremendous. The noninjured spouse may remain more integrally involved in the life of the person with a head injury than is usual following divorce; the relationship may become more paternal or maternal. In cases where the marriage was leading to divorce at the time of the injury and the noninjured person remains in the marriage to help the spouse with a head injury, there is often a feeling of being trapped. Resentment generally builds when the life crises are over; later, these marriages frequently do end in the divorce that would have occurred much sooner.

Spouses of persons with head injuries face an unusual, very complicated dilemma because they have permanently lost their partners as they knew them when they first chose them. Spouses have occasionally admitted, cautiously, that they never would have chosen for a mate the individual who resulted after the effect of head injury. Yet, they remain in the marriage. Lezak (1978) explains:

> The spouse cannot divorce with dignity or in good conscience. Gratitude, fond memories, feelings of responsibility, guilt and fear of social condemnation contribute to the reluctance of a once happily married spouse to divorce his hapless mate. Moreover, brain injury not infrequently prolongs an unhappy marriage, bonds of guilt and fear of disapproval tying the caretaking spouse to the patient as nothing could were the patient well. (p. 593)

The often unpredictable behavior of persons with head injuries presents considerable anxiety for their children. Children of a parent with a head injury report feeling deprived of a parent who can nurture them as their friends' parents do. This situation is described poignantly in Chapter 4 by Hope Hardgrove, a 14-year-old girl reflecting on her life after her father's head injury. Moreover, in cases where the parent with the head injury is home with children and the other spouse works full time, the children may end up assuming a parental role or, in some cases, a surrogate spouse role. In cases where the person with the head injury is a sibling, the other siblings may experience resentment over the need to help care for the person and may worry about how his or her friends will react to the person. Individuals with head injuries are frequently upset by having a younger sibling who has more privileges (e.g., a 17-year-old sibling who can drive, when the 21-year-old sibling with a head injury is unable to because of seizures). Developmental problems and/or acting out may occur.

When one considers the amount of disruption to the family system, it is remarkable that families cope as well as they do. There are families, particularly those whose communication has always been open and direct, who require minimal intervention and who cope well with the changes forced upon them. Others experience varying degrees of inability to cope with the alterations in the family system. Rosenthal and Muir (1983) suggest that certain kinds of high-risk families can be expected to experience the most dysfunction; they are families with a history of maladaptive behavior patterns (e.g., marital discord); prolonged use of denial; and/or a member with persistent, severe chronic, physical, and/or mental impairments.

Community reentry issues for families of persons with head injuries are complex, as they reflect the uniqueness of both the person with the head injury and the family as a unit. They also vary as a function of the point in the community reentry process. When the individual with a head injury is returning to his or her parents' home, any anxiety over the responsibility for care of the individual is tempered or outweighed by the euphoria at reaching this point in the process. Later, family members may resent the responsibility for care, particularly when, as is often the case, the individual is exceedingly egocentric; the individual may persist in making demands on family members, without a word of thanks for their efforts. Family members may intellectually understand that such behavior is organically-based, but emotionally they may be weary of this behavior. Most people wish to have their efforts appreciated or at least acknowledged. Still later, family members may feel detached. Detachment may be a healthy coping strategy that allows the family member to take charge of his or her own life again. To an extreme degree, however, it may reflect a desire to avoid the entire situation and may result in the loss of a relationship that, although altered, still offers some inherent satisfactions.

McKinlay et al. (1981) studied the "10 most frequent symptoms reported as problems by relatives of head-injured men" at 3, 6, and 12 months post-injury. They found that stress in families was usually attributable to specific kinds of problems rather than the severity of the injury. After 6 months post-injury, the dependency of the men was felt to be a burden; emotional and behavioral changes were a source of significant stress. Bad temper and mood swings were thought to reflect the persons' reactions to their traumas, their growing awareness of their handicaps, and their diminished productivity. Brooks and McKinlay (1983) emphasized that, after 6 months post-injury, "attempts should be made to classify, to understand, to predict, and importantly, to modify the changes in personality and behavior in the patient which may have such an impact upon the family" (p. 343).

Lezak (1978) summarizes the "characterological alterations" of adults with brain injury as including an impaired capacity for social perceptiveness, an impaired capacity for control and self-regulation, stimulus-bound behavior, and inability to profit from experiences. She identified the most common specific emotional alterations as apathy, silliness, lability, irritability, and either greatly increased sexual interest or a virtual loss of the sex drive. These characterological changes result in more family stress than do physical disabilities or impaired intellectual capacity following head trauma.

Characterological changes are not always constant. One family member described her responses to her son's characterological changes as "an emotional roller coaster." Following is a description of that situation:

Robert, a single male from a middle-class Catholic family, sustained a head injury in a motor vehicle crash on his way home from his 20th birthday party; he was a passenger in a car driven by an acquaintance. He remained in a coma for 2 weeks and, following comprehensive rehabilitation therapies, continued to exhibit noticeable gait deviations and speech impairments as well as significant cognitive and behavioral changes.

Robert reported that, prior to his injury, he had been "pretty wild and irresponsible." He had dropped out of high school just months before his high school graduation, abused alcohol and drugs, and held a series of jobs for a week or two (as he explained it, just long enough to get a paycheck and quit, or "rip off" his employer and leave). He hung out with a gang of boys whose favorite pastime was to steal cars, strip away the parts they wanted, and then ram the cars into trees in a dense wooded lot near Robert's home. Robert often slept in the woods following arguments with his father.

After his head injury, Robert's behavior changed dramatically. He became the "model patient," and the dutiful and loving son. He expressed a strong sense of morality; in fact, he was very rigid and self-righteous about smoking, drinking and drugs, stating repeatedly that, if he were president (of the United States), he would ban all alcohol and drugs.

Robert was discharged to his home to live with his parents and three sisters. Over the next few years, Robert continued to receive outpatient and community-based therapies. He worked extremely hard in his therapies. Significantly, he passed the state high school equivalency test and earned his General Education Diploma. With job placement assistance, he obtained a volunteer job which led to part-time and then full-time paid employment as a library aide, earning union wages of $8.00 per hour—more than double the minimum wage he had earned pre-injury. He passed a driver's evaluation and began driving again. His family was very proud of the "new Robert."

Two years later, Robert was still employed, but he was feeling socially isolated. He attended church, occasionally engaged in bowling and golfing with family members and went out socially with his siblings and their friends sometimes; however, he did not initiate contacts with people and expressed finding it hard to relate to his former friends. He had one "friend" whom he met at the rehabilitation hospital. That friend, also with a history of drug and alcohol abuse, started spending time with Robert. Robert began missing work or showing up late and then quit his job. Robert's parents were distraught, and relayed with dismay, "The old Robert is back."

During the community reentry process, the needs of family members differ depending on whether their family member with a head injury is participating in a day treatment program at a facility, receiving at-home and/or community-based treatment, or receiving no treatment or services. The family's needs must be taken into account in assessment, goal setting, and intervention.

ASSESSMENT

The need for long-term supportive services for persons with head injuries and their families is being recognized increasingly. Yet, assessments by professionals still usually remain focused only on the family member with the head injury. While the results of the assessments of the member with the head injury may include, by implication, recommendations for the family, systematic assessments of the family's needs during the community reentry process are conducted very infrequently. In retrospect, professionals may acknowledge that their failure to adequately consider the family dynamics precluded a successful outcome for the individual with the head injury and perpetuated dysfunction within the family. For example:

An individual with a head injury was the vice president of an engineering firm at the time of his injury. His job required that he wine and dine prospective clients.

He did this 3 or 4 nights a week and had quite a reputation as a womanizer as well. His wife was never quite certain where he was, or with whom. Following his injury he could no longer drive, and his cognitive impairments were severe enough that he needed supervision. He became quite dependent on his wife and was rarely out of her sight. She appeared to enjoy this change. When he subsequently enrolled in a community reentry program and made considerable progress, she began to find fault with the program and terminated his involvement in it. This happened with three different programs, at the point where more independence for him, and possibly driving, was recommended. It became evident that she preferred his dependence on her.

Rosenthal and Muir (1983) recommend an assessment process with three major components: 1) an analysis of the pre-morbid history of the individual and family; 2) accurate estimate of the likely severity and duration of the physical and mental sequelae; and 3) identification of signals from the family that suggest need for intervention. Guth, Lasseter, and Harward (1988) comment on the importance of reassessment of families post-discharge because of changes in the family system itself, the progress of the family member with a head injury, and/or external stresses on the family such as marital problems. They state that the purpose of a comprehensive family assessment is to identify family members and their level of involvement, family interaction patterns and roles, the level of family knowledge and adjustment to head trauma, the types and availability of support and resources, and sources of stress to the family system. They suggest structured interviews, measurement questionnaires (self-report mechanisms), and observation. They indicate that observations could be made in either the natural home setting or in an artificial, laboratory environment. They add that observation in the home setting may provide an index of more normalized family interactions, but that it may be difficult to standardize tasks across different families. In this author's opinion, standardization of tasks across different families is not the most important clinical consideration; establishing an intra-family baseline is what is needed to evaluate change and the effectiveness of interventions.

Schwentor and Brown (1989) discuss the need for a comprehensive family assessment to gauge "the extent of the family's involvement in the rehabilitation process during treatment and after discharge." They describe the functions of a family assessment:

1) to obtain background information about the patient's pre-trauma functioning, extent and scope of problems, and other demographic information for agency records
2) to determine the extent to which the family can support and follow-through with specific therapy interventions in the home or other environments, and determine whether the family will be capable of providing long-term aftercare
3) to determine the family's reaction to this traumatic event, pre-trauma family functioning, current functioning, their expectations for recovery, their needs for services, and their coping capability (p. 8)

In particular, determining the extent to which family members can carry out or support therapy interventions is essential. Deutsch (1988) recommends that family members be trained to become disability managers for individuals needing extended care. While the objective of giving the person with a head injury and his or her family as much control as possible over their lives is desirable, there are families who simply do not have the resources to perform the caretaking role and would not choose it. It is important to respect the right of the family to decide the amount of involvement they wish in the rehabilitation of their family member and to determine how to provide the support needed. They may wish to decide *what services* are needed, *who* is to provide the services, and *what setting* is preferred, and to then rely on professionals to assume the day-to-day responsibility for treatment. Other families may wish to be the careproviders. Whether or not families take an active role in the treatment of their family member with a head injury, their ideas and feelings about treatment should be solicited. This way the family's needs are more evident.

It is the author's conviction that there is no better way to assess the needs of the family during the community reentry process than to actually spend time in the home, on a basis frequent and consistent enough to reveal how the family actually functions. Observations by an astute clinician will yield a wealth of data on which to base goal setting and intervention that encompasses the family's needs as well as the needs of the individual with a head injury. Through observations of, or casual conversation with, family members in their homes, clinicians have acquired information that made the individual's behavior understandable, shed light on why a compensatory strategy that seemed well-conceived was not working, made obvious the pitfalls in a treatment plan, and made clear what steps needed to be taken. The following illustrate:

> With the referral material received by a community reentry program was an excellent, detailed social summary that provided a wealth of information about the family resources and roles of family members. What was not known until time was spent with this family was that there was one less bed in the home than the number of people residing there when the member with a head injury was discharged home. The last person home would sleep on the couch in the living room. This arrangement meant that the 21 year old male with a head injury would usually share a bedroom with his 19, 17, or 16 year old sister, precluding not only the privacy needed by these siblings, but also consistency in the routine of the family member with the head injury. The inconsistency was unsettling to him and resulted in an increase in his irritability, which affected his interactions with family members.

> One goal for a young woman with a head injury, insisted upon by her mother, was that she be assisted in organizing her room. While the neuropsychological testing had revealed that she had *mild* difficulty with categorization skills, her impairments were far more obvious on "real" tasks. Observing her as she began to tackle the organization of her personal belongings yielded a better understanding

of why the mother was so focused on this issue. In the same dresser drawer were candy wrappers, batteries for her portable tape player, dirty underwear, clean underwear, shoes, photographs of her accident, scraps of food and a tube of toothpaste without the top.

While sitting with a young male with a head injury and his father, in the family room of their home, the therapist observed him taking out his appointment book and looking at it. The therapist was silently observing this with great pleasure, having waited a long time for him to master the use of his appointment book. (Without this aide, his memory problems precluded his being able to get to appointments on time, if he even remembered them at all.) The father, also observing him look at his appointment book, questioned the therapist in a very exasperated tone, "Can't you *do* something about this? He takes his appointment book out and looks at it about ten times a day!"

After arriving early in the morning at the home of a young man with a head injury, the therapist was sitting in the kitchen talking with his younger sister, who was setting the table for breakfast for him and herself. When he entered the kitchen, he immediately threw a temper tantrum because she had not reversed the placement of his knife and fork in order to accommodate his left-handedness.

It is when the family becomes accustomed to the therapist being present in the home during the community reentry process that such interactions are observed. A single home visit or periodic visits at widely spaced intervals do not yield the same kind of information. However, given constraints that prohibit extensive assessment (or intervention) at home, other assessment techniques or strategies are indicated.

Not only should the assessment take into account the cultural context of the family, but also the norms and mores of the community in which the family resides. Moreover, assessment of the individual with a head injury must be based on age-related norms, not simply progress since the onset of the injury. When attempting to reenter the community, an individual's behavior is evaluated by persons in the community in relation to that expected of someone his or her age. When looking at age-related behavior, it is important to distinguish between what is organically-based and what is developmental. For example, is the argumentative behavior of a 16-year-old with a head injury a function of organicity or adolescent rebellion? Is the energy level of a 4-year-old with a head injury characteristic of children that age, or is it hyperactivity secondary to head trauma?

Often overlooked in assessments are the seemingly minute details of family life that have significant impact on the treatment for individuals with head injuries and, consequently, on the family. For example, it may seem a simple matter for a therapist to ask a mother to assist her son with a head injury by seeing that he leaves for work on time, at 6:30 A.M. However, if that mother is the wife of a husband who works a 3:00 P.M. to 11:00 P.M. shift and she prepares dinner for him when he comes home from work at midnight (and does not get to bed herself until 1:00 A.M., after doing the dishes), she may not be able to get up in time to provide assistance to her son. It is important that professionals look realistically and sensitively at what family members can provide.

GOAL SETTING

If one accepts that the impact of a head injury is felt by all family members, then the needs of family members (including the one with a head injury) must be considered in setting realistic, attainable goals for community reentry. The process of goal setting is often exceedingly difficult. Family members who become aware of the individual's areas of dysfunction may disagree on the priorities for treatment, or they may want attention given to all issues simultaneously, even though the individual may not have the capacity to address them all at the same time. This is frequently a time when family members "shop around" for programs that will provide "the cure." Family members may believe that it is the inadequacy of the community reentry program that is responsible for the persistence of the impairments rather than acknowledge the severity of the injury and permanent dysfunction. Behavioral problems are understandably unsettling for family members, particularly as reminders of the changes that have occurred. Family members become frustrated and dwell on the impairments, failing to recognize improvements. In other cases, family members continue to exhibit considerable denial even many years post-injury. In fact, Romano (1974) found that relatives of persons with head injuries tended to imagine measurable progress when there had been none.

Family members, as well as the individual with a head injury, must be provided with as much information as is pertinent, and must be assisted in setting goals that are within the reach of the individual. Due to the nature of head injury, the individual may have difficulty perceiving his or her own strengths and limitations and, therefore, have difficulty setting realistic goals. The family may also still be in a period of denial and, consequently, set goals that exceed the individual's potential. This can be psychologically damaging to the individual. Following is an example of how:

> Nine years post-injury, the mother of a 27-year-old woman kept insisting that speech therapy continue, stating that she had observed many occasions when people avoided her daughter because they could not understand her. She would emphatically say, "It is *essential* that she learn to speak clearly; if she cannot, she will *never* be accepted by other people." The mother would also remind the rehabilitation team that it was through her hard work and persistence that her daughter had achieved her current level of independence; she emphasized that additional hard work and persistence would lead to more clarity in her daughter's speech. However, repeated reevaluations of her speech indicated that was not the case. Despite her best efforts, the daughter found that she was unable to consistently speak with greater intelligibility. The message to her, given the insistence that she "speak better or never be accepted," was that she was not worthwhile. Knowing that she had been making a monumental effort to speak clearly, the only

conclusion she could draw was that she never would be accepted. In this case, goal setting included helping her and her family to appreciate her abilities and worth as an individual even though her speech would never be as clear as she or others would like.

Goal setting that fails to take into account the family's needs as well as those of the person with a head injury is often a result of inflexible service delivery systems that overlook the obvious. For example, when planning for discharge of someone from the hospital to the family home, it is important to appreciate the roles and functions family members held at the time of the injury and at the time of discharge. It is advisable to try to preserve the family members' roles and functions to the extent possible. For instance, if an individual with a head injury is unable to remain at home without supervision, it could be considered necessary for one of two working parents to stop working in order to provide supervision. However, flexible programming can result in scheduling that allows both parents to work while their son or daughter continues to receive needed therapies. This simple attention to family members' needs prevents resentment over caregiving, which is certain to build if a family member has to give up a career in which he or she has invested. Flexible programming can prevent other stresses. For example, a father recently commented that he was fearful that, when he came home from work at the end of a long day, his 27-year-old son with a head injury would be waiting for him to take him out somewhere, to get out of the house. An obvious solution was to schedule treatment time encompassing social activities for his son in the evenings, enabling the father to get needed rest and not worry about disappointing him.

Often individuals with head injuries, their family members, and the professionals involved do not agree on what the focus of intervention should be. The person with the head injury may want to focus on employment goals, while the rest of the family members may want to concentrate on maladaptive socio-sexual behavior because it is often a source of embarrassment in public. The professionals may believe that cognitive remediation should be the priority. If the individual with the head injury, family members, and professionals are not in agreement on the intervention goals, progress can be undermined. It is crucial that communication between all involved parties take place so that mutual goals can be established. Professionals must be cognizant of their own values and guard against imposing them on the family.

In looking at family dynamics, it is crucial that professionals understand the cultural milieu. In particular, perceptions of the culture in relation to illness and disability must be taken into account to understand the family's reaction to the rehabilitation process, and how to intervene appropriately. For example, where there is cultural emphasis on the extended family, professionals must consider the extended family, not just the immediate family, in assessing and treating the individual with a head injury. They must be able to work within the cultural framework of the family.

SUMMARY

Family members as well as individuals with head injuries are usually unaware of the problems they will face during the process of community reentry. In particular, personality changes contribute to long-term stress in families and often result in significant changes in the roles and functions of family members. If rehabilitation of the individual with the head injury is to be successful, the entire family's needs must be addressed. During the process of community reentry, the person with the head injury, family members, and professionals must work together to identify problems and to set goals that will address the needs of all family members. In doing this, professionals must be mindful of the need to work within the frame of reference of each particular family and community.

The process of community reentry presents enormous challenges for the individual with a head injury and his or her family. Families have expressed both positive and negative experiences in facing these challenges. While some families report that living from day to day is a continual struggle, others report immense satisfaction from renewed commitments to each other and from discovering their capacities to cope with circumstances that they certainly would not have chosen. Most seem to be somewhere in between, working to solve problems as they arise and reporting varying degrees of satisfaction with their solutions.

REFERENCES

Brooks, D.N., & McKinlay, W. (1983). Personality and behavioral change after severe blunt head injury—A relative's view. *Journal of Neurology, Neurosurgery and Psychiatry, 46,* 336–344.

Condeluci, A., & Gretz-Lasky, S. (1987). Social role valorization: A model for community reentry. *Journal of Head Trauma Rehabilitation, 2*(1), 49–56.

DePompei, R., Zarksi, J.J., & Hall, D.E. (1988). Cognitive communication impairments: A family-focused viewpoint. *Journal of Head Trauma Rehabilitation, 3*(2), 13–22.

Deutsch, P.M. (1988). Family-centered rehabilitation. In P.M. Deutsch & K. Fralish (Eds.), *Innovations in head injury rehabilitation* (pp. 2-1–2-10). Albany: Matthew Bender.

Guth, M., Lasseter, S.A., & Harward, M. (1988). *Head injury rehabilitation: The role of the family in TBI rehabilitation.* (Vol. 19 in the HDI Professional Series on Traumatic Brain Injury edited by Burke, W.H., Wesolowsi, M., & Blackerby, W.F.) Houston: HDI Publishers.

Hendryx, P.M. (1989). Psychosocial changes perceived by closed head-injured adults and their families. *Archives of Physical Medicine and Rehabilitation, 70*(7), 526–530.

Lezak, M.D. (1978). Living with the characterologically altered brain-injured patient. *Journal of Clinical Psychiatry, 39,* 592–598.

Lezak, M.D. (1986). Psychological implications of traumatic brain damage for the patient's family. *Rehabilitation Psychology, 31*(4), 241–250.

McLaughlin, A.M., & Schaffer, V. (1985). Rehabilitate or remold?: Family involvement in head trauma recovery. *Cognitive Rehabilitation, 3*(1), 14–17.

Oddy, M., Humphrey, M., & Uttley, D. (1978). Stresses upon the relatives of head-injured patients. *British Journal of Psychiatry, 133,* 507–513.

Panting, A., & Merry, P.H. (1972). The long-term rehabilitation of severe head injuries with particular reference to the need for social and medical support for the patient's family. *Rehabilitation, 38,* 33–37.

Romano, M.D. (1974). Family response to traumatic head injury. *Scandinavian Journal of Rehabilitation Medicine, 6,* 1–4.

Rosenthal, M., & Muir, C. (1983). Methods of family intervention. In M. Rosenthal, E.R. Griffith, M.R. Bond, & J.D. Miller. (Eds.), *Rehabilitation of the head injured adult* (pp. 407–419). Philadelphia: F.A. Davis.

Schwentor, D., & Brown, P. (1989). Assessment of families with a traumatically brain-injured relative. *Cognitive Rehabilitation, 7*(3), 8–20.

Thomsen, I.V. (1984). Late outcome of very severe blunt head trauma: A 10–15 year second follow-up. *Journal of Neurology, Neurosurgery and Psychiatry, 46,* 260–268.

Weddell, R., Oddy, M., & Jenkins, D. (1980). Social adjustment after rehabilitation: A two year follow-up of patients with severe head injury. *Psychological Medicine, 10,* 257–263.

Zarski, J.J., Hall, D.E., & DePompei, R. (1987). Closed head injury patients: A family therapy approach to the rehabilitation process. *The American Journal of Family Therapy, 15*(1), 62–68.

13

FAMILY AND RETURN TO WORK

SARALYN M. SILVER

PATRICIA L. PRICE

ANASTASIA BARRETT

The ultimate goal of rehabilitation is the restoration of the person to the maximum level of functional competency attainable. This includes, ideally, community reintegration of the person as a contributing, self-sustaining member of society. Persons with traumatic brain injuries are not different from persons with other disabilities in terms of outcome goals. However, their journey towards achieving these goals is different and, because of the nature of the disability, can never be considered complete. In order to achieve and sustain accomplishments, the person with head injury requires varying degrees of support for the remainder of his or her life.

The process of vocational rehabilitation occurs generally as part of the final phase of a lengthy rehabilitation process, which may involve multiple hospitalizations and transitions. Most likely the process will also include a return to home and family. Recruitment of family support in the vocational rehabilitation process is essential, for it is family members, those intimately involved with the person with head injury, who will form the first line of support necessary to the process of return.

Timing, and the manner in which vital services are delivered to people with traumatic head injury, remain critical considerations in the course of rehabilitation (Silver & Kay, 1989). While different models of vocational rehabilitation have been proposed, it is the authors' clinical experience that persons with head injury often require intensive preparation before they are ready for this final phase of rehabilitation. The family (including all significant others) requires similar well-timed periods of preparation. Without this preparation, families may unintentionally subvert successful vocational rehabilitation.

The word *timing* is not meant to imply a timetable. The pace at which a person with a head injury and his or her family move towards rehabilitation goals is highly individualized. Practitioners involved in promoting this movement can do so by being attentive listeners and observers, sensitive to the signals being relayed by those involved. Information should be delivered only as people are ready to hear it. The determination of readiness is the responsibility of the therapists most closely involved in the process. These professionals will make judgments about appropriate timing based upon continuing assessments.

The vocational rehabilitation counselor must remain mindful that degrees of readiness are not always displayed positively. In this chapter, case studies dealing primarily with problematic issues are presented, followed by suggestions for turning negative reactions into more positive ones.

THE NEED FOR FAMILY
INVOLVEMENT IN THE VOCATIONAL PROCESS

As part of this continuum of preparatory stages, therapists and other rehabilitation professionals spend months and even years providing intervention designed to enhance the physical, cognitive, and behavioral skills that the person needs to return to the community and a job. Yet the vocational aspect of the rehabilitation process often remains shrouded in mystery, full of surprises, and least understood by the consumers (i.e., clients, families, referral sources), who often feel that their needs have not been adequately met. To a large extent, this reflects the failure of the rehabilitation system to involve the family in a process of gradually understanding the nature and implications of the newly imposed limitation on the person with the head injury (as well as the fact that families often go through a number of stages before they can integrate this information, which is discussed later in this chapter). If families were actively enlisted throughout the entire recuperative process, that is, exposed to (and offered explanations about) the person's strengths and weaknesses, they would be in a better position to accept more realistic vocational goals.

A range of factors are the basis of the family's expressed dissatisfaction with the goals and outcomes of this final phase of rehabilitation, not the least of which is the family's emotional inability to accept and support vocational planning that falls short of their family values and anticipated goals. Romano (1974), describing the early reactions of families of people with head injuries, found a process of prolonged family denial of disability particularly noteworthy. In many families this stage extends throughout the formal rehabilitation process, including return to work. The continual hope for total recovery presents barriers to readiness to set realistic vocational goals.

While much has been written in the 1970s and 1980s detailing the impact of traumatic brain injury on family systems (see Chapter 10), very little has appeared in the literature describing the impact of family systems on the process of reintegration for persons with head injuries. The burden on the family has been acknowledged, discussed, researched, and documented. Lezak (1978, 1986), Bond (1984), Brooks and McKinlay (1983), Mauss-Clum and Ryan (1981), and a host of others tend to be in agreement that behavioral dysfunction as a consequence of traumatic brain injury is most closely associated with the disruption of and loss of cohesion within family constellations.

Since the early 1980s, model rehabilitation programs have recognized the importance of including families in a formal way in the rehabilitation process. As far back as 1978, Ben-Yishay and colleagues (in their Head Trauma Program at New York University Medical Center), through their experience in Israel, included the requirement of family participation as part of their original research design (Ross et al., 1983). The important role played by the family throughout the initial and interim phases of recuperation is continually addressed by Lezak (1978). Family support as essential during the vocational rehabilitation process is noted by Rosenbaum, Lipsitz, Abraham, & Najenson (1978) in their description of rehabilitation services for a group of Israeli war veterans with head injuries.

While there is general acknowledgment of the importance of including families in the rehabilitation process, not all families produce positive influences during the vocational rehabilitation phase. Seldom addressed is the touchy issue of how to work productively with families who are pushing for unrealistic vocational goals, or who, because of conflict and lack of cohesiveness within their own system, are unable to carry out a plan of action that is conducive to optimal vocational outcome. One of the authors' primary purposes in this chapter is to present information, gathered experientially, on the impact of disrupted family systems on the vocational rehabilitation process, and how to work productively with these family systems. An appreciation of how the family contributes to rehabilitation of a person with head injury must be based upon knowledge of family dynamics, as well as an appreciation of the role that the family's value system plays in determining the response to projected vocational goals.

WORK AS A REFLECTION OF CULTURE AND FAMILY VALUES

Rehabilitation professionals can best understand the satisfaction or dissatisfaction expressed by people with head injuries and their families regarding vocational rehabilitation services and outcomes by asking the question, "What are your expectations?". The answer to this question often reveals a great deal of information about the family system, their needs, their values, their adjustment to and accommodation of the family member with a head injury, and their individual and collective resources.

The American work ethic connotes that the harder one works, the more one deserves, not only in terms of material goods and possessions, but in terms of respect as well. In other words, respect is something that is earned. The most common vehicle each of us has through which to earn respect is work. Overs (1975) concluded, "Most of us have been almost altogether indoctrinated by the work ethic, so that we continually interpret all data *solely* in terms of work careers. We are so subtly controlled by this thought structure that we frequently are not even aware of the limitations within which we operate" (p. 151).

Though not true in all societies, in American society work is most often the foundation of an individual's identity, within the community and within the immediate and extended family. One needs only to reflect on the opening conversation of people first meeting to realize the impact of this concept. The first or second question most often asked of new acquaintances is, "What do you do?" Identifying a person's work provides a general idea of how much one has in common with a new acquaintance. We can make fairly accurate assumptions about the individual's level of education, earnings, living environment, life-style and even leisure interests. For example, upon meeting both a physician and a grocery clerk at the same party, one would draw very different conclusions about each regarding these life-style aspects. Also one would be likely to make some decision about which of these individuals, if either, to become better acquainted with, either personally or professionally.

This "Who I am = What I do" (Price & Schmidt, 1987) attitude reflects the importance work holds for people in terms of addressing strong, deeply felt needs and values, and eliciting psychological protective mechanisms. It follows that work serves to justify one's value, identify one's worth in society. While the most obvious purpose of working is providing financial support, most individuals do not work for financial support alone, nor is this necessarily the biggest reason for choice of work. Rather, most individuals choose certain jobs because they fulfill certain needs and address values that the individual with his or her family have developed over a lifetime. Altruism, status, creativity, security, relationships with co-workers, and utilization of abilities are all examples of important components of job satisfaction. Each individual defines job satisfaction differently, depending on his or her unique set of talents, interests, and familial and cultural values. The larger the discrepancy between the individual's and family's value systems and vocational status, the greater the emotional conflict that will arise.

The part that family members play as role models in the process of adjustment to work is important to consider at all times. At one end of the spectrum are families determined to be productive and self-supporting (described as possessing a work ethic). At the other end are families with little or no investment in work as a way of life. These latter families may subtly (or more obviously) transfer their attitude toward work as non-essential and valueless to the member of their family who has a head injury. Certainly the person who comes from a family with firmly established work ethics is a better vocational rehabilitation candidate than the one whose family is not motivated to work. While professionals certainly should not judge the value systems of individual families, including those who place other rewards above the value of conventional work, it is of pragmatic importance to recognize the influence of such value systems on the person with the head injury and adjust vocational rehabilitation accordingly.

ABILITY OF VOCATIONAL SYSTEMS TO INTEGRATE FAMILIES

In spite of a somewhat vague acknowledgment by vocational specialists that the unique constellation of cultural values, personal values, attitudes, and priorities of families affects the vocational outcome of the person with a disability, historically there has been a passive resistance toward incorporating these elements into vocational programs and services. Several practical reasons exist for professionals' hesitancy to seek out and use ecological information in the vocational process. Traditionally, the vocational rehabilitation system emphasizes the right of the person with a disability to make life choices and maintain the dignity of risk; individuals are encouraged to take responsibility for their successes and failures. As with the clients of independent living agencies, the public vocational rehabilitation system's client's rights are ensured through federal and state mandated policies. Though collecting ecological information (i.e., actively seeking out relevant information from the person's home and community environment) does not necessarily infringe upon an individual's privacy, boundaries can be unclear, particularly to those whose job it is to advocate for the person. Consequently, vocational counselors may mistakenly feel the need to exclude family input from the vocational planning and placement process. Familial influence on the vocational development of persons with developmental disabilities may not be as dramatic as familial influence on individuals who have had regular vocational development patterns. Vocational counselors may not recognize the substantial difference vocational development patterns make in the vocational process because, in most public and private vocational rehabilitation agencies, vocational counselors are rarely assigned to work with a specific disability group. Rather they may carry a case load of individuals with a variety of disabilities, and as a rule most will be developmental or congenital in nature. Consequently, vocational counselors may not have enough awareness of or experience with persons with a particular disability to recognize and understand the impact or importance of including ecological and familial information in the development of a vocational preparation plan.

Another issue that is a practical consideration is job placement. The placement of persons with disabilities into the competitive job market is typically an arduous process. Job placement personnel conduct their search for available competitive jobs under a certain amount of pressure to produce a defined number of placements in a given amount of time. Often, the performance of job placement personnel is judged by the number of placements obtained. In a difficult job market with limited resources professionals may feel that considering another layer of confounding information, such as familial characteristics, which may further complicate the placement process, is unrealistic.

THE CHANGED VOCATIONAL STATUS OF A MEMBER: IMPACT ON FAMILY SYSTEMS

The ability of a family to come to terms with the inescapable effects on and changes within the family system has enormous implications for future adjustment. The position held and the role played by the person with head injury prior to injury must be one of the first considerations in vocational rehabilitation.

Vocational Status and the Income Provider

When the person with a head injury is the income provider, there is likely to be a loss of family income, economic stability, and perhaps a perceived and/or real loss of social status. This crisis will be more or less devastating depending on the number, ages, and social maturity of other family members. The need to arrive at a revised economy carries with it the need to change roles. One or more family members, including perhaps extended family members, may be forced to assume the role of the provider. Emotionally it is difficult for other family members to accept a change in the family authority figure, who may be the income provider. Often cultural and ethnic heritage not only contribute to the preparedness of another to take on the new role, but also contribute in a significant way to the emotional conflict that is likely to develop for the new provider. Commonly the family member who assumes responsibility for the financial support of the family is the same person who assumes the case manager/caretaker role for the family member with a head injury.

Vocational Status and the Homemaker

When the family member with a head injury is the homemaker, role revision again becomes the focus of the unanticipated transition. Duties must be assumed by other family members and responsibilities must be shared. Depending on the ages and levels of maturity of members of the family constellation, there may be the need to select a new and different homemaker/family caretaker. Often, identifying and incorporating a new and different homemaker leads not only to additional expense, but also to emotional conflict for all family members. Superficially, this role revision is probably the most easily accomplished initially, especially with the presence of helping others, including extended family, friends, and neighbors. However, with greater realization of the long-term consequences of the head injury, these helping others generally withdraw from the family (Lezak, 1978).

Vocational Status and Children

When the family member with a head injury is a child, parents are faced not only with the loss of dreams, but also with the eventual realization that lifelong caretaking may be necessary. The family has a significant investment in the career aspirations of a child with a head injury. Years of familial encouragement and financial planning support a child/young adult's involvement in activities such as supplementary courses, extracurricular activities, clubs, sports, and part-time jobs, which most often precede and influence choices of lifelong endeavors. With the realization of the long-term consequences of their child's head injury comes not only the loss of dreams, but also the task of considering how to provide technical, emotional, and financial support for their child for a lifetime.

CASE EXAMPLES OF THE IMPACT OF FAMILIAL RESPONSES ON VOCATIONAL ADJUSTMENT

Ideally, by the time individuals with head injuries approach vocational rehabilitation, they and their families should have developed a sense of the permanence of the limitations imposed by the injury. Unfortunately, this does not always happen. It has been well documented (Lezak, 1986; Romano, 1974) that families persist in viewing the changes they experience as transitory in nature. Too frequently rehabilitation practitioners *neglect* to provide information realistically in their tendency to avoid what would be painful to the family.

Families need help to develop an awareness of the permanence of the limitations of their member with a head injury; with this awareness they can be more realistic in their expectations. The direct result of professional neglect (i.e., lack of informed participation) is that the family continues to anticipate complete return of the person as he or she was pre-injury, and is unable to supply appropriate support.

Another origin of the attitude that the person with head injury will recover fully is the family's need to view the person as essentially the same loved, well-remembered, familiar individual. The fact that families continue to deny a family member's limitations or minimize the limitations' effects has been noted by Prigatano (1986). In spite of what is considered by many professionals as ongoing confrontation with limitations throughout the process of recuperation, it may be that, out of emotional self-protection, families need to continue this denial even into the final phases of rehabilitation.

If the gap between the reality of permanent disabling conditions and the families' ability to acknowledge them as such remains large, then it is incumbent upon rehabilitation professionals to examine carefully the content of the information they provide and the manner in which they convey it. Many persons providing care for individuals with head injury continue to give family members only helpful and kind messages. Well-intentioned, but seriously misguided, these people may provide platitudes meant to soothe that actually just fuel the family's hope for total recovery. This way the family is set up for disillusionment, which provides a serious impediment to the vocational rehabilitation process.

Transitions

Transitions, or life changes, are an inevitable and recurrent part of adulthood. Normal transitional events can be expected to alter familial roles, relationships, routines, and assumptions. Schlossberg (1987) characterized transitional events as those: 1) that can be anticipated and, therefore, planned; 2) the unanticipated transitions, those events that occur unexpectedly and often disrupt or drastically change established patterns of living; and 3) the nonevent transitions, that is, when expected events (such as marriage and having children) do not occur. The sudden shifts in roles, goals, and responsibilities that affect all family members after traumatic brain injury are certainly unanticipated transitions.

Case Example #1

Vocational goals that suggest a significant, permanent change in life-style or threaten an anticipated return to economic stability can create distressed reactions in family members. Spouses seem to be especially vulnerable to anxiety and depression. The greater the family members' dependency on the person with a head injury for economic sustenance, social status, or intrafamilial stability, the greater the likelihood of distressed reactions.

A Spouse's Adjustment   Sue is married to an almost tenured professor of business at a well-known university in the northeast. She became obviously disturbed when her husband Tom joined a vocational development group in the rehabilitation hospital. Tom was nearly 18 months post-injury, and his progress was quite slow. He had severe language impairments and needed a wheelchair for mobility. Sue increased the frequency of her visits from monthly to weekly. Each weekend after driving nearly 200 miles she would work with Tom practicing math, writing, and reading using materials from her elementary school classroom. Her complaints about therapies increased, and she requested that her husband be seen more often during the week. She reported to the vocational counselor that Tom would be able to return to the university on a part-time basis for awhile and felt that he could work on research rather than teach, for a semester or two. During the next 4 months Sue lost weight, appeared fatigued, and frequently complained of headaches.

Sue's inability to come to terms with the reality of her husband's diminished skill repertoire and the implications requires intervention by a responsive counselor skilled in gentle confrontation. The agitated behavior observed by staff members indicates some degree of realization (or readiness) on Sue's part. She has reached a crisis point in her life and it is crucial that her needs be addressed. So focused has she become on what she perceives as her husband's needs that she put aside her own personal issues. Though she has tried to push them aside, Sue's anxieties show themselves continually in the desperate quality of her efforts. Her attentions have actually become counterproductive for Tom.

Sue needs to be drawn into the rehabilitation process as an effective collaborator. She will be able to do this only following a period of intensive counseling, designed to lessen her fearful anticipation. The anxiety she has built centers around what she foresees as an impossible transition. Through counseling, she will have her feelings validated—the fear, the sense of foreboding are real and overwhelming; through the therapeutic process she will be able to place these feelings in perspective.

Case Example # 2

The *unanticipated* transition precipitated by traumatic head injury finds families ill-prepared to cope effectively in terms of both their own needs and those of the person with head injury. In response to their own emerging sense of despair (plans and hopes are dashed), and their emotional inability to acknowledge and accept limitations, families may adopt a pejorative view of the vocational rehabilitation process. A well-defined vocational rehabilitation plan, based upon observed limitations that cannot be denied, can be extremely threatening because it serves to remove all pretense. This process forces the ultimate painful confrontation with the reality of the implications of brain damage on the resumption of meaningful productivity.

Self-protective denial produces the difficult familial responses that vocational rehabilitation counselors must often deal with as they provide services for people with head injuries. Sometimes in response to efforts to realistically plan the approach to vocational reintegration, families declare suggested vocational rehabilitation goals unacceptable: "This is not what we had planned." They convince themselves that the professionals are wrong in their assessment and then search for other professionals, therapies, or programs that will share their point of view: the so-called "shopping around" syndrome. This pattern may be unwittingly fueled by well-intentioned professionals who continue to imply that they will be able to accomplish for the person what no one else has (which is not to deny the fact that some programs are simply more effective than others).

A Family's Readiness for Change   Robert, the 21-year-old son of a successful Connecticut attorney, was 12 months post-injury when he was referred for vocational services. Upon completion of a vocational evaluation, the rehabilitation counselor reported that Robert's skills indicated that he would most likely be successful in an occupation such as office clerk. The counselor also indicated that entering law school in the fall was unrealistic for Robert because he did not have the memory or problem-solving skills necessary to manage the rigorous curriculum. Shortly after first meeting with the rehabilitation counselor, Robert's family initiated his discharge from the facility stating that they had found another program that, "knew how to work with their son so that he could finish law school."

Despite the fact that the counselor may have been correct in evaluating Robert's vocational potential, the information presented was in complete disaccord with the family's plan for Robert to one day become a partner in the family-owned firm. Their inability to make at least some acknowledgment of their son's limitations and the impact on his career goals is more a reflection of their lack of preparation to receive and assimilate the information, than an inability to understand or be realistic about the situation. Pronouncements about work or educational potential that conflict with a long-held dream or goal often precipitate an emotional crisis for the family system.

The direct and confrontational style of reporting the results of the vocational assessment was not appropriate for Robert and his family. Part of effective vocational counseling is being able to deliver negative messages in a well-cushioned and hopeful fashion. Instead of consigning the young man to a lifetime of what his family of achievers viewed as menial service, the counselor would have done better to assess family needs and then pose the clerk position as a type of interim placement during which Robert could habituate himself to mnemonic devices to support his memory functions. Additionally, the family should have been told that Robert's poor problem-solving skills might prove responsive to environmentally imposed structure and counselor designed strategies, which could be put in place in an employment setting. The counselor could have immediately followed this information with the *suggestion* that perhaps it would be in Robert's best interest, at this point, to place return to school on hold.

It has been the authors' experience that, assuming a basic level of appropriate behavior, actual job placement lends itself over time to the acceptance of redesigned, more realistic goals. Certainly within the context of real work, both Robert and his family will be able to develop a better understanding of his limited skills and the impact on his aspirations.

STAGES IN THE PROCESS OF AWARENESS AND ACCEPTANCE

Some families maintain the view that any indication by the person with head injury of acceptance of disability is tantamount to giving up. They cling to the notion that determination alone (or sheer will) produces the desired results. This type of family assumes the role of a "cheering squad" and bombards the person with head injury with exhortations to keep up the good fight. In this way, without intent, they often sabotage vocational rehabilitation efforts. Awareness and acceptance, or at least acknowledgment of limitations imposed by the injury is fundamental to the vocational rehabilitation process (Ben-Yishay, Silver, Piasetsky, & Rattock, 1987). Persons with head injury are unable to become effectively engaged in vocational rehabilitation without acceptance of the support mechanisms (e.g., mnemonic devices, strategies for accomplishment) that they will require for adequate job performance, probably for the rest of their lives. This acceptance is based upon their ability to recognize (perhaps after persuasion by a trusted other) the need for these support systems. Even when family members are provided with the rationale that accompanies the introduction of compensatory mechanisms, some continue to view them as crutches and will continue to encourage the person with head injury to test his or her ability to perform without them. The differing messages from the professional and family are confusing to the person with head injury.

Lezak (1986) defines six stages in an evolutionary process of family awareness and acceptance. In Stage 1, the family member with injury returns home and the family experiences an almost euphoric period. In Stage 2 the family's optimism and energy begin to wane. During this stage growing uneasiness attests to the family's confusion and need for counseling. However, it is not until Stage 3 that families begin to entertain the thought that the effects of head injury may be permanent. It is during this 3rd stage that family conflict becomes especially evident. Stage 4 brings some recognition of the chronicity of their loved ones' limitations. The 5th stage is one of active mourning, during which the family is generally able to acknowledge that their member with a head injury will never totally recover from the injury. The 6th stage represents the point when families begin to disengage from the situation emotionally.

Denial

Many of the families that the authors see during the course of vocational rehabilitation appear to be stuck somewhere between Stages 3 and 4, or are, as

Romano (1974) described, in a prolonged phase of denial. This continuing need to resist the intrusion of reality, as represented by reduced vocational reintegration plans, leads families to align themselves almost oppositionally to the person with a head injury, against the messages of the vocational counselor. When the person with the head injury offers resistance to beginning the vocational rehabilitation process at an entry level in order to rebuild skills and ensure success, the family supports that resistance. People with head injuries have clear memory of how they performed before the injury. Many are reluctant to engage in what they view as boring or nonchallenging tasks. Families may support this attitude and offer idealized goals as alternatives and suggest that these are the only work areas in which the family member will feel productive.

This discussion of denial suggests an analogy to the stages of facing death and dying defined by Kubler-Ross (1969): denial, anger, bargaining, depression, and accommodation. While we are aware that a mechanical application of these stages to adjustment after head injury reduces the family's complex process of coping to a cookbook formula, we nevertheless believe that families pass through many of these stages in struggling to hold on to their identities. More important, an understanding of why families react as they do may be extremely helpful to professionals in working with families and facilitating their growth.

An experience (the shopping around syndrome) corresponding to the anger stage was discussed under Case Example #2. The following sections discuss analogies to the remaining stages of denial, bargaining, depression, and accommodation.

Bargaining

Bargaining is a stage of adjustment that vocational counselors must learn to manage, particularly when working in rehabilitation hospitals or other settings where the individual is living away from home. Frequently, this stage is initiated by the person with a head injury and centers around the individual's desire to terminate treatment because he or she feels ready to return to the previous life-style, including work. Often, this stage will occur when the individual has made substantial physical improvement such as regaining the ability to walk or talk. The individual feels that it is now time to be "rewarded" for his or her efforts and achievements in rehabilitation. Though the individual does recognize some limitations, he or she selectively denies and minimizes many others, especially those less tangible (i.e., organization, problem-solving, reasoning, safety, and personal judgment limitations) and those that are critical for community survival and employment adaptation.

Family members and rehabilitation team members, both of whom desire to see the individual function at a higher level and have an investment in that goal, can be drawn into the individual's convoluted thinking. Most frequently, family members will begin identifying idiosyncratic characteristics or skills the individual continues to possess. For example, "John was always good with people," or "Mary really has a way with children." Also, it is not uncommon for rehabilitation team members to begin identifying splintered skills that the individual has demonstrated in therapy. For example, "I asked Bob to determine how much the grocery bill would be and he was able to do this without the help of a calculator," or "Gene had no problem using tools to fix his roommate's wheelchair." The suggestion, subtly or more obviously implicit in these reports is that vocational counselors should find jobs that rely on these idiosyncratic or splintered skills. The unacknowledged dilemma of vocational counselors is that jobs do not exist that rely on only one or two splintered skills. Nor is there an abundance of benevolent employers, who are willing or can afford to reconstruct a job so the individual can do only those tasks that rely on one or two limited skills. Even if the vocational counselor were able to find that one perfect job, the individual would still need work readiness skills for punctuality, safety and personal judgment, self-monitoring, and communication and interpersonal relations to get along with co-workers and supervisors.

Placing an individual with a head injury in a job for which he or she does not possess the skills may cause embarrassment or ridicule at the job site or eventually cause the person to be ostracized. The risk to the individual is a loss of self-esteem, which may take much time to rebuild. Also, certain jobs could expose the individual to danger. In a dangerous environment, cognitive limitations, especially a vulnerability to distraction or reduced safety judgment, could result in an accident or injury. Another detrimental result of placing an individual on a job when he or she possesses only splintered skills is the possibility of a critical mistake costing the employer much time, effort, and/or money to correct, or an irreparable mistake. In the worst case the program or professional could be held liable for restitution; at the least, a valuable employment resource could be lost.

Vocational counselors will need to remain neutral if they are to be helpful in managing the delicate situations of families attempting bargaining. Helping the individual and family to put into perspective the progress that has been made is a good first step. Encouraging them to list the pros and cons to terminating rehabilitation or trying a job placement may be the next step. By assisting them with discussion, the counselor can facilitate movement toward acceptance of the situation, while maintaining an objective and supportive role. The counselor can also ask for the assistance of the individual, the family members, and the rest of the rehabilitation team in identifying jobs that demand the skills the individual currently possesses. The counselor may also begin preparing a list of jobs in which the individual may be successful with an expanded repertoire of skills. A list of potential job options can help all parties to refocus and remain hopeful when the reality of the market viability of splintered skills is recognized.

Depression

One of the major focuses of vocational rehabilitation is to determine how an individual's work skills compare with the industrial norm. In other words, how able is the individual with a disability to compete with nondisabled individuals for a position in the work place? While earlier phases of rehabilitation measure an individual's progress against his or her own previous functional levels (i.e., improved strength or endurance from last month, or improved ability in meal preparation from making only cold meals to microwave cooking), vocational rehabilitation must compare an individual's functioning with the demands of the work place. Though individuals may make marked improvement while participating in vocational programs, it is likely that these gains will not be substantial enough to make a real difference in the individual's ability to compete for a job. It is this measurable and quantifiable aspect of work and vocational rehabilitation that presents the stimulus that can trigger depression in both individuals with head injury and their family members. For the individual with a head injury the central issues are the loss of self-esteem that accompanies the loss of a career or unemployment, the lack of societal identity generally defined by one's work, and guilt created by reduced earning capacity and subsequent financial burden on the family. Family members may become depressed as they anticipate their own loss of independence as they realize their own future goals and plans will have to be readjusted to accommodate the caretaking needs of their family member with a head injury.

Vocational counselors need to use both supportive and exploratory counseling approaches with the depressed individual with a head injury and his or her family members. Counselors should help these individuals to examine and challenge some of their long held ideas about what aspirations one must have and what goals one must reach in order to be worthwhile. Counselors may also need to explore the individual's premorbid feelings and attitudes towards persons with disability. Frequently, these feelings will have been based on stereotypical ideas of disability being equated with helplessness and the sick/patient identity. Helping both the individual and family members to identify their feeling of losing control over their lives and assisting them in developing ways to regain control, including establishing worthwhile, contributing roles in the home and community, can diminish depressive reactions. Vocational counselors will also need to provide active listening support and confirmation as the individual and family members express their sadness about their losses.

Accommodation

For the individual with a head injury and his or her family members, the last stage of the adjustment process is marked when the dreams and possibilities of the past are put aside and their goals turn to, "Where do we go from here?". Even if reality dictates that competitive paid employment is not a likely option, individuals will demonstrate interest and motivation to explore other ways to create for themselves a niche that provides structure, meaning, and a sense of contribution to their lives.

The vocational rehabilitation process can be viewed and used by professionals not only as the culmination of a successful rehabilitation program, but as a psychotherapeutic tool to facilitate movement through stages of emotional adjustment. The skillful use of vocational tools and situations in the rehabilitation process should facilitate emotional adjustment to limitations resulting from head injury, while encouraging the use of practical accommodation strategies. If vocational counselors are to be successful in assisting individuals with head injury in becoming gainfully employed, they will need not only to focus on the desired outcome, but also to become knowledgeable and sensitive to the adjustment issues and process that must first occur. The adapted Kubler-Ross model (Kubler-Ross, 1969) is a conceptual framework counselors can use to become better prepared and more sensitive in responding to the adjustment needs of individuals with head injury and their families.

MOVING TOWARD RESOLUTION

Integrating the Family into the Vocational Process

Clearly, family involvement and participation in the rehabilitation process of individuals with head injury should not be considered an optional part of a program, or a program addendum, if professionals are to effect the best possible outcomes (Rosenthal et al., 1984). Just as the needs of individuals with head injuries are assessed, so should the needs of their family members be assessed, and education around their needs should be provided on a continuous basis. Family members need to be provided with explanations regarding the nature of the individual's injury, including organically-based limitations on the ability to function. If family members can be provided with clearly stated status reports throughout the rehabilitation process, it is very likely that a more collaborative effort between the professional team members, the individual with a head injury, and family members will evolve. Professionals need to develop their skills so that they can prepare family members for the rehabilitation outcome or prognosis with information that is well-timed, understandable, and helpful. As with any partnership, the collaboration of professionals, family members, and the individual with a head injury is based on honest communication, trust, and empathy.

One of the techniques that the authors (and others, see Rosenthal & Young, 1988) have successfully used in assessing a family's readiness to become engaged in the vocational reintegration process is a family interview. Bringing all family members together allows careful analysis of the family's values, strengths, and weaknesses, and individual capacities to become part of the supportive structure that the person with head injury will need. Much can be learned by observing family interactions and attitudes. In addition, a series of meetings affords the opportunity to reshape family dynamics in a way that may be conducive to the process of vocational rehabilitation.

Case Example

Mark is a 34-year-old man whose wife died in the accident in which he was injured. He was called in for a conference with his family. The family constellation consisted of the mother, who was a widow, and two sisters. Mark's mother sat next to him. One sister, younger and less involved, seated herself some distance from the other family members and remained there in spite of the counselor's invitation to sit closer. While Mark lived with his mother and this younger sister, it was the older sister who had assumed the role of case manager. Initially, she also sat next to Mark. A family history was taken, and after disagreeing with the mother's presentation, the older sister moved to a far corner of the room where she lit a cigarette; this in spite of (or perhaps as a result of) the fact that the mother had just finished with a description of how difficult her life had become, especially because she suffered from acute asthmatic attacks.

The dynamics seen in just the first few minutes of this family encounter provided the counselor with a fund of observational data. The older sister, as might be expected from her track record as case manager, proved most dependable in providing Mark with the support he required. With her help, Mark moved into his own independent living situation while he was still engaged in the vocational assessment process. This gave his mother a much needed respite (although she continued to complain), and from this distance Mark's appreciation of his mother's efforts on his behalf grew appreciably.

Suggested Approaches

Barrer (1988) developed a systems approach to working with families, which provides a framework with which to view family response as well as suggestions for family intervention. What follows is examples of levels of family participation and suggested strategies for maximizing even limited family engagement in the vocational rehabilitation process; these examples are gleaned from the authors' clinical experiences using the Barrer model.

The Involved and Supportive Family

The Involved and Supportive Family approaches the vocational process armed with a substantial knowledge of head injury, having availed themselves of the literature and current intervention methods, as well as documentation of each therapy and procedure in which their loved one has been involved since initial hospitalization. These are the case managers; they are advocates who have carefully researched what their family member needs, as well as what professionals are expected to provide. These families can be a tremendous resource and should be informed about goals and the assessments and measures used to determine rehabilitation goals. The difficulties that the Involved and Supportive Family experiences during the rehabilitation process relate to the intensity with which they have involved themselves. There is the potential for an overdependent individual and a family system that may align itself with their loved one's needs at the expense of their physical and psychological health, or that of others in the family constellation. Often, a by-product of this intensity is unrealistic expectations regarding vocational outcome. This creates a pressure that is draining for the individual with a head injury, who, during the vocational assessment, is confronted with concrete evidence of limitations and a reintroduction (or induction, depending on the individual's age at injury) to the demands and standards of the work world.

To relieve the pressure, for both the family members and the individual with a head injury, the following approach is recommended. Before beginning any vocational assessment, openly discuss the activity with the individual with a head injury and explain the rationale for each activity. After each activity, lay out for the person, verbally and in a written or graphic format, strengths and weaknesses demonstrated by his or her performance. If the individual is many years post-injury, information on limitations, though painful, may be a relief. The idea of not being able to return to school or work at the pre-injury level probably has been entertained but not verbalized by the individual before, especially to over-involved, encouraging family members. The technique of laying out information on limitations validates the individual's feelings. Armed with the knowledge of the vocational strengths he or she still possesses, the individual can begin to explore with the counselor other vocational options. Many individuals are uninformed about the wide range of occupations that exist and the various levels of jobs included in each occupational category. The process of vocational rehabilitation includes assisting an individual with a head injury in becoming aware of the vocational options and exploring and matching the skills needed for success at the person's current level of ability.

Concurrently, regular family meetings should be scheduled during which the counselor, in the presence of the individual with a head injury, discusses with the family that information already discussed with the individual. This type of meeting structure serves two purposes. First, it allows the individual with a head injury to be more in control since he or she already has the information that will be shared with the family members. Equally important is the fact that the individual with a head injury may feel not only supported, but perhaps even protected by the counselor when it is likely that the information discussed either is less positive or is a departure from what the person feels is anticipated by the family members. Again, it is critical that meetings of this nature be scheduled regularly throughout the evaluation and vocational process. Regularly scheduled meetings prevent the counselor from reporting that therapy is in progress that the family has had no time to come to understand, which could lead to a catastrophic reaction from the family. Regular meetings give the family time to understand and assimilate information piece by piece, so that they can come to a conclusion regarding appropriateness of the therapy that is similar to that of the vocational counselor and the individual with a head injury. It is important that as many members of the family as possible be present so everyone hears the same message. The individual who is ready should have the opportunity to explain to the family how he or she understands what is being discussed. It is also helpful to have an agenda. Prior to the initial meeting, the counselor should encourage the family to write down questions, concerns, and comments; the counselor and the individual should do this also. With the Involved and Supportive Family, the counselor may suggest ways the family can assist in the vocational exploration process. Contacting some of the local resources, tracking down names of key individuals in state agencies who may be helpful, even something as simple as obtaining a copy of their local telephone directory for the counselor, are all ways in which the energy of this type of family can be directed so that they are part of the team process. The counselor may suggest ways the family can obtain respite. Counselors should avoid an expert profile; rather they should stress that the vocational process continually tries to gauge to what degree the person can adequately self-manage and be independent, and that the family is an important source of information in making these determinations.

The Uninvolved and Supportive Family

The second category of family identified by the Barrer model is the Uninvolved and Supportive Family. This family keeps a distance from the vocational rehabilitation process. They do not interfere with intervention, nor do they ask questions. They seem to bestow implicit trust upon the professional. The vocational counselor may find it difficult to identify the family member to whom concerns should be directed. Professionals may even have the impression that they are working with the individual in a vacuum. The reasons a family is uninvolved are varied. For some it is because of financial or geographic constraints. For others it is other familial obligations. Some families are simply overwhelmed or exhausted. Uninvolved and Supportive Families relinquish the case management of their loved one to the professional.

The family who is uninvolved in the rehabilitation process may only serve to emphasize feelings of isolation from peers and community in the individual with a head injury. Rehabilitation recommendations and strategies (e.g., keeping a log book, which the individual uses during the assessment process) are usually not reinforced or carried over at home by the family. This type of reinforcement is key because, to make the transition from the structured environment of the program to a home or work situation, the individual must have the opportunity to become habituated to compensatory mechanisms by practicing them whenever possible.

Steps the counselor can take to maximize family involvement include establishing guidelines for communication. Ideally, regular meetings or telephone contact should be established. Unfortunately, the Uninvolved and Supportive Family tends to miss appointments. Excuses made are varied; typically family members are busy "putting out other fires" and will name a multitude of family, work, and health crises that keep interfering with their ability to address the concerns of their family member with a head injury. If it appears that regular meetings are not viable, the counselor should establish a written format for communicating the vocational process. It should be brief and concisely written, excluding all professional jargon. This report should be shared with the individual and can become a regular tool for providing feedback. The report should be sent to the family through the mail with the promise that a follow-up call will be coming to answer any questions. Through this process the counselor can identify a family contact who will serve as the major relayer of information.

The Involved and Unsupportive Family

The third category of family identified in the Barrer model is the Involved and Unsupportive Family. The most obvious characteristic of this family type is anger, which colors most if not all interactions with the rehabilitation professional. It is in this category that one encounters the "shopping around" syndrome. Usually this type of family takes their member with a head injury to many programs, with which they always find fault, being quite vocal about their dissatisfaction as they move on to the next program. Guilt is predominant among the many factors contributing to adoption of this approach.

These are the families that most often focus on the physical limitations of the individual, often ignoring or minimizing the behavioral and cognitive issues. It is common for the family to dismiss evidence of difficulties with assurances such as "he always had a bad temper," or "she was always forgetful." The rehabilitation of an individual with a head injury whose family is involved in this unsupportive way is fragmented. The individual's loyalties are divided between the family who loves him or her and insists they have the person's best interests at heart, and a series of brief involvements with programs or professionals, many of whom the individual also believes has his or her best interests in mind. When the individual enters the vocational rehabilitation process, he or she is usually physically and medically stable. It is not unusual for the family to take credit for both the medical recovery and the progress achieved through rehabilitation efforts. Typically, the family will attribute the individual's progress in recovery to their critical monitoring of rehabilitation and their efforts and willingness to change programs or professionals when they felt it was necessary. Upon embarking on the vocational rehabilitation process, the family may be very verbose in presenting their vocational expectations for their loved one. Often, the family's stated expectations are that their loved one return to work or school at a level that matches or exceeds the pre-injury level. The unstated message communicated is that if the program or professionals cannot accomplish this, the family will continue to seek "more competent treatment." These expectations are also communicated to the individual with a head injury. Frequently, the individual feels depressed or powerless, knowing that these expectations are unrealistic, but not knowing how to handle the situation without appearing to be a loser or ungrateful for the support the family has provided. Sometimes the individual may not be emotionally ready to engage in vocational activities that by nature are concrete and confrontational. These individuals demonstrate that they are unprepared by being unwilling to engage in any activity that they perceive as mental or too challenging, thereby avoiding substantiation of the worst fear of not being the same as he or she was pre-injury. Frequently, the result is that the efforts of the professional to establish a level of vocational skill are undermined.

The vocational counselor's best recourse is to establish a written, working contract with the individual with a head injury and his or her family. It must be stressed that it is in the individual's best interest that the rehabilitation process be approached in a systematic manner by a cohesive team. The contract must explain the expectations the workplace holds for all workers as well as the particular work goals established with the individual and family. For example, a basic rule of the workplace is that a worker should cooperate with co-workers and follow through with job performance without arguing. For an individual who tends to debate and argue, this workplace expectation can be translated into a specific goal that stresses more appropriate ways the individual can ask for clarification or more information about instructions. In working with the Involved and Unsupportive Family it is critical that the counselor not only acknowledge his or her vocational dream for the member with head injury, but also really take time to listen and understand the meaning of this dream. Under no circumstance should the counselor's view of vocational reality be forced on either the individual or the family members. Rather, the counselor needs to encourage both the individual and the family to focus their attentions on the basic, fundamental rules and expectations prerequisite for any productive activity. The counselor should provide ways and tools to help the individual draw his or her own conclusions about the reality of vocational dreams. The counselor should concurrently develop a counseling plan that guides both the individual and the family through a step-by-step discovery process, during which the counselor supports them with professional confirmation of their discovery; refocuses their attentions to strengths uncovered, while de-emphasizing limitations; and, perhaps most important, provides possible vocational alternatives that emphasize strengths and de-emphasize limitations.

The Uninvolved and Unsupportive Family

The fourth and final type of family identified in the Barrer model is the Uninvolved and Unsupportive Family. This category of family is characterized by detachment and rejection of responsibility in the rehabilitation of the individual with a head injury. While there can be many reasons family members may be uninvolved and unsupportive, two of the most common are a history of uninvolvement in the life of the individual prior to injury, and current litigation. In the case of an individual who was not particularly close with the family prior to injury, family members may demonstrate resentment toward the professional who now expects their involvement. Reasons for a history of minimal involvement or uninvolvement between the individual and family members may range from an argument or falling out to a longstanding familial interaction style. Though it might be helpful for the professional to understand the reasons family members are not willing to become involved, it is probably unrealistic to expect significant change. Sometimes a change in the relationship between the individual with a head injury and some or all of the family members will occur, but again, it is unlikely within the rehabilitation planning period.

Litigation is sometimes overemphasized as a barrier to vocational rehabilitation of persons with head injury; however, it can be a true cause of reticent family involvement. Family members are frequently unaware of the extensive time frames of and possibly limited financial gain by the litigation process. They do not always understand that the thousands and sometimes millions of dollars won through a lawsuit are quickly reduced by attorney's fees, trial and court expenses, and reimbursement of medical costs covered by the insurance company. They also do not always understand that the real cost of their financial gain is the time lost in postponing intervention at critical recovery periods. Most often families do understand that the litigation outcome and size of settlement is commensurate with the individual's level of disability and that level of disability is often defined by a formula based on premorbid earning capacity. Where litigation is involved, the family may truly believe they are acting in the individual's best interest by discouraging the vocational interests and ambitions of their loved one.

Regardless of the causes for a family's uninvolvement and lack of support of the individual with a head injury, it is unlikely that they will carry through with intervention efforts and recommendations made by professionals. Though it is unlikely that the family can be encouraged to become involved in vocational rehabilitation, vocational professionals nonetheless should communicate clearly and honestly the goals of the vocational rehabilitation process. Again, providing regular written reports detailing goals and progress, as described above, to the family, and attorney, if appropriate, is recommended if the family does not attend conferences, so that there is no surprise information for the family.

The families encountered by the vocational counselor will rarely fit neatly into one of the categories discussed above, but they may exhibit several of the characteristics noted, which may change as time goes on. For the vocational process to make any long-term impact on the individual with a head injury the valuable resources in the family must be included. In maximizing their contributions and the individual's investment in vocational rehabilitation, the key when working with any family system is open communication exchanged consistently and clearly.

SUMMARY

Head injury and return to work is truly a family matter. At no point in the rehabilitation process is it more important to consider, understand, and include cultural, familial, and ecological information in rehabilitation planning than when the individual with a head injury begins planning for return to work. Professionals can no longer afford to take a myopic view of vocational rehabilitation, focusing their energies only on the identification and placement of an individual in a job for the sole purpose of financial support. Experience has shown that not only is this an ineffective approach to achieving desired vocational outcomes, but physical, cognitive, and behavioral gains made in earlier phases of rehabilitation can be jeopardized when placements do not work. In order to effect the long-term and lifetime career success that individuals with head injury and their families need, professionals must provide vocational services that are more comprehensive. Professionals must become more skilled in identifying individual, familial, and systemic adjustment issues that affect vocational rehabilitation. Professionals must also become more sensitive and skilled in designing interventions that are helpful, timely, and culturally and ecologically appropriate. Vocational rehabilitation success for individuals with head injury will be commensurate with the degree to which professionals successfully involve and consider family members as a needed and valued part of the rehabilitation team.

REFERENCES

Barrer, A. (1988, August). *A systems approach to working with families.* Paper presented at the annual meeting of the American Psychological Association, Atlanta.

Ben-Yishay, Y., Silver, S. M., Piasetsky, E. B., & Rattock, J. (1987). Relationship between employability and vocational outcome after intensive holistic cognitive rehabilitation. *Journal of Head Trauma Rehabilitation* 2(1), 35–48.

Bond, M.R. (1984). The psychiatry of closed head injury. In D.N. Brooks (Ed.), *Closed head injury: Psychological, social, and family consequences* (pp. 148–178). Oxford: Oxford University Press.

Brooks, D.N., & McKinlay, W. (1983). Personality and behavioral change after severe blunt head injury—A relative's view. *Journal of Neurology, Neurosurgery and Psychiatry, 46,* 336–344.

Kubler-Ross, E. (1969). *On death and dying.* New York: MacMillan.

Lezak, M.D. (1978). Living with the characterologically altered brain injured patient. *Journal of Clinical Psychiatry, 39,* 592–598.

Lezak, M. (1986). Psychological implications of traumatic brain damage for the patient's family. *Rehabilitation Psychology, 31*(4), 241–250.

Mauss-Clum, N., & Ryan, M. (1981). Brain injury in the family. *Journal of Neurosurgical Nursing, 13,* 165–169.

Overs, R.P. (1980). Avocational exploration and work adjustment. In B. Bolton & D.W. Cook (Eds.), *The rehabilitation client* (p. 141). Baltimore: University Park Press.

Price, P.L., & Schmidt, N.D. (1987). *The vocational readiness manual for families: A home program for persons with head injuries.* Waltham: Massachusetts Head Injury Association.

Prigatano, G.R. (1986). *Neuropsychological rehabilitation after brain injury.* Baltimore: Johns Hopkins University Press.

Romano, M.D. (1974). Family response to traumatic head injury, *Scandinavian Journal of Rehabilitation Medicine, 6,* 1–4.

Rosenbaum, M., Lipsitz, N., Abraham, J., & Najenson, T. (1978). A description of an intensive treatment project for the rehabilitation of severely brain injured soldiers. *Scandinavian Journal of Rehabilitation Medicine, 10,* 1–6.

Rosenthal, M., & Muir, C. (1984). In M. Rosenthal, E. Griffith, M. Bond, & J. Miller (Eds.), *Rehabilitation of the head injured adult* (pp. 407–419). Philadelphia: F.A. Davis.

Rosenthal, M., & Young, T. (1988). Effective family intervention after traumatic brain injury: Theory and practice. Journal of Head Trauma Rehabilitation, *3*(4), 42–50.

Ross, B., Ben Yishay, Y., Lakin, P., Piasestsky, E., Rattok, J., & Diller, L. (1983). The role of family therapy in the treatment of the severely brain injured. *New York University Medical Center, Rehabilitation Monograph,* No. 66.

Schlossberg, N.K. (1987). Taking the mystery out of change. *Psychology Today, 21*(5), 74–75.

Silver, S.M., & Kay, T. (1989). Closed head injury: vocational assessment. In M. Lezak (Ed.), *Assessment of the behavioral consequences of head trauma* (pp. 171–194). New York: Alan R. Liss Publishers.

14

FAMILY AND
RETURN TO SCHOOL

RONALD C. SAVAGE
ROBERT R. CARTER

Each year in the United States as many as one million children sustain traumatic brain injuries (TBI) from motor vehicle accidents, falls, sports, and abuse (Bush, 1986). Approximately 165,000 of these youngsters will be hospitalized, with 16,000–20,000 having moderate to severe symptoms (Bush, 1986; Kalsbeek, McLaurin, & Harris, 1980; Rosen & Gerring, 1986). Unfortunately, many of these children with TBI are only seen by acute care specialists since the number of rehabilitation programs for children with TBI has not paralleled the dramatic increase in rehabilitation programs for adults from 1985 to 1990. However, many of these children will later experience transition problems when they return to school (Savage & Carter, 1984).

Parents face several critical overlapping problems when their child reenters the school system. They must resume the role of being their child's first and most important teacher, and they must assume the responsibility of becoming an advocate for their child. Typically, parents relinquish the "teacher role" once the child is established in school as an independent learner. To the parents of children who do not have disabilities the advocate role is one of little significance and rarely necessary. When a child has a head injury, returning to school may be considered an important milestone in the recovery process, and parents often mistakenly think their child is back to normal when he or she finally returns to school. However, parents who have experienced aggressive medical intervention in a hospital or rehabilitation facility may not be prepared for the passive attitude of school personnel. Parents are often caught up during this period with the need to acknowledge that what once was primarily a bio-physical problem is now being viewed as primarily a psycho-dynamic problem. The role of teacher and advocate now takes on more critical dimensions, and parents and families may find themselves revisiting the problems of coping and adjusting that they experienced in the early post-injury days. Unfortunately, fewer support services are available to parents and families during return to school. Many families confront, for the first time, the reality of the long-term nature of a traumatic brain injury.

In addition, school-age siblings of the child with TBI may see reentry as a disruption of the only part of their lives not yet touched by the stress of a traumatic injury on the family system. Inappropriate expectations for the injured child or his or her siblings can lead to increased familial tension (Slater & Rubenstein, 1987). Parents and rehabilitation personnel should keep all family members informed not only of the child's educational status, but of potential problems that may arise from cognitive and behavioral changes that may call negative attention to the child with TBI and his or her siblings. The resources of the educational systems must be mobilized by the parents acting in their capacity as the child's advocate.

Hospital and rehabilitation personnel should assist parents by helping them to identify, by title and function, all the professionals who should serve as part of an interdisciplinary team that could help them bridge the gap between the hospital services and the school system's services. To this end, the educational program must be a logical extension of the rehabilitation plan. Children with TBI and their families are best served when they are provided with a range of options. Schools must provide a continuum of services and individualized education program (IEP) based upon areas of concern and need. Assisting families in gaining access to these services is best done by providing them with clear information on their child's unmet needs and their rights and entitlements to having these needs met in the community and the school (NHIF, 1988).

School reentry is compounded by ongoing family adjustments to the traumatic brain injury. Family resources and strengths are tested during a severe crisis. Slater and Rubenstein (1987) found research reports showing that the worst periods of stress for relatives of children with traumatic injuries range from the months immediately following the accident to as long as a year after the accident. It is likely, therefore, that the family will approach school reentry at a point in time when they are least well prepared to engage in a complex and demanding process.

It is particularly important that parents be cognizant of the rights granted to handicapped children under Public Law 94-142, the Education for All Handicapped Children Act, 1975. Parents of students with TBI are somewhat unique in that their need for special education services is the result of a sudden, traumatic interruption of what had been a normal, generally uneventful school career. As previously stated, most parents feel that once their child returns to school, she or he is "safe and back to normal." However, the majority of children, especially those with moderate or severe traumatic brain injuries, will have quite the opposite experience. The student with TBI often returns to a school system that is unprepared for her or his needs and unfamiliar with the sequalae of traumatic brain injury. The conflict of the parents' relief that their child is out of the hospital and back to school and the school not knowing what to do with students with traumatic brain injuries presents a host of problems that can easily overwhelm both parents and school personnel. This chapter is written to help parents gain access to special education services for their children by providing guidelines they can use to contact school personnel, initiate and coordinate school/hospital visits, support in-service training for educators, design appropriate educational programs and related services, and secure follow-up service.

Successful transition of a child with TBI into the educational system should involve the following four steps:

1. Involvement of the school-based special education team in the rehabilitation setting
2. In-service training for all school-based staff who will have contact with the child
3. Short- and long-term program planning for the student's IEP and related services
4. Continued follow-up of the child by the rehabilitation facility and the school system

INVOLVEMENT OF THE SPECIAL EDUCATION TEAM

Schools are generally ideal places for continued cognitive and social rehabilitation of students with traumatic brain injuries. Schools on the whole are structured and organized mini-communities that provide a framework for successful learning and positive socialization. Schools contain different types of educational specialists (including classroom teachers, special educators, administrative and guidance personnel, speech and language teachers, physical educators, art/music teachers) who can serve the student through a coordinated team approach.

Most school systems will know when one of their students has been injured outside of school. Yet, few schools are kept informed about the status or progress of the injured child. Once the child is medically stable, the hospital should contact the child's school and inform the school that the child has left acute care and is now receiving rehabilitation services at home or in a specialized facility. Both the school and the hospital often assume that the parents will keep the school informed of the child's progress. However, with all the major stresses and changes resulting since the injury, parents often forget to keep the school notified; they are concentrating their energies on their child's physical recovery.

Next, parents are best advised to contact the Special Education Director for their school district. Some larger school districts may have a program designed specifically to meet the needs of hospitalized children or those who must remain at home. If this is the case, contact should be made with this program as early as possible. Parents need to keep in mind that hospitalized children or those who must remain at home are equally entitled to special education services.

In addition to the Special Education Director, the parents may also want to speak to the local school special education teacher and the school nurse. Both of these professionals are in direct everyday contact with the child's former teachers and will be able to share key information with them and eliminate misinformation about "a child with brain injury."

Besides knowing whom to contact, parents need to understand the parameters of PL 94-142. This law requires that a free and appropriate education be provided for all children regardless of the degree or nature of their handicapping condition. Parents need to be well versed in this law since they will not only be helping plan the student's educational program, but they also may be put in a position of advocating on behalf of their child. Following is a summary of the major issues addressed by PL 94-142 that parents need to know about:

1. Guaranteeing the availability of special education programming to handicapped children and youth who require it
2. Ensuring fairness and appropriateness in decision-making with regard to providing special education
3. Establishing clear management and auditing requirements and procedures regarding special education at all levels
4. Financially assisting the effort of state and local governments through the use of federal funds

The responsibilities of parents advocating for their children are based on the law, the school's role, and the rights of the child. To this end, the following principles must be considered:

1. *Zero Reject:* Simply put, the zero reject concept means that no child between the ages of 3 and 21, regardless of the nature of his/her handicapping condition, can be denied a free and appropriate public education.
2. *Nondiscriminatory Testing and Classification:* Testing procedures used by many school systems, while effective in diagnosing the unmet educational needs of children with learning impairments and disabilities, may not originally have been designed and/or normed to assess the learning

and behavioral styles of children with traumatic brain injuries. It is important that assessment and evaluation procedures be comprehensive and that those specialists administering such tests be acquainted with the unique needs of these children. Parents can and should insist on new or different approaches in testing, especially for neuropsychological and general cognitive assessment.

3. *Appropriate Individualized Education:* The intent of PL 94-142 is to clearly involve parents, teachers, administrators, and other necessary professionals as equal partners in the process of developing an individualized education program (IEP). Parents must be particularity concerned with the IEP (see list on p. 211) since it determines the appropriateness of the educational experience and spells out exactly what will be provided to the child.

4. *Least Restrictive Environment:* This legal mandate maintains that, to the maximum extent possible, handicapped students must be educated in the company of their nonhandicapped peers. This may sometimes work against children with TBI who need a very structured and monitored environment in order to make the best progress with minimal distractions. In some cases, it may also mean that the least restrictive environment is residential placement in a private school/facility with programs for students with TBI.

5. *Due Process:* While it is to be expected that in most instances school-parent partnerships will result in the appropriate placement and education of the child with TBI, parents must be ready to challenge decisions seen as being inappropriate or counterproductive to the child's development. Parents should ask schools for the due process procedures for their state and the local district prior to reentering the child (Carter & Savage, 1985).

After contacting the special education director, the school-based special educator, and school nurse, parents and the rehabilitation staff can invite these people to visit the hospital/facility, to observe the child, and to confer with the rehabilitation professionals. Not only does such practice provide the school professional with an opportunity to see the child and better understand the sequelae of traumatic brain injury, it also allows the rehabilitation staff a chance to show educators the various rehabilitation techniques, materials, and assessment instruments being utilized. This is also an excellent opportunity to clarify the terminology commonly used in medical facilities, which may not readily translate into educationally relevant language. All too often terms like cognitive rehabilitation, neuropsychology, subdural hematoma, and many others are foreign to education professionals, whose work has focused mainly on academic skills such as reading, mathematics, and content subjects.

Hence, a glossary of terms commonly used by rehabilitation professionals is an excellent resource for education personnel.

In addition to regular visits by the special educator and/or school nurse, the rehabilitation facility should make every effort to document through videotape the child's progress and the various cognitive activities used in the child's rehabilitation. This videotape will greatly benefit the classroom teacher later when the child is transitioned into school, since teachers do not see the child until many weeks after the injury and often do not realize the tremendous progress the child has made since then. The videotape provides the school with a series of taped reports from which the teacher gains a better sense of the cognitive processes disrupted by the brain injury and areas of need that still exist even though in a less prominent form.

It is also sound practice for the family and the rehabilitation team to visit the school prior to the child's reentry. By walking around the school and observing instructional areas, the family and rehabilitation professionals are able to spot potential problem areas that could interfere with the child's continued progress. Rehabilitation staff need to be aware of potential mobility problems for the child within the school's physical plant, classroom environments that may be overly stimulating, and instructional components that may need to be adapted to eliminate frustration for the child. For many children with TBI, fatigue is a major factor in cognitive recovery, and a student may need a place to rest during the day. These situations and others can best be recognized by those who have been working with the child since his or her injury.

IN-SERVICE TRAINING PRIOR TO REENTRY

Prior to the child reentering school, the rehabilitation team and the special educator or school nurse should conduct in-service training for all the teachers and school staff, including teacher aides, secretaries/clerks, student support services, and, when applicable, the child's peers. During training the rehabilitation team needs to carefully present not only information on traumatic brain injury and its effects on this particular child, but also an overview of how the brain works. In one survey it was found that only 5% of the special educators in a particular state had received any information on TBI in their undergraduate program and only 8% of the special educators had received information in their graduate studies (Savage, 1985). Therefore, TBI will be a new disability area for the majority of special educators and certainly for the general classroom teacher. In fact, many educators may even confuse the term "minimal brain dysfunction" (a precursor to the term "learning disability") with "traumatic brain injury," and rehabilitation professionals need to clarify the differences. It will also be beneficial for the teachers to receive a copy of the definition of traumatic brain injury as adopted by the National Head Injury Foundation.

Since few educators receive training on the brain and how the brain works, rehabilitation professionals need to conduct their training in such a way that educators can make the most of the information in a brief amount of in-service time. Teachers need to know how the brain processes information, some basic neuroanatomy, and what happens to the brain when it is injured. With this information, teachers will be better able to understand the effects of a traumatic brain injury on a child and be able to integrate what they know about how children learn.

In-service training is also an excellent opportunity to share the videotape that the hospital/facility has compiled on the child. Teachers will be able to see the progress the child has made to date and understand the instructional program recommendations made by the rehabilitation professionals. Carefully organized in-service training efforts will provide educational personnel with information on traumatic brain injury, and on the child and his or her family, which will provide for easier transition of the child from hospital/facility to school.

REENTRY AND IEP PLANNING

Transition is often mistakenly thought of as a 1-day activity. In fact, effective transition of the student with TBI into the mainstream of school may take several days, weeks, or months. The student most likely will need a comprehensive educational plan which will need continual adjustment and flexibility in order to best meet the student's needs.

Parents and rehabilitation professionals need to keep in mind three very important general questions in the transition process: 1) when is the child ready to reenter school-based programs, 2) where should the child initially be placed, and 3) what does an individualized education program include?

Six questions parents should ask the school include:

1. Do your personnel know what traumatic brain injury is?
2. What can my child do now?
3. What should my child do next?
4. What environmental or program changes does my child need?
5. Who should do "what" with my child?
6. How will I know that the program is working for my child?

As previously mentioned, many children reenter school without the teachers having a firm understanding of traumatic brain injury. Equally important, many children with TBI all too often are placed back into school before they are ready. Rehabilitation professionals have identified several factors that need to be considered before a child reenters school. To benefit from a school experience, students with TBI should be able to do the following (Cohen, Joyce, Rhoades, & Welks, 1985):

1. Attend to a task for 10–15 minutes.
2. Tolerate 20–30 minutes of general classroom stimulation (movement, distractions, noises).
3. Function within a group of two or more students.
4. Engage in some type of meaningful communication.
5. Follow simple directions.
6. Show evidence of learning potential.

Such factors greatly contribute to the success or failure of the transition process. In addition, the initial placement of the student needs to be carefully considered by the parents, the rehabilitation professionals, and the school-based special educator. The student with TBI may be placed initially in one of the following education options:

1. Regular class placement with no direct or indirect special education services
2. Regular class placement with a range of support services including special education consultation, cognitive rehabilitation, speech and language therapy, occupational therapy, physical therapy, adaptive physical education, psychological counseling, and tutoring in reading or mathematics
3. Resource room services
4. Self-contained classes
5. Residential programs

The educational placement decision must be based on the strengths and needs of each student, and as these needs change the placement of the child must also change. Students with TBI often make rapid gains at the beginning of their recovery and will need to have their placements in the school reevaluated more often than other special needs students. Of course it would be preferable for each child to return to his or her original peer group. However, after being in a hospital environment for several weeks or months, the challenge of returning to an academic program would be difficult for the best of students. Hence, the initial placement and subsequent reevaluation constitute a major component in successful transition.

Paramount to the educational welfare of students with TBI is the specific, focused, nondiscriminatory assessment of the child's strengths and needs. Experience has shown that test results may be used to classify children for educational purposes on the assumption that labeling children is a necessary part of the administration and organization of work done with special needs students. While some administrative need for labeling may exist, the process may be problematic for students with TBI since there is at present no discrete category of education disability that best fits traumatic brain injury. In the absence of such a category, these student are often assigned to a category of convenience such as having mental retardation (MR), learning disabilities

(LD), emotional disturbance (ED), health impairments (HI), developmental disabilities (DD), and so forth. Parents need to understand that placement decisions based on reasons other than individual needs are contrary to both the letter and spirit of the law (Carter & Savage, 1985). The use of the definition of traumatic brain injury adopted by the National Head Injury Foundation provides schools with a "categorical labeling" of the student with TBI without the risk of mislabeling for administrative convenience.

Another area of concern for parents is not knowing exactly what an IEP should comprise. The child's IEP is essentially the contract between the parents and the school for services to be rendered. In this sense, the parents are the consumer and the IEP is not acceptable until they agree to its contents, specifically the educational goals and objectives it sets forth. Thus, when advocating for their child, parents may find they need to consult with rehabilitation professionals before agreeing to and signing off on the IEP. Following is a list of the major features the IEP is required to incorporate:

1. The child's present level of educational performance
2. Yearly goals and short-term objectives
3. The specific special education services to be provided
4. The extent to which the child will participate in the regular classroom programs
5. The projected dates for beginning such special services
6. The evaluation procedures to be used to measure the child's progress
7. A schedule to determine if the child is achieving the IEP objectives, including an annual evaluation of the program and revision as necessary

Generally, the IEP team will consist of the parents, school personnel, and the child when appropriate. In addition, the parents may wish to recommend the names of other professionals to the team. Depending on the age of the child, a representative from the Department of Vocational Rehabilitation (VR) may need to be assigned to the child. The cooperative agreements being worked out between individual state head injury foundations and departments of vocational rehabilitation allow students at any age to be referred to VR services for monitoring. Students who will be leaving secondary school and continuing into employment or postsecondary training need to have a VR counselor assigned as soon as possible to ensure successful transition between school and community.

The initial IEP for the student with TBI should be written for a short term (4–6 weeks). Often, for other special needs students the IEP is written to cover an extended period of time such as 6 months or longer. Some states provide for the development of multi-year plans for some special needs students. Regardless of the time frame, IEPs must be reviewed at least once a year. Since the child with TBI often makes rapid gains in the first year following the brain injury, it is important that the IEP be flexible enough not to restrict the changing needs of the child. Also, schools often make the mistake of writing the objectives for the IEP in academic areas only rather than focusing upon cognitive processes and thinking skills. In the case of one student, the IEP initially written by the school focused on having the student make up all the academic work she had missed while she was in coma for 6 weeks. This IEP did not focus on the child's needs; it focused on the school's needs instead. Parents will need support from rehabilitation personnel to make sure the IEP meets the guidelines set forth by PL 94-142, and that the IEP is focused on the cognitive processes the child needs to work on as part of the rehabilitation plan, rather than merely on the academic work the child has missed.

FOLLOW-UP

It is important for parents to note that the case should not be closed by the members of the rehabilitation team when the IEP and/or the vocational re-habilitation plan is finalized. The rehabilitation team and the school system should identify liaison persons who will continue to work cooperatively until both the rehabilitation facility and the school agree that the transition is complete. It may be practical, for example, to consider utilizing the physical or occupational therapists from both the school district and the rehabilitation program since these are common interdisciplinary professionals.

Providing an appropriate education for children with TBI requires a tremendous amount of teamwork. Specific guidelines and practices vary throughout the nation and in some instances throughout a given state; how-ever, it is required in every jurisdiction that planning and placement decisions be team decisions. The advantages of the multidisciplinary team are apparent, and every effort should be made towards increasing the effectiveness of this approach. By utilization of the expertise of the rehabilitation professionals, the educational specialists, the families, and, where appropriate, the student, the unique needs of the child with TBI can be met more readily.

RECOMMENDATIONS

Following is a list of specific recommendations for the family in educational planning:

1. The student with TBI needs a place to check into and check out of each school day. Frequently, the special educator or guidance counselor is best able to help the student get organized before the beginning of each day and to make sure the student has everything needed before leaving school. The key is to set up an organizational structure before the student becomes confused or overwhelmed. This will provide the family with a sense of security.

2. Test scores, both on standardized and teacher made tests, do not

necessarily provide accurate measurements of how well or how poorly a student is performing. While standardized tests provide valuable information on how the child is receiving, processing, and utilizing information, test scores per se (grade equivalents, stanines, percentiles, standard scores) can place the child above or below actual level of functioning. Caution is required in the interpretation of such test scores and in communicating test results to families.

3.   The physical layout of the school must be carefully considered. The student placed in an "open concept" school may have attention and concentration problems compounded by the additional distractions possible in such an environment. In addition, students with problems negotiating spatially may have difficulty trying to find their way around the classroom or school.

4.   Personnel must be aware that increased visual and auditory distractions at recess, lunch, and in the hallway may confuse the student and cause self-monitoring problems when the student is not aware of sensory misinformation he or she is receiving and of subsequent inappropriate behaviors he or she may exhibit.

5.   Students reentering school may need schedule adjustments or an abbreviated school day in order to allow for fatigue or therapies (physical/occupational therapy) necessary outside of the school itself. Many students need a time-out period during the day to allow for rest periods or opportunities for the child to work with a particular educational specialist.

6.   The student should keep a daily journal of activities to which he or she can continually refer whenever necessary. Teachers and parents should check and review the journal frequently to make sure the student is organizing and keeping track of assignments, appointments, and activities. The journal can be used for three-way communication among teachers, parents, and students.

7.   Every effort should be made to educate the student's peers about traumatic brain injury, especially at the upper grade levels. Socialization for the adolescent is compounded by the traumatic brain injury. If the student's peers are aware of what their friend and his or her family are going through, they can be an asset in rebuilding appropriate social and behavioral skills.

8.   Lack of initiative and motivation and difficulty with planning frequently accompany a traumatic brain injury. Teachers need to reinforce the student constantly and help the student to concentrate on success rather than failure.

9.   Flexibility in classroom work and differentiated assignments will help the student rebuild the cognitive processes necessary to experience success independently. Teachers should present new information in such a way that the student uses all the sensory modalities and teachers should call upon the student's prior knowledge when introducing new information.

10.   The family should be kept informed and be an integral part of the education team. Educators need to share with families the techniques and strategies that they have found successful when working with the student.

CONSIDERATIONS

Following is a list of considerations for educational planning:

1.   The transition from hospital/rehabilitation facility to the school requires involvement of the family and personnel from both institutions. Representatives from the medical arena and educators from the school system need to meet prior to the student's reentry to the educational environment. Information about the student must be shared and recommendations need to be made in order to ensure proper transition of services.

2.   Teachers and staff in the school need in-service training about traumatic brain injury and all its ramifications. Literature and videotape materials that focus on the special problems and needs of students with TBI are available from the National Head Injury Foundation.

3.   The school needs a team approach in order for the student to best continue recovery. Parents, regular classroom teachers, the special educators, the guidance counselor, the reading and art and music teachers, the school nurse, and administrators must be involved. Traumatic brain injury is too complicated for one individual teacher to address, and the splintering of instruction without integration causes additional confusion for the student. Thus, a multidisciplinary approach is necessary for continued recovery.

4.   The needs of the student must be carefully considered in all domains—cognitive, psycho-motor, and social/behavioral. The student's problems may be pervasive and complicated, and rehabilitation for each problem should be integrated with rehabilitation for all the others.

5.   The student should be placed in an educational service category that is appropriate. Students with traumatic brain injury do not have mental retardation, learning disabilities, or emotional disturbances. Placement into special programs designed exclusively for students with these conditions may not meet the special needs of students with TBI and may even further hinder their recovery.

6.   Programs for students with TBI need to concentrate on cognitive processes as academic skills are learned. Focus should be made on the interaction between the teacher and the student; the material is not as important as the evidence of the student's attempt to learn.

While the needs of children with traumatic brain injury are often extraordinary and the ability of educational systems to meet these needs often underdeveloped, parents can gain access to and coordinate programs that will enable continued recovery for the child. In order to accomplish educational goals, parents must understand the complexities of the special education laws and be committed to helping educators better understand the effects of traumatic brain injury. The issues and ideas presented in this chapter are a first step in developing a truly interdisciplinary network that will ensure that children with TBI are not lost between the cracks that presently exist between schools and hospitals.

REFERENCES

Bush, G. (1986). *Coma to community*. Paper presented at the Santa Clara Conference of Traumatic Head Injury. Available from Southborough, MA: National Head Injury Foundation, Inc.
Carter, R., & Savage, R. (1985). Education and the traumatically brain injured: Rights, protections, and responsibilities. *Cognitive Rehabilitation, 3*(5), 14–17.
Cohen, S., Joyce, C., Rhoades, K., & Welks, D. (1985). Educational programming for head injured students. In M. Ylvisaker (Ed.), *Head injury rehabilitation: Children and adolescents* (pp. 383–409). San Diego: College-Hill.
Kalsbeek, W., McLaurin, R., & Harris, B. (1980). The national head and spinal cord injury survey: Major findings. *Journal of Neurosurgery, 53*, 19–31.
National Head Injury Foundation Task Force on Special Education. (1988). *An educator's manual: What educators need to know about students with traumatic brain injury*. Southborough, MA: National Head Injury Foundation.
Rosen, C., & Gerring, J. (1986). *Head trauma: Educational reintegration*. San Diego: College-Hill.
Savage, R. (1985). *A survey of traumatically brain injured children within school-based special education programs*. Available from the Head Injury/Stroke Independence Project, Rutland, VT.
Savage, R.C. (1987). Educational issues for the head injured adolescent and young adult. *The Journal of Head Trauma Rehabilitation, 2*(1), 1–10.
Savage, R.C., & Carter, R.R. (1984). Re-entry: The head injured student returns to school. *Cognitive Rehabilitation, 2*(6), 28–33.
Slater, E.J., & Rubenstein, E. (1987). Family coping with trauma in adolescents. *Psychiatric Annals, 17*(12), 786–790.

OTHER READINGS

Begali, V. (1987). *Head injury in children and adolescents: Resource and review for schools and allied professionals*. Brandon, VT: Clinical Psychology Publishing.
Boll, T. (1983). Minor head injury in children. *Journal of Clinical Child Psychology, 12*(1), 74–80.
Boll, T. (1983). *Minor head injury in children: Out of sight but not out of mind*. Southborough, MA: National Head Injury Foundation.
Boyce, B.B., & Gaspard, N.J. (1986). *Effects of major and minor head injury in children*. Southborough, MA: National Head Injury Foundation.
Burns, P.G., & Gianutsos, R. (1987). Re-entry of the head-injured survivor into the educational system: First steps. *Journal of Community Health Nursing, 4*(3), 145–152.
Carberry, H. (1985). Psychological methods for helping the adolescent rehabilitation patient. *Cognitive Rehabilitation, 3*(2), 24–25.

Cook, J. (Ed.). (1986). *The ABI handbook: Serving students with aquired brain injury.* Thousand Oaks, CA: Consortium for the Study of Programs for the Brain Injured in California Community Colleges.

Deaton, A.V. (1987). Pediatric head trauma: A guide for families. New Kent, VA: Healthcare International, Inc. (Cumberland Hospital).

Hock, R. (1984). The rehabilitation of a child with a traumatic brain injury. Springfield, IL: Charles C Thomas.

Jaffe, K.M. (Ed.). Pediatric head injury. *The Journal of Head Trauma Rehabilitation, 1*(4).

Mehanes, F. (1985). *A child's courage, A doctor's devotion.* Southborough, MA: National Head Injury Foundation.

Savage, R.C., & Allen, M.G. (1987). Educational issues for the traumatically brain injured early adolescent. *Teaching Early Adolescents Magazine, 1*(4), 23–27.

Shapiro, K. (1985). *Head injury in children.* Southborough, MA: National Head Injury Foundation.

Ylvisaker, M. (Ed.). (1985). *Head injury rehabilitation: Children and adolescents.* San Diego: College-Hill.

IV

SPECIAL
ISSUES FOR FAMILIES

Section IV presents specific issues that are encountered by families after a person experiences a head injury. The effect of culture, child development, behavioral issues, and sexuality issues on the family and its support system are important aspects of the individual's and the family's experience that cannot be overlooked at any given time. Specific situations are presented to exemplify the importance of each issue in a family's life.

✓ 15

FAMILY, CULTURE, AND CHILD DEVELOPMENT

JANET M. WILLIAMS
RONALD C. SAVAGE

The family has the greatest influence on how children grow up and become adults (Lidz, 1976). The influence is evident in how families make decisions and translate those decisions into action. Often, the decisions are based upon ethnic and cultural values and beliefs. While the values may not be evident every time a family makes a decision, they are present nonetheless.

To understand child development and the experience of head injury, it is also important to understand family development and the experience of head injury. The effect of the head injury on the child, the ethnic background of the family, and the family life cycle are three important components of understanding the future implications of a head injury on the entire family that includes a child as one of its members.

CHILD DEVELOPMENT, ETHNICITY, AND THE FAMILY LIFE CYCLE

Critical aspects of child development are divided into phases commonly referred to as infancy, toddlerhood, preschool, school age, adolescence, and young adulthood (Lidz, 1976). The tasks of development are not clearly demarcated by when one phase ends and another begins, but the overall schema allows one to understand the process of growing through childhood into adulthood.

Presenting information about ethnicity is difficult at best. Trying to identify ethnic trends may create simplified pictures of a culture, and one runs the risk of presenting stereotypes. This chapter in no way attempts to stereotype ethnic groups. Its purpose is to sensitize people to ethnic trends that may affect the ways in which families react to the intervention for a child with a head injury.

The cultural background of a family encompasses many different components, including socioeconomic status, geographic location, and religion (Turnbull & Turnbull, 1986). Ethnicity is also a major component and can influence all other factors. Ethnicity is commonly handed from generation to generation through the family and is reinforced by the interpretation of the family and the surrounding community (McGoldrick, 1982a). Different values that a family draws from their ethnic background are important in interpreting how the family understands a member's head injury and the goals that the family aims to achieve. Ethnicity can also influence how a family grows and develops through the life cycle.

The family life cycle comprises the tasks a family achieves in their development through time. As with the development of a child, the development of a family is difficult to categorize. The stages of newly married couple, the family with young children, the family with adolescents, and the family with children launching and moving on are useful in understanding general life cycle theory (McGoldrick & Carter, 1982). Each family life cycle stage is affected if a member of the family experiences a head injury. For some families, a life cycle stage may be prolonged as in the case of a person who experiences a head injury and continues in childlike dependence on the family for prolonged periods of time. For the independent young adult, the event of head injury may cause a return to a previously mastered life cycle stage. For parents, when a child experiences severe head injury at any age, the life cycle stage of launching and moving on may never be realized.

This chapter gives a broad overview of child development, ethnicity, and the family life cycle. A family situation is presented for each of the child development stages: infancy, toddlerhood, preschool age, school age, adolescence, and young adulthood. Each situation is discussed in light of child development, the ethnic background of the family, and the current life cycle stage of the family. Future implications for the child and family are drawn based upon information presented.

INFANCY

Sharon and Bob Ward have been married 8 years and decided after 5 years to have a child. Six months ago, their now 12-month-old son Peter was dropped and fell down a flight of stairs while in daycare. He experienced a severe head injury and did not respond to anyone for an entire month. After 6 months, Peter still needs a tracheostomy to allow him to breathe and a gastrostomy tube in his stomach for feeding.

Both parents are from upper-middle-class, Protestant, white families and were raised with very high expectations of themselves and others. Sharon is a successful real estate investor and Bob a successful tax attorney. They live on the West Coast and their parents live on the East Coast. Sharon's younger sister is the only family member who lives near them. They talk to their parents every week and try to make it home at least twice a year. When they were married at 28, there was no question that they would wait to have children because they wanted to be sure that their children could have all that they had growing up.

When Peter was 3 months old, Sharon returned to work full time. She had chosen the daycare center based upon a friend's recommendation and the location; it was around the corner from her office, and she was sometimes able to stop by and see Peter during the day. She really liked the people and was especially pleased that it had a homelike environment. Peter had been going to daycare for 3 months when the accident occurred. Sharon was devastated when the hospital called to tell her what had happened. She and Bob had felt that they had all that they could want and suddenly it was all taken away.

Sharon's mother came and stayed with them for the first month but had to return home before Peter started to respond to them. All of Peter's grandparents have taken turns being with the family since the accident. He was in intensive care for 2 months and was then moved to the children's unit. The family is beginning to think about where Peter will go next. The medical staff have recommended a rehabilitation program 100 miles from their home, and their family is urging Sharon and Bob to take him home.

Traditional Developmental Milestone

Prior to his injury, Peter was a normally developing infant. He could stand when holding on to an object or person for support and he was beginning to pull himself to a standing position. He was feeding normally and able to drink from a cup held by an adult. His parents said that Peter understood his name, could shake his head "no," and waved "bye-bye." Since his brain injury involved the frontal-parietal lobes and the motor strip, the therapists on the children's unit were working with him on basic psycho-motor skills and prespeech activities. However, Peter will need extensive rehabilitation and long-term therapy in order to redevelop past skills and to ensure the continuity in new skill development. Of particular concern is whether Peter can be cared for at home and through outpatient therapy or if he should be admitted to a rehabilitation hospital.

Severity of Injury and Effect on Milestone

Many infants who sustain brain injuries as severe as Peter's generally need intensive rehabilitation. It is also not unusual for such infants to recover fairly rapidly after their injury, only to display additional problems with cognition and behavior when they reach age 2. Such problems often continue and even become worse as the child is called upon to use more of his or her brain and enters the school system. In addition, children who must receive extensive rehabilitation in specialized hospitals a long way from home often are unable to see their parent(s) frequently. Thus, some of these children experience serious psychological problems associated with being uprooted from their family, and these problems can be exacerbated by their head injuries.

Ethnicity

The values of white, Anglo-Saxon Protestants have been characterized as emphasizing self-reliance, self-control, achievement, and self-determinism (McGoldrick, 1982b). Sharon and Bob could certainly be considered to hold these values. Both are college educated and followed their predicted career paths to reach the point of success. Like their parents, they had dreams of successful, independent children. They were proud to have a first-born son to follow in their footsteps. Now, they see that the previous dreams they had for Peter may not be realized, and they have begun to focus their goals on maximum independence for Peter. Most of the rehabilitation professionals working with the Wards have the same goal of independence for Peter, stressing the need for intensive rehabilitation.

Family Life Cycle

Sharon and Bob successfully negotiated the task of joining two families through marriage and waited 5 years before they faced the next life cycle transition of having children. The transition of adjusting to a young child in the family was relatively easy, and parenting roles were established early on. Since both parents were working, household chores and responsibility for Peter were shared equally. Sharon and Bob had adjusted their marital system to make room for Peter and had taken on their parenting roles with excitement. In addition, both sets of grandparents doted over Peter, celebrating each developmental milestone he reached.

While in the hospital, both parents spent as much time as possible with Peter, taking all of the time they could away from work. They spoke with their parents daily on the telephone. Peter would have a prolonged infancy and they had to shift their parenting roles once again. They began to wonder about the impact that caring for a child with a disability would have on their careers and future plans to have more children. Since their parents lived so far away, Sharon and Bob could look to them for emotional support, but could not receive assistance with caregiving.

Future Implications

The goals for Peter present a dilemma for the family and the rehabilitation team who both share many of the same values and expectations. Should the family push for the independence they so greatly value at the expense of uprooting Peter from his home and familiar surroundings? Would intensive rehabilitation away from home leading to greater independence outweigh the possible psychological consequences? Could they set up a rehabilitation program at home, meaning that one parent would give up employment?

With a decision to be made about Peter's future care, Sharon and Bob also need to make some crucial decisions about their current roles and decide how to handle the next life cycle stage they will face. If Peter goes to rehabilitation, can they continue to have flexible hours at work? They know that Peter will eventually come home, and they need to make decisions about whether Sharon or Bob will give up employment to care for him. Sharon thought of quitting her job, as so many women do when caring for a family member with a disability, but she can see that Peter needs more therapy, and the loss of an income presents a difficult choice.

TODDLERHOOD

The Ruocco family has three children with a fourth on the way. Tina Ruocco is the third child and only daughter of Sonny and Mary Ruocco. Her brothers Tony and Sam are 6 and 8 respectively. When Tina was 2½ she and her brother were playing in the yard with their father. Tina wandered into the street as their father was retrieving the ball during a game of whiffle ball. She was hit by a car and thrown about 30 feet. Along with several broken bones, Tina experienced a head injury. Her 3 months in coma seemed endless to the family, who maintained a vigil at her bedside. Sonny felt responsible for the accident and prayed that she would be alright. The time Tina's parents spent at the hospital limited time with the boys. There was no question about who would care for the boys because there is a large extended family, and both sets of grandparents lived nearby.

Before Tina's accident, the Ruocco family lived in what they referred to as constant happy turmoil. Both Sonny and Mary are from large Italian families, and all of their siblings live within 10 minutes of their house in an Italian section of an eastern city. Both sets of parents live on the same street. There was never a time that someone was not visiting. In their family, children are allowed to be free of responsibility until they are 10, and then they are expected to take on responsibility around the house. Chores have always been divided strictly by traditional gender roles. Most of the family gatherings are social events centered around food and meals. Every Sunday afternoon one of Sonny's or Mary's sisters or brothers has all of the families over to their house for Sunday dinner.

Three years ago Sonny and two of his brothers started their own construction business. They had all been union carpenters, knew their trade, and decided to work for themselves. Business was good, mostly because they relied on their extensive network of friends and family for contacts. Within a year everyone wanted the Ruocco brothers to work on their additions or build their porches. Because it took some time to build up equity in the business, they had not been able to get large health insurance policies. As the Ruocco's learned, you never know what you really need until you need it.

Four months after the accident, Tina was recognizing her family and was beginning to take trips home on Sunday to the big family gatherings. The rehabilitation team told the family that she would be overstimulated by the number of people at the gatherings, but Tina seemed to love the attention and the family loved having her there. She had not started talking again and could not walk, but the family thought she seemed to understand what they were saying to her. She still lives at the hospital and spends most of her day in rehabilitation. The family is beginning to ask about the possibility of having Tina live at home and travel to rehabilitation each day for therapy. They would love to celebrate her 3rd birthday with a coming home party.

Traditional Developmental Milestone

At the time of her injury, Tina was a precocious toddler who had always tried to keep up with her brothers. Tina could kick and throw a ball, pedal her bicycle, name the major parts of her body, count to 20, and was always talking a "mile a minute." After she began to emerge from coma, Tina's behaviors were very infantile, and she was overwhelmed if more than one unfamiliar person was with her at a time. She seemed to be able to tolerate several family members at one time. Tina's injury was massive and diffuse, she had experienced several seizures in the hospital, and she had a shunt placed in her brain to reduce fluid build up and reduce brain swelling. Magnetic Resonance Imaging (MRI) scans showed a great deal of injury in her left frontal-temporal lobes. Tina has not tried to vocalize at all, but she sometimes nods approval or disapproval. Her parents are concerned that Tina will remain a baby and never be able to walk or talk again.

Severity of Injury and Effect on Milestone

Because Tina's injury is so diffuse, her problems with language and movement seem to be compounded by her inability to filter extraneous information and her growing problems with spatial confusion. These behaviors are further complicated by Tina's extensive stay in a hospital and the amount of fatigue she experiences as a result of her head injury. Her therapists are concerned that as Tina develops she will need very structured and organized home and, eventually, school environments in order to continue rehabilitation and be successful. More than likely, Tina will continue to have language problems for a long time. Delays in speech and language will hinder her ability to learn to read, and spatial problems could inhibit her learning of mathematics. In addition, she will require outpatient physical and occupational therapy.

Ethnicity

In Italian culture the family is seen as one's greatest resource and protection against all troubles (Rotunno & McGoldrick, 1982). Education and advanced training are seen as secondary to the security, affection, and sense of relatedness found in the family. Identity has more to do with a person's affiliation to family than with one's occupation or personal success. The network of significant others is often large, with extended family often residing in geographic proximity. The Ruocco family is so characterized and is very proud of their heritage. Their extended family is not considered by them to be extended at all, as they all live within shouting distance in the same neighborhood.

The construction business reinforced the sense of "family," allowing them to provide for their immediate families and the rest of their kin. Women take care of the home and family and the men provide the economic security. As the only girl in the family, Tina was regarded by Sonny as Daddy's little girl, which increased Sonny's sense of guilt about the circumstances of the injury. He found his support through the church, which he attended daily after the accident, and through his family. The entire family rallied to support Sonny and urged him to look to the future and plan for providing for his family.

In the rehabilitation setting, the family's goals did not always agree with the rehabilitation team's goals. The family believed that the sooner Tina was back in the family, the sooner they could get on with life. They did not see the large family gatherings as a problem. Quite the opposite, they saw them as vital to Tina's continued enculturation and sense of belonging to the family. The team believed that the family should set up the same structured environment for Tina at home as she had in the rehabilitation hospital, and they did not want her to return home permanently until the family had an appreciation for the need for structure in the home. They felt that they had "failed" to reach the family and became increasingly frustrated with the family's inability to see the need for Tina's independence.

The family met with the rehabilitation team and decided to take Tina home even though the rehabilitation team recommended against it. The clash between the family's values and the rehabilitation team's values created increasing tension, and the rehabilitation hospital did not support the family to the maximum extent possible upon discharge. They continued to insist that Tina needed more rehabilitation and stressed the goal of independence.

Family Life Cycle

The Ruocco's are well into the life cycle of having young children to care for, with three children and one on the way. Mary and Sonny Ruocco are good parents who take pride in their children's accomplishments and place their children's needs above their own in all situations. They had not only adjusted to having the extended family involved with them, they could not imagine life without them. They did not spend a lot of time thinking about what their children would grow up to be; they were more concerned about their current happiness.

Tina's two brothers saw the accident and both experienced nightmares after the crash. They missed Tina terribly. They went to the hospital once a week after school and looked forward to Tina's home visits. The social worker at the hospital gave them coloring books and suggested to their parents that they receive some counseling. The family did not see the need for counseling; they felt the boys would do better if they spent more time with Tina. They talked about the accident openly and encouraged the boys to ask questions.

The impending birth of their fourth child also presented concern for the family. A new baby demands a lot of time and attention, attention that is also critical to Tina. As with many families after head injury, the other children are not seen as needing the immediate attention that the child with the injury needs, and chances are that they will not receive the same attention for long periods of time. Parental attention may be replaced by attention from the extended family, which was the best adjustment this family could see at this time.

Future Implications

The future implications in this situation revolve around what is best for Tina and what is best for the rest of her family. The rehabilitation team should keep this in mind as they prepare for Tina's discharge. Although they do not agree with the family, they should do all they can to support the family. A home visit should be set up by the therapist most familiar with and accepted by the family. A structure should be suggested to the family, although in their need to discover for themselves what works best, they may not use the structure. As time passes, if the family becomes frustrated with their situation, the rehabilitation team should be available to do a follow-up visit. It is natural for families to try what has worked in the past, asking for help when they realize that new strategies are needed. It is also quite possible that the family will figure out new strategies on their own. In any case, the therapist should also plan a home visit after Tina has been home for a few weeks.

Given the involvement of the extended family, they should also be enlisted to help out. The therapist can meet with the entire family in the home, fielding questions and suggesting supportive techniques. It might also be helpful to introduce the family to another family who is also caring for a toddler with head injury at home and is able to offer resources and information as well as support. The extended family and parents should be encouraged to plan for the needs of Tina's brothers.

PRESCHOOL

Sam Willis is a 4-year-old boy in a black family who has an older brother Leo Jr., 8, and a younger sister Tanya, 2. One day when he was at his brother's T-ball practice, Sam was hit in the head with a bat. His father was with him and rushed him to the hospital where he had a few stitches above his right temple and was sent home with a list of instructions for his parents. They were told that if he started to show any symptoms of concussion they should take him to his pediatrician. Sam did indeed show signs of concussion, and his mother brought him to the pediatrician's office the next day. The parents were instructed to keep an eye on him and wait and see what happened.

The Willis family lives in a nice suburb outside of a Midwestern city. Leo Willis, Sr. grew up in a rough neighborhood in an inner city. His parents and two brothers still live in the old neighborhood. His grades were good in high school, and he wanted to go to college and play basketball. When he went to college he met Tara, and they were married shortly after graduation. Tara grew up outside of the city, and her parents were both lawyers. Leo and Tara decided early on that they wanted to raise their children in a nice suburban community. They go to visit his parents about once a month and enjoy having his parents come stay with them.

Leo works as an insurance salesman and Tara works half time as a writer at a local newspaper. They enjoy spending time together as a family and are really beginning to feel that their life is becoming more hectic. Their children can now express choices about the kinds of things they want to do, and it seems that if there is not a little league game, there is karate practice or dance lesson. Sam usually enjoys all of the activity, but lately he has been more irritable.

Leo and Tara notice that Sam has not been himself since the concussion. In addition to being irritable, he becomes tired more easily than before and is having more difficulty reading the bedtime stories he usually enjoys. They have called the pediatrician who has said he will grow out of it over time. Still, Tara worries. She and Leo hope that when he starts preschool in 2 weeks the teacher will be able to help.

Traditional Developmental Milestone

As a toddler, Sam demonstrated delayed speech and did not begin to verbalize until he was 3 years old. He has difficulty dressing himself and often throws temper tantrums to get what he wants. His mother reports that since his injury

Sam constantly loses his temper and has even struck her a few times. She notes that Sam is "OK talking," but that he is "always forgetting to do things I ask him to do."

Severity of Injury and Effect on Milestone

Even though Sam's injury was mild, he was still experiencing difficulties 4 weeks after being hit by the bat. Since his injury involved the right frontal lobe, many of the inappropriate behaviors that Sam has exhibited are predictable. He is irritable and short-tempered, has short-term memory problems, and is unable to control his anger. Such behaviors are typical in persons with mild head injuries and often are exaggerated if there is a history of such behaviors pre-injury. In many children with mild head injuries difficult behaviors tend to clear up in 3–4 weeks; behaviors that persist after this period may develop into long-term psychological issues if not addressed. Many preschool children who have experienced mild or moderate brain injuries are often misclassified by educational systems as having attention deficit disorder, being hyperactive, or having learning disabilities. Consequently, many of these children rarely receive the cognitive therapy they need to recover from or compensate for their brain injuries.

Ethnicity

Prejudice and the assumption that all black families fit one negative stereotype obscure true cultural meaning (Hines & Boyd-Franklin, 1982). In addition, social, economic, and political hardships often faced by black families force them to face every situation with three possible obstacles to overcome. The Willises had certainly experienced their share of discrimination and prejudice. Now, because they have been so successful, the Willises usually find people making statements to the effect that they are not "like the others." The Willises resent these statements because they firmly believe in their cultural values of loyalty and strong kinship bonds (Hines & Boyd-Franklin, 1982). They keep close contacts with their family and in their other personal relationships. The Willises have many close friends through their children's activities and through their own interest in the town's recreation activities. These friends are considered as close as family.

For Sam and his siblings, the experience with prejudice was minimal. Tara always dreamed of protecting her children from discrimination and hatred but she knew the chances were slim. When Sam entered school, Tara secretly feared that Sam's behavior problem would be attributed to race rather than his head injury. She did not vocalize these fears and approached the situation with documentation of his concussion and a complete description of his behavior before and after his head injury. When she approached the family doctor with this information he was receptive, and she hoped the school would be also.

Family Life Cycle

The Willis family is currently focused on raising their children and has a very busy schedule revolving around the children's activities. Leo and Tara have talked about their dreams of college for their children and place great emphasis on education and hard work. They hope that Sam's opportunities to get ahead are not hampered by his head injury. They plan to watch him closely and spend extra time with him on his school work.

Future Implications

As mentioned previously, the major dilemma in minor head injury is the fact that people know little about its consequences and often assume that a minor head injury causes only minor problems. Because minor head injury does not require that a person be hospitalized and take on the sick role in a traditional sense, society seldom understands its effects. This is especially true with young children who cannot always describe the problems they are having. Additionally, they are often supervised by several adults in 1 day. The adults are not always aware of the problems that could be caused by the injury, and parents might not be informed of such incidents.

Add to the poor understanding of minor head injury, the poor understanding of ethnic backgrounds and it becomes clearer why Tara may have a justified fear about intervention for her son, Sam. Families are the unquestioned experts about their members, and professionals should always take their concerns seriously. Clinical skills and observation can be used to measure the validity of their concerns. By acknowledging the family as expert, professionals can discover important information for their work.

SCHOOL AGE

The Rodriguez family moved to the Southwestern part of the United States 2 years ago from Mexico. After only 2 months, Mr. Rodriguez was killed in an accident on the farm where he worked. Maria Rodriguez and her four children, 8-year-old Rosa, 6-year-old Tina, 5-year-old Carlos Jr., and 3-year-old Juan, have lived on food stamps and odd jobs that Maria is able to find around their small town. She has learned a few words of English but most of the jobs she has taken have been with other Spanish speaking people. Rosa and Tina have been learning to speak English in school but have not been able to practice at home with their mother.

One day on the way home from school there was a school bus accident. Rosa and Tina were both on the bus, but Rosa was the only one of the two who was hurt. She experienced a severe brain injury and was hospitalized for several months. The family had no insurance so Rosa was not able to receive inpatient rehabilitation. The local church donated a wheelchair to the family and Rosa is now at home.

The day is now filled with tasks centered around caring for Rosa. Maria has been unable to work since Rosa came home because she has to provide care for her. Their house is not accessible for a wheelchair so Maria carries her daughter from room to room. Rosa has not returned to school because Maria is not sure how to get her there now that she cannot board the bus.

Rosa is able to feed herself and can communicate with the few words she has relearned in Spanish. She is not able to move her wheelchair around very much, but her mother has been bringing her outside more, and she is starting to move herself around on the gravel driveway. Her younger sister helps a little but usually becomes frustrated with her mother for giving Rosa so much attention.

Despite the many challenges Maria now faces, she continues to take great pride in caring for her children. There are strong affectionate ties and the children always listen when their mother tells them to do something. She has started to sing with Rosa and thinks that this might help her learn to talk again. At least Rosa enjoys it and will laugh.

The language barrier has been difficult for Maria. She never did understand exactly what they told her in the hospital. The family does not have a telephone, and the only communication Maria has received from the school is a letter written in English encouraging her to call the school counselor if she needs help.

Traditional Developmental Milestone

Rosa was considered an average student by her second grade teacher, but a child with a great deal of potential. Not only had Rosa learned English with minimal difficulty, but she had been in the top math group. She had good socialization skills, a solid foundation of general knowledge, and excellent motor development. She was reading at the first-grade level, could tell time, and had excellent listening and comprehension skills.

Severity of Injury and Effect on Milestone

The whole school was deeply upset over the schoolbus accident. Several children had sustained serious injuries; however, Rosa's was the most severe. She had been thrown against the metal rail on the seat in front of her (school buses do not require seat belts) and sustained a deep brain injury to her limbic area and parietal lobes. She was comatose for 46 days and had a great deal of internal bleeding and brain swelling. While the school knew that Rosa was in the hospital for over 4 months, neither the hospital nor Maria ever informed the school of her discharge. By the time the special educator heard that Rosa was home and not receiving any rehabilitation or educational services, summer vacation had started, and the school chose to wait until fall to see how Rosa was doing. Unfortunately, the lack of rehabilitation services and the length of time between the hospital stay and the beginning of the new school year would only compound Rosa's problems and would more than likely complicate her long-term recovery.

Ethnicity

Mexican American families have been characterized as valuing cooperation, interdependence, collectivism, and cohesiveness (McGoldrick, 1982a). The Rodriguez family values each of these attributes, with special emphasis on interdependence. Maria never questions putting a great deal of energy into caring for her children. Although, in caring for Rosa she does find that she is tired most of the time and is not able to plan beyond the following day. She had not yet recovered from the death of her husband, and Rosa's injury seemed to set her back even further. She dreams of moving back to Mexico to live with her younger sister and her family but has not been able to work to earn the money to move.

The language barrier also poses problems for the Rodriguez family. Maria cannot communicate with people who can help with returning to Mexico or putting Rosa back in school. Before her injury, Rosa had taken on the role of interpreter for her mother when they went out in public. At one time the school did have a special education teacher who spoke Spanish, but she left after Rosa had been in school only for several months.

Family Life Cycle

Maria and her husband were living a traditional family life when Mr. Rodriguez was killed. They lived hand-to-mouth before his death and their situation became worse after his death. Rosa, as the oldest child, took on more responsibility, caring for her younger brothers and sisters at the early age of 8. When roles in the family were being redefined and Maria realized that she would be a single parent indefinitely, Rosa's head injury occurred.

Future Implications

The implications of Rosa's head injury reach far beyond the need for her to have additional rehabilitation and return to school. The entire family system has been altered for a second time by Rosa's accident. Not only is Rosa unable to help care for her brothers and sister and act as interpreter for her family, she is also unable to care for herself. The family does not have an extended family to look to, and they are not accustomed to looking beyond their family in times of need.

The community and the family's limited social network are their greatest sources of support. Perhaps the church that provided the wheelchair will recognize that the family has further needs and help them enlist a professional. Perhaps if Maria works with anyone who speaks Spanish, she could ask that person to act as interpreter for the family. When school starts, the special education teacher should contact the family right away. An interpreter should be provided for the family. In addition, a social worker should work with Maria to develop strategies to meet her communication needs, perhaps an evening course in English as a second language. If Maria cannot arrange childcare, the social worker should help her find a language teacher willing to come to her home. Reaching beyond the school to community resources through the church and other advocacy organizations should be a priority. The state protection and advocacy center and the regional parent center along with the local head injury foundation are possible sources of assistance.

ADOLESCENCE

Jason McCormick, 15, was drinking with his buddies and decided to borrow his father's car to visit another friend. The car struck a telephone pole at a high speed, resulting in Jason's severe brain injury. No one else was hurt in the crash.

After a brief hospital stay, Jason moved to a rehabilitation hospital. Within 4 months he was walking without help, and his father Pat decided it was time for him to return home and "get back to work." The rehabilitation team predicted disaster if Jason's behavior problems were not addressed.

Jason is the fourth of seven children in this large Irish Catholic family. Six of the children live with their parents. Jason's accident was one of three incidents of drinking and driving for Jason. Still his father believed that "boys will be boys." His older brothers were no different. The males in the family believed there was nothing wrong with drinking. Mrs. McCormick privately worried about Jason; she deferred to her husband's attitude, although she did wish that none of the men in the house would drink. Mr. McCormick's drinking had become progressively worse over the previous 3 years, and Mrs. McCormick was beginning to think he might be an alcoholic.

Jason returned to high school and had a lot of difficulty concentrating on his work. He also seemed to become involved in more and more fights. At first, Mrs. McCormick would go up to the school by herself to talk to the principle because she thought it better that her husband not become more upset than he already was. Now, Jason faced his second suspension and was in jeopardy of failing.

Traditional Developmental Milestone

Prior to his accident, Jason had a normal childhood and was well-liked by his peers. He had never been an outstanding student in school but had always managed to maintain a "C" average, with an occasional "B" here and there. Jason was a member of the football and baseball teams and was considered a good athlete. In his junior high school years, Jason started drinking after games and on weekends with his friends. His blood-alcohol level at the time of his accident was 1.8. This level of intoxication tended to disguise the severity of his brain injury, as is often the case for injured drunk drivers.

Severity of Injury and Effect on Milestone

When Jason first returned to school, he was given a hero's welcome. But he soon found himself wandering the hallways trying to remember where his locker was and forgetting which class to go to next. One week after his return to school, his teachers met with him and gave him all the assignments he had missed while he had been in the hospital. As soon as Jason saw the stacks of books and papers he went into a rage and refused to do ". . . all this stupid crap!" As the weeks went by, Jason found that he was easily confused and overwhelmed; had no way to remember what was being taught in his classes; and had little control over his behavior or what he inappropriately said to his friends. The injury to his frontal lobes inhibited Jason's ability to control and monitor his behavior. He needed intensive therapy to learn compensatory strategies, therapy which the public school could not provide. His friends began to avoid him and mock him behind his back. It wasn't long before Jason faced his first suspension from school for punching several students (male and female) in the cafeteria.

Ethnicity

Many Irish American families have been characterized by strong mother-son relationships, emotional distance, and close ties with the Catholic church (McGoldrick, 1982b). Common consumption of alcohol, especially by males, is considered socially acceptable. Irish women often dominate family life, and fathers have been characterized as playing a more distant role (McGoldrick, 1982b). The McCormick family strongly identifies with their Irish roots. Mrs. McCormick, while outwardly deferring to her husband in the decision about Jason's discharge, is very much in control of the family's life. While Mr. McCormick may talk a lot about what is best for Jason, it will most likely be Mrs. McCormick who takes action. Like many Irish families, the McCormicks value good outward appearances; Jason's inappropriate behavior will not be tolerated for extended periods of time. If Jason is to have help, it will likely be a result of his mother's insistence. His brothers and sisters may exert pressure on him to conform to make their mother's life more tolerable. They may also cover up some of his odd behaviors to spare his mother or spare themselves from their father's wrath.

Family Life Cycle

The family with adolescents undergoes a shift from exerting complete control over their children to allowing more flexibility in family boundaries (McGoldrick & Carter, 1982). The adolescent is pushing away from parental influence and control, while the parents are wondering how much independence to allow. Until Jason's injury the McCormick family had adapted to having five adolescents in the house without significant event. Jason's older brothers and sisters had done their share of being rowdy, and there was some truth to Mr. McCormick's statement that Jason is no different from his older brothers, but Jason's behavior was the family's first experience with a major problem.

It has become clear to Mrs. McCormick that her usual influence over her son Jason is not going to resolve the problems he faces. She knows that she has to tell her husband, and she will have to deal with his temper while trying to find Jason the help he needs. She does not expect her husband to help. He may discipline Jason, but he will not become involved in active problem-solving. Mrs. McCormick will take on that responsibility by herself.

Future Implications

For Jason and his family, it has become clear that his current difficulties cannot be attributed to "normal adolescent behavior." His father may see "getting back to work" as the best course of action, but his mother may take charge and find Jason the help he needs. In the intervention setting, the therapists may underestimate the influence Mrs. McCormick has in the family. They may interpret her agreeing with her husband as compliance rather than her desire to present a good front in public.

It is important to give Mrs. McCormick as many resources as possible, knowing that she may never call the therapist to report her results with the information. Information about alcoholism and rehabilitation would also be beneficial. Information is also important for the school setting. The teachers should offer Mrs. McCormick information and recommendations and encourage her to follow through. However, they should not anticipate feedback.

YOUNG ADULTHOOD

Amy and Howard Klein have one son, Barry, who sustained a head injury at age 18. The car he was driving was hit broadside at an intersection when someone ran a red light. Although Barry was wearing a seat belt, he experienced a brain injury. The emergency medical team was surprised he was alive.

The Klein family is Jewish and celebrates all traditional Jewish holidays. Howard is a lawyer and Amy is a social worker. Howard's father is a rabbi and his mother is a homemaker. Both of Amy's parents are physicians. Barry was an exemplary student in high school, valedictorian of his class, and president of the debate team. He was scheduled to attend Harvard University in the fall, and with 3 weeks left of summer, the family was very excited. The crash changed everything.

When Barry arrived at the hospital, the shift was changing and the information from the emergency medical team was misplaced for several hours. His parents were on vacation in Hawaii, and when the hospital finally contacted his grandparents they all came to the hospital immediately. His parents flew in from their vacation and waited.

Barry was in intensive care for 5 weeks. He began to recognize his family within 2 weeks after the crash. His most severe problems were physical. He fell and hit the floor one day, which caused him to need back surgery and experience some paralysis. The family decided to sue the hospital and were hoping the additional money would help Barry when it was time for him to live independently.

Three months after the accident Barry was in a rehabilitation hospital approximately 200 miles from the family's home. Amy and Howard spent weekends visiting Barry, and every Monday morning Amy called the hospital to report their observations and ask questions. When requested treatment or procedures were not carried out, the family usually wrote to the hospital and sent a copy of the letter to the administrator of the hospital.

Since Barry was so far from home, and his high school class had gone off to college, he had few visitors aside from his parents and grandparents. He came home around the new year and was able to see many of his friends, but he seemed to become depressed knowing that he too should have been in college. The family seemed to handle the situation by obtaining every bit of information available about head injury and all possible intervention options. The rehabilitation team felt the family was looking for a cure when in fact they were just trying to identify all the assistance available for Barry.

Traditional Developmental Milestone

Barry sustained a coup-contracoup injury, which resulted in shearing and twisting of the neural tissue in his frontal-temporal lobes. After the injury his mother would report that even though Barry was able to "talk again and think again, he was not the same person; he was not himself." Like many people with traumatic brain injuries, Barry's "loss of self" was significant despite what the results of the neuropsychological tests said about his cognitive abilities. He could not seem to redevelop a sense of who he was or to manage himself independently.

Severity of Injury and Effect on Milestone

Barry's parents took him to specialist after specialist to be tested. He was pulled from one therapy program and placed in another and then pulled again by his parents. Amy became Barry's case manager, mother, and counselor all in one. She read everything on brain injury she could find and questioned the professionals on their diagnoses. Barry, unfortunately, became more confused and depressed and would greatly depend on his mother for support. He no longer sought out his former friends, and he was afraid to go to college or even leave his own house. He had become, as one therapist said, "a psychological mess as the result of a neurological injury; he was 'sick' rather than injured." That sickness would become progressively worse if not addressed properly.

Ethnicity

Jewish families have been characterized by primary emphasis on centrality of the family, intellectual achievement, financial success, the sharing of problems, and verbal expression of feelings (Herz & Rosen, 1982). The Klein family has kept these values in their everyday life, with intellectual achievement and financial success being the basis for all other values. They had been extremely proud of Barry and felt that all of their dreams had come true the day his acceptance letter came from Harvard.

The experience with the medical system was eye opening. Amy and Howard had always been on the providing end of treatment and thus in control. They had never felt so out of control and vulnerable as they did after Barry's accident.

Family Life Cycle

The goal of young adulthood is regarded as emotional, physical, and financial independence from one's family (Walsh & McGoldrick, 1988). Barry Klein and his family were looking forward to this life cycle change with great anticipation of his successful career. The last thing they expected was to be thrown back into the life cycle stage of having a dependent member at the time when Amy and Howard were looking forward to retirement. The lack of control they felt in the medical setting heightened their need to control Barry's life. Barry felt confused and did not object to his parents' protectiveness. The rehabilitation team tried to help Barry achieve some independence from his parents. The more they raised questions about Amy's role in Barry's life, the more the family struggled to maintain control.

Future Implications

After previously holding great expectations for Barry's future the Kleins found themselves facing a future of daily struggle. At the same time, the rehabilitation team was questioning the family's motives and actions. It is important that the family and team understand one another's motives and goals. A conference with the family to discuss issues of communication would help establish consistent rules about the role of each person involved. The team should have asked the family to clarify their urgency about receiving information on Monday mornings. Also, the team should have given realistic timelines for delivery of that information. The loss that the family feels because of the head injury should be discussed openly, and Barry and his family should be encouraged to share their vision of his future. The team might be surprised to realize that the family is not looking for a cure at all. They may share the team's goal of maximum independence for Barry but choose an approach to that goal that is different from what the team is comfortable with and accustomed to.

CONCLUSION

This chapter has attempted to illustrate how, in addition to understanding the consequences of head injury on a child's development, it is also important to understand the consequences of head injury on the family life cycle and how ethnic and cultural background will affect intervention planning.

There is no valid family stereotype based purely upon ethnic background and culture. Families are as different from one another as individuals are from one another. There are many variables to consider; ethnicity is only one. By understanding a family's cultural background professionals can understand what implications cultural values can have on the intervention planned for the family.

Not all families have independence and success in work as a primary goal. Often in the rehabilitation process, the team can lose sight of the family's goals and values and strive for independence at all costs. The intervention should reflect the values that shaped the person's and the family's life before the head injury. Chances are these values will remain relevant.

It is important for professionals working with people with head injuries to understand their own ethnic background and how their cultural values affect their own lives. This will also help therapists to be aware of the effect of their own values on the intervention plans they recommend. Therapists must guard against imposing their own values on a family. Therapists must acknowledge to themselves conflicts between their own values and those of families and consciously try to resolve them. Talking with other therapists is often helpful. Maintaining a nonjudgmental attitude toward families is important in striving to discover what is truly in their best interest.

A family's behavior with professionals and in the therapeutic environment may not be indicative of their natural behavior. Medical settings are often intimidating, and families may find themselves taking on different behaviors to cope. For example, some families appear completely in control in the team conference and ask good questions, only to leave the setting and forget most of what took place because they were so intimidated. Other families appear disorganized and confused but feel in charge once they leave the therapeutic setting. In addition, cultural norms and values may dictate one set of behavior in public settings and another at home.

A crisis in the family, such as a head injury, may cause families to identify more with their cultural heritage than they did previously. This is not surprising given the importance of family in the life of someone who has experienced a head injury.

REFERENCES

Falicov, C.J. (1982). Mexican families. In M. McGoldrick, J.K. Pearce, & J. Giordano (Eds.), *Ethnicity and family therapy* (pp. 134–163). New York: The Guilford Press.

Herz, F.M., & Rosen, E.J. (1982). Jewish families. In M. McGoldrick, J.K. Pearce, & J. Giordano (Eds.), *Ethnicity and family therapy* (pp. 364–392). New York: The Guilford Press.

Hines, P.M., & Boyd-Franklin, N. (1982). Black families. In M. McGoldrick, J.K. Pearce, & J. Giordano (Eds.), *Ethnicity and family therapy* (pp. 84–107). New York: The Guilford Press.

Lidz, T. (1976). *The person: His and her development throughout the life cycle.* New York: Basic Books.

McGoldrick, M. (1982a). Ethnicity and family therapy: An overview. In M. McGoldrick, J.K. Pearce, & J. Giordano (Eds.), *Ethnicity and family therapy* (pp. 3–30). New York: The Guilford Press.

McGoldrick, M. (1982b). Irish families. In M. McGoldrick, J.K. Pearce, & J. Giordano (Eds.), *Ethnicity and family therapy* (pp. 84–107). New York: The Guilford Press.

McGoldrick, M., & Carter, E.A. (1982). The family life cycle. In F. Walsh (Ed.), *Normal family processes* (pp. 167–195). New York: The Guilford Press.

Rotunno, M., & McGoldrick, M. (1982). Italian families. In M. McGoldrick, J.K. Pearce, & J. Giordano (Eds.), *Ethnicity and family therapy* (pp. 340–363). New York: The Guilford Press.

Turnbull, A.P., & Turnbull, H.R. (1986). *Families, professionals, and exceptionality: A special partnership.* Columbus: Charles E. Merrill.

Walsh, F., & McGoldrick, M. (1988). Loss and the family life cycle. In C.J. Falicov (Ed.), *Family transitions: Continuity and change over the life cycle* (pp. 311–336). New York: The Guilford Press.

16

FAMILY AND BEHAVIORAL ISSUES

HARVEY E. JACOBS

PREVALENCE OF BEHAVIOR DISORDERS FOLLOWING TRAUMATIC BRAIN INJURY

Behavioral issues remain among the most prominent sequelae following traumatic brain injury. First noted in early outcome studies, behavior disorders remain prevalent in later findings. Effects have been noted for both the person who experienced a traumatic head injury (Benton, 1979; Bond, 1976; Brooks & Aughton, 1979; Brooks & McKinlay, 1983; Drudge, Rosen, Peyser, & Pieniadz, 1986; Garoutte & Aird, 1984; Jacobs, 1987, 1988b; Levin & Grossman, 1978) and people who surround the individual, most notably family members (Jacobs, 1988a; Jacobs, Muir, & Cline, 1986; Livingston, Brooks, & Bond, 1985; Oddy, Humphrey, & Uttley, 1978; Panting & Merry, 1972; Romano, 1974; Sbordone, 1983).

Similar to other aspects of head injury effects and outcome, behavior disorders are specific to each individual and his or her family members. The range of deficits is as broad as the people who sustain injuries. Lishman (1968) noted that 86% of those surveyed experienced psychiatric or emotional problems, which was comparable to the 84% noted in Thomsen's (1974) study. In the Los Angeles Head Injury Survey (Jacobs, 1987, 1988b) at least 90% of the participants experienced at least one of the 50 listed behavioral disorders post-injury and approximately 25% experienced severe behavior disorders that significantly interfered with daily life. Similar levels of emotional or behavior disorder have been noted by Najenson, Groswasser, Mendelson, and Hackett (1980) and Lezak, Cosgrove, O'Brien, and Wooster (1980). Issues of greatest incidence have included anxiety, depression, withdrawal, aggressive behavior, changed temperament, decreased initiation, poor self-control, and attention seeking.

Family members also experience a variety of serious consequences post-injury. These include separation, divorce, alienation of specific family members, and increased psychosomatic, emotional, and physical illness (Lezak, 1978; Mauss-Clum & Ryan, 1981; Oddy, Humphrey, & Uttley, 1978; Thomsen, 1974). Some of these challenges may be due to the emotional stress and strain that people experience when a loved one has a catastrophic injury. Other challenges may be due specifically to changes in roles and expectations that occur in post-injury life. Still other issues may reflect the exacerbation of premorbid problems.

FACTORS CONTRIBUTING TO BEHAVIOR DISORDERS

Family reactions to behavior sequelae help to demonstrate the dynamic systems in which behavior occurs. Whether one considers behavior a product or a reaction, it is not a solitary phenomenon. Behavior relies on a diverse set of salient factors for its occurrence (Jacobs, 1988c; Wood, 1987), including at a minimum neurological/physical presentation and environmental/social variables.

Neurological deficits resulting from the traumatic head injury play an important but not exclusive role. A broad base of behavioral and psychiatric syndromes have been ascribed to lesions in selected areas of the brain, especially the frontal and temporal lobes. However, indirect effects from other lesions also contribute to behavioral changes. Thus, a person with visual field cut demonstrates neglect, or persons with hypersensitivity may respond with avoidance and protective aggression to prevent further pain. Cognitive deficits are noted for their influence on behavior, especially in areas of learning, memory, initiation, attention, processing speed, and stimulus overload. Other deficits related to associated injuries indirectly incurred in the incident (e.g., skeletal loss, organ removal, amputation) may also affect a person's behavior. Issues of lethargy, amotivation, and other impoverishments of behavior must also be considered. Too frequently the concept of behavior disorder is equated with aggressive tendencies, rather than a person's inability to respond competently in identified situations.

Behavior is also a function of its environment (Skinner, 1953), and it is the interaction between the person and the immediate setting that often determines the course and judgment of behavior. Family settings and family members are very prominent in post-injury life. It is therefore important to understand the comprehensive effects of family systems on the person who experienced the head injury, as well as the converse. This requires a detailed analysis of the people in the situation, the rules and expectations of the environment (contingencies), the antecedents and consequences for the person's actions, the consistency of the social setting, and a host of other variables. Assessment of behavioral competence without consideration of the prevailing environment is meaningless.

For example, a stress-diathesis model of personal competence notes that behavior is a balance between the demands of the environment and the person's ability to perform under increasing pressure. Thus, a supportive environment, may be less judgmental of a person's actions than a nonsupportive environment and present fewer stressors. Fewer demands and stressors may also promote fewer adverse behavioral episodes than a more intense situation. Two individuals with the same behavioral repertoires may act differently because of different environmental influences. Under a nondemanding environment, one individual may be perceived as performing competently and effectively within the prevailing social milieu. A second and neurobehaviorally equal individual may decompensate under the rigors of a more demanding and stressful situation.

Finally, it is also critical to note that the label of behavior disorder is a social judgment. In a society, or in a smaller social group such as a family, people may identify different forms of behavior as acceptable or unacceptable (i.e., disordered) because of the effect that the behavior has on them or other members of the community. These definitions can also change with changes in social mores or individual abilities. For example, following a prolonged coma, any vocal behavior on the part of the patient is most welcome, including the type of language that previously would have been admonished. As the individual progresses, new rules for acceptable and unacceptable behavior will again take hold.

Ultimately, behavior itself is lawful and orderly; a product of the environment and organism from which it emanates (Skinner, 1938, 1953). Thus, an incapacity to identify the salient factors and the contingencies effecting a behavior demonstrates the absence of skilled inquiry by the observer rather than the logic or illogic of the behavior in question.

WHEN ARE BEHAVIOR DISORDERS LIKELY TO OCCUR?

There are several key epochs when behavior disorders are most likely to occur within a family setting. Transitions and stimulus changes, such as returning home following hospitalization or changes in housing arrangements, often increase the likelihood of behavioral decompensation. Persons who are stimulus bound, or who have trouble generalizing skills from one environment to another are highly susceptible. When cues in the new environment or social situation do not match previous structure, the individual may have difficulty adapting to the new surroundings and develop new patterns of behavior, some of which may be considered maladaptive.

Changes for caregivers can also cause disruption for dependent individuals. Thus, the family member who leaves home may also leave an important gap in the daily life of the person who experienced the head injury. Changes in health, business, or personal relationships may require a close friend to alter their level of involvement, tilting the overall balance of the person's social support system. Loss of counseling support for a spouse may make a marginal marriage unbearable, leading to its dissolution. The likelihood of behavioral impact following each of these changes may be determined in part by the level of involvement and support that the caregiver provides and whether the loss can be suitably compensated for.

Passage of life milestones may also potentiate disruption. Not graduating from school or getting married, and so forth, when one's friends are having these experiences can promote disorders. Failure can easily cause decompensation, but so can success, especially when the success places the person in an environment or situation beyond his or her capacity to manage.

Finally, not all behavior disorders are reactive. Some are insidious, and demonstrate gradual decompensation over time such as when friendships gradually diminish over the years until there is no one left except the television. Loneliness is perhaps the most chronic long-term challenge that people with severe disabilities face (Jacobs, 1989).

ROLE OF FAMILY MEMBERS

The prevalence of family reports of behavior disorders is not surprising given the role of family members in the lives of dependent persons with brain injuries. As noted in a number of studies (Jacobs, 1987, 1988b; Lezak, 1978, 1987; Romano, 1974), family members assume the bulk of responsibility for caring for their member with an injury after discharge from formal rehabilitation, often with few if any resources and little knowledge. This responsibility is often thrust upon them due to a lack of other resources and makes discussions about what the role of family members should be, moot. In the absence of alternatives, they are often the only source. In addition to attempting to reestablish the continuity of life that existed prior to the injury, family members must also reconcile with a variety of sequelae that are foreign to the person they once knew.

Similarly, the person who experienced the injury finds that the other members of the family have also changed. Part of this change is the result of the individual experiences and reactions that individual family members face as a result of the person's injury and course of treatment. Part of this change is related to the manner in which the person who experienced the head injury perceives and interacts with the environment, secondary to the neurobehavioral sequelae. Part of this change is due to general role confusion and incompetency in dealing with a new and unexpected situation. Hence, behavior disorders are interactive and a function of all individuals involved in the situation, not just the person with the injury.

BASIC PREREQUISITES FOR FAMILY INTERVENTION

When working with family members it is important to acknowledge some basic guidelines prior to any form of behavioral intervention. First, there is no such thing as *THE* family. Families are composed of individuals, each of whom plays a different role according to personal interest, ability, need, and expectations. The importance of involving different family members when addressing behavioral issues will depend on the identified issue and each person's role. Often too much time is spent trying to encourage an unwilling family member to help with a specific challenge, or trying to enlist the help of someone who is overwhelmed and feels guilty about their lack of involvement, but can provide only lip service. It is more important for family members to be open and honest about their contributions, expectations, and limitations, allowing then those who can and will be active to go on to problem identification and intervention. This may mean working without a member who is perceived as critical to the process, but general experience has indicated that it is more important to work within established resources than to count on tenuous promises.

It is also not the role of the professional to decide what the role of individual family members should be. As persons who happen to be professionals, we must always remember that we are present to provide service to the person with the injury and their family, not to determine their roles, patterns of responsibility, and future.

Second, the person who experienced the brain injury is also a family member and deserves an active role in any intervention process. Too often, this individual is left out of case formulation and intervention because of assumptions of disinterest or ineptitude. These often fatal mistakes help to highlight what may be the real problems facing family members and promoting the behavior disorder, that is, poor communication and neglecting personal rights of determination among all participants.

Third, because of the dynamic nature of behavior, it is important to focus on the specific challenges facing the family unit before beginning any intervention. Individual family members often present different challenges or different variations of the same challenges. Establishing concurrence on the specific goal to be addressed can take considerable time, but intervention without a directed goal is unlikely to be successful. Good goal formulation is likely to follow good therapeutic process intervention. This type of process intervention need not be cumbersome or long, if properly directed. It can be a valuable investment before attempting problem-solving or other goal oriented interventions. When involved and interested people cannot agree on what direction to move in, their efforts often become diluted and contradictory because each person goes in a different direction.

Fourth, attempting to ascribe responsibility for or ownership of a problem to a specific family member (usually the person who experienced the brain injury) is generally unsuccessful and rarely productive. The behavior problem affects all who are involved, and all who are involved generally contribute to the problem! The fact that the individual who experienced the injury may have changed the most does not place the responsibility for change on that person only. In general that person, just like every other family member, is acting in a personally logical fashion. In addition, the person who is perceived as having the behavior problem may have no problem with his or her behavior; it is the other family members who do. Their reaction to this person may contribute to or be the actual cause of the problem.

For example, a mother recently complained that her son was argumentative and would throw things whenever she tried to help him. She sought help for her son's temper tantrums and it was readily evident that the son displayed the precise behaviors that the mother had described. However, these behaviors occurred whenever the mother made decisions for the son that he was still capable of making. Frustrated, the son would act out, which caused the mother to back off and give him his way. These two individuals were locked in a vicious circle. The mother, increasingly concerned about her son's inability to manage daily affairs, as evidenced by his temper tantrums and low frustration tolerance, became more domineering, which increased his outbursts. The son, unable to identify alternative approaches to addressing the problem, would manage his mother through this anger. Successful resolution was facilitated by promoting behavior change in both individuals. The mother learned to give her son more autonomy and respect him for his abilities. The son practiced alternative problem-solving strategies and learned how to cue his mother when he felt that she was becoming too obtrusive.

Fifth, it is important to direct family members towards the development of prospective goals rather than the amelioration of presenting deficits. Too often goals of decreasing some undesirable behavior without identifying the pro-social alternative are not viable. Thus, a person who successfully decreases some form of aggressive behavior may find the result less than satisfying if it means the person just sits or otherwise has a poorer quality of life than before. Focusing on the development of pro-social goals, in conjunction with the amelioration of a behavioral excess, is often more successful and more satisfying.

BEHAVIORAL FAMILY TRAINING

Most behavioral family interventions occur through training programs and generally focus on an outcome and problem-solving orientation. This is in contrast to the process oriented approach of more traditional therapeutic models. Some professionals argue that both models incorporate support and skill development and that the difference is semantical. However, identifying the emphasis in each provides important distinctions.

By emphasizing problem-solving techniques and outcomes, rather than process, participants take a stronger role in the development of selected interventions and can more concretely measure their accomplishments by the progress they make on specific issues. They also learn critical skills that can be applied to future problems as they develop. In contrast, many therapeutic models place the responsibility and control of such processes on the therapist. Obviously professional direction, support, and guidance through the training process is crucial, but most training models place a greater emphasis on the transfer of knowledge and control from the professional to the participant.

A number of behavioral family training models have been developed for various groups of people including persons with developmental disabilities (Baker, Brightman, Heifetz, & Murphy, 1983), persons with psychiatric disability (Fallon et al., 1982), children (Becker, 1971; Patterson, 1975) and persons with dementia (Mace & Rabins, 1982). Most programs follow similar training formats but are specialized in terms of the specific populations that they serve.

One of the earliest applications of behavioral family training in head injury was the UCLA/Robert Wood Johnson Foundation Family Training Project (Jacobs, 1988a; Jacobs & Muir, 1988; Muir, Jacobs, & Martel, 1987). The program is based on the principle of managed intervention. A key assumption of the project was that most of the long-term challenges that persons who have experienced head injuries and their family members face are greater than the knowledge and resources at their disposal. Thus, it is necessary for family participants to be good case evaluators as well as interventionists. Prior to any type of intervention, family members are required to prioritize presenting challenges and compare this list to available resources. Those challenges that are less responsive to successful intervention require deferral to those that are likely to be responsive to the intervention, within each family's available resources. In essence, the program taught family members to work smarter rather than harder.

The overall training model was based on the seven components of education, problem identification/problem selection, resource assessment, behavioral assessment, intervention, evaluation, and maintenance/generalization.

During early developmental phases of the project, education was discovered to be critical before any realistic goal setting or decision-making could occur. Most family members presented only limited knowledge about brain injury and long-term needs, along with substantial misinformation. While most family members could identify the cause of the brain injury, few could identify localization of the damage or its effects on physical, cognitive, or behavioral issues. Most family members also had incorrect knowledge about neurological recovery and rehabilitative processes, with some people expecting substantial neurological repair 5–10 years post-injury.

Without basic knowledge about brain injury and outcomes, it was not possible for participants to make concise or even rational decisions about intervention needs or priorities. A basic educational program was developed to teach participants about brain and behavior relationships, neurological recovery, treatment alternatives, and resource options. Armed with this knowledge, participants could make more informed decisions about goals and priorities.

Problem prioritization was the next step of the training process. Most families faced an overwhelming number of challenges which could not be simultaneously addressed. By requiring participating family members to list all challenges and develop a list of priorities, communication and consensus were facilitated, along with several other important benefits. First, as problems were identified and prioritized, participants discovered the interrelationships between each of the individual challenges. Expectations about magic bullet cures, simple interventions that could solve all problems, quickly faded. Second, participants quickly began to understand the complexity of their challenges and the effort and resources required even for the simplest changes. Support from other participants in the group and group leaders helped bolster against feelings of hopelessness and discouragement during this process. Third, participants learned the distinction between problem identification and problem-solving; identifying a problem provides the opportunity but not necessarily the means to address the issue.

Resource assessment, the next step in the training process, helped to match prioritized problems with available means. Most training program participants assumed that money and insurance coverage were the only resources at their disposal. However, time from individual family members, family influence, knowledge, community resources, contacts and other means are also vital resources. By listing these resources by priority or availability, it was possible to systematically identify a broad base of support. The final step in this process was to match precise resources to selected priorities. This helped family members determine what challenges they had the greatest success in addressing. These became the problems targeted for intervention.

Behavior assessment, the next step, was a critical prerequisite to intervention. In many situations a problem's perceived prominence and its actual presentation varied substantially. For example, general clinical experience demonstrates that most behavior problems occur less often than perceived, but make a marked impression each time they occur. As a result, participants confused the intensity of a behavior with its frequency. A similar problem occurred when the definition of the behavior differed from its actual presentation. Thus the problem being measured could be different from the problem that was identified during the previous step of prioritization. This made it appear that the problem vanished once data collection began. In both situations, it was necessary to determine how important the original problem was in light of the new data. Sometimes the original problem was determined to be less important than one identified later, which caused a shift in emphasis. This determination was far better made at that earlier point than after substantial time and resources had been directed toward intervention.

Determining the relationship between the targeted behavior and the salient factors assumed to be responsible for its occurrence was also critical. Many times participants made assumptions about why behavior occurred that had little relationship to the controlling variables. If the correct relationships were not properly identified, effective intervention strategies could not be developed. This information was collected at the same time that data on the presence and magnitude of the target behavior were recorded. Discrepancies between perceived reasons for the occurrence of behavior and its actual controlling variables had to be addressed before effective intervention could be implemented. Without this step, most intervention strategies were doomed to failure from the start.

For example, in one family training group, a mother had identified her daughter's slovenly appearance as the problem to be addressed. Early into behavioral assessment of this issue, the mother stopped taking data. Assured by her hunch that an increase in allowance money would change her daughter's dressing habits, the mother began intervention. Initial results were impressive. The daughter began taking a greater interest in what she wore, the care of her clothing, and even went on a diet. Results were maintained for 3 weeks and the mother was ecstatic. Then all of a sudden, the daughter returned to her pre-intervention levels of self-care.

Retrospective investigation revealed that the mother's intervention had little to do with the change in her daughter's grooming behavior. At the same time that the program was started, the daughter found a boyfriend. The relationship lasted for 3 weeks before he left her for someone else. The changes in the daughter's behavior were related to these events. The mother had made two mistakes. First, she did not involve her daughter in the identification of the behavioral issue. Second, she established intervention without proper assessment of controlling factors.

Once the magnitude and intensity of the targeted behavior had been documented, as well as the salient factors responsible for its occurrence, effective intervention programs could be implemented. In most situations, the actual intervention was fairly simple because the precise controlling variables, their relationship to the targeted behavior, and the resources needed to effect the desired change had been well established. This made most interventions a realignment of resources, goals, and expectations. Thus, although the initial processes of problem identification, resource identification, and assessment appeared laborious, intervention brought reward.

Continuous evaluation was also a key element of the intervention program. Participants continued the data collection efforts they began during the assessment phase to help guide intervention. These data did not determine unitary success or failure, but helped to guide participants in the management of the intervention. Thus, favorable results confirmed sustained intervention efforts, while less successful results indicated need for changes in approach and intervention strategies, until the desired outcomes were attained. This goal-oriented method of intervention was consistent with general behavioral approaches.

Finally, maintenance of behavior change was also critical to program success. Most problems with long-term gains involved therapeutic changes reverting to earlier (pre-intervention) forms of behavior, once a successful change had been facilitated. Not surprisingly, when the variables responsible for a given behavior reverted to pre-intervention relationships, behavior reverted as well. Also, expecting family members to maintain the consistency and intensity that many behavioral programs require for long periods of time is unrealistic. However, it was often easy to use the momentum developed in the intervention to develop less intrusive maintenance programs. Overall program success was determined by the length of time the goals were maintained.

Teaching participants these seven steps required persistent effort. With weekly 3-hour training sessions, between 15 and 20 weeks of training were required. However, once the steps were mastered, they could be applied to a broad range of challenges. Participants in the behavioral family training groups noted success with traditionally recognized behavior problems such as excessive talking, temper outbursts, personal hygiene, verbal abuse, self-care, behavioral self-monitoring, interpersonal relations, as well as other long-term challenges, such as vocational training, money management, independent living, and education. The type of challenges that trained individuals could address was unique to each person according to his or her resources and circumstances. Because of this, it is important that all training participants demonstrate credible decision-making skills.

BEYOND FAMILY TRAINING

Behavioral training programs can teach people some but not all of the skills required for the successful resolution of some challenges. Not all post-injury challenges are amenable to behavioral intervention. Skills and knowledge vary across individual families and family members and problems can vary in their persistence and severity and whom they affect. The assumption that behavior problems are the sole domain of the person who experienced the traumatic head injury is patently false.

In those situations where family resources are not adequate to meet presenting problems, there is still the need to be able to identify and define the presenting issue as clearly as possible when seeking the services of others. As is all too evident in this field, this ability is not a guarantee that needed services are available or accessible, but it will help to increase access to available opportunities.

Managing the more difficult problems is often a compromise between what resources are available and what is needed. It has been recognized that there are insufficient resources in the community to effectively address presenting challenges. Many people in need go without services; they and their social support systems continue in various states of disarray and stress. When behavior becomes extreme, the individual may come to the attention of psychiatric treatment or come before the criminal justice system; these two alternatives are often counterproductive to the management of neurobehavioral disorders.

For most people, addressing long-term behavior problems must begin with a focus on the individual's abilities. In a society where each person is evaluated by his or her societal contributions, an emphasis on deficits is counterproductive. Thus a person who is labeled noncompliant may also be an excellent cook. A person labeled aggressive must have other behaviors in his or her repertoire. It is physiologically impossible to sustain intense aggression for more than 5%–10% of the time! Amelioration of a behavioral deficit alone is not sufficient treatment. It is the amelioration of a deficit in combination with the development of pro-social skills within a functional social environment that determines the success or failure of intervention.

Building from a person's strengths early on is a hallmark of modern rehabilitative intervention. By carrying this focus to family programs, it may be possible to avoid the development of many of the insidious behavior problems that appear over time.

REFERENCES

Baker, B.L., Brightman, A.J., Heifetz, L.J., & Murphy, D.M. (1983). *Behavior problems*, Champaign, IL: Research Press.

Becker, W. (1971). *Parents are teachers*. Champaign, IL: Research Press.

Benton, A. (1979). Behavioral consequences of closed head injury. *Central nervous system trauma research status report*. National Institute of Neurological and Communicative Disorders and Stroke. Distributed by the National Head Injury Foundation.

Bond, M.R. (1976). Assessment of the psychosocial outcome of severe head injury. *Acta Neurochirurgica, 34,* 57–70.

Brooks, D.N., & Aughton, M.E. (1979). Psychological consequences of blunt head injury. *International Rehabilitation Medicine, 1,* 160–165.

Brooks, D.N., & McKinlay, W. (1983). Personality and behavioral change after severe blunt head injury—A relative's view. *Journal of Neurology, Neurosurgery and Psychiatry, 46,* 336–344.

Drudge, O.W., Rosen, J.C., Peyser, J.M., & Pieniadz, J. (1986). Behavioral and emotional problems and treatment in chronically brain-impaired adults. *Annals of Behavioral Medicine, 8,* 9–14.

Fallon, I.R.H., Boyd, J.L., McGill, C.W., Razani, J., Moss, H.B., & Gilderman, A.M. (1982). Family management in the prevention of exacerbations of schizophrenia: A controlled study. *New England Journal of Medicine, 306,* 1437–1440.

Garoutte, B., & Aird, R.B. (1984). Behavioral effects of head injury. *Psychiatric Annals, 14*(7).

Jacobs, H.E. (1987). The Los Angeles head injury survey: Project rationale and design implications. *Journal of Head Trauma Rehabilitation, 2,* 37–50.

Jacobs, H.E. (1988a). Family reaction and treatment. In A. Christensen & D. Ellis (Eds.), *Neuropsychological treatment of head injury.* Boston: Martinus Nijhoff Publishing.

Jacobs, H.E. (1988b). The Los Angeles head injury survey: Procedures and preliminary findings. *Archives of Physical Medicine and Rehabilitation, 69,* 425–431.

Jacobs, H.E. (1988c). Yes, behavior analysis can help, but do you know how to harness it? *Brain Injury, 4,* 339–346.

Jacobs, H.E. (1989). Adult community integration. In Paul Bach-y-Rita. (Ed.), *Traumatic brain injury: Current status and a research agenda.* New York: Demos Publications.

Jacobs, H.E., & Muir, C.A. (1988, September). *From family systems to family outcomes.* Paper presented at the second annual conference, Cognitive Rehabilitation: Community Integration Through Scientifically Based Practice, Richmond.

Jacobs, H.E., Muir, C.A., & Cline, J. (1986). Family reactions to persistent vegetative state. *Journal of Head Trauma Rehabilitation, 1,* 55–62.

Levin, H.S., & Grossman, R.G. (1978). Behavior sequelae of closed head injury. *Archives of Neurology, 35,* 720–729.

Lezak, M.D. (1978). Living with the characterologically altered brain injured patient. *Journal of Clinical Psychiatry, 39,* 592–598.

Lezak, M.D. (1987). Psychological implications of traumatic brain damage for the patient's family. *Rehabilitation Psychology, 31,* 241–250.

Lezak, M.D., Cosgrove, J.N., O'Brien, K., & Wooster, N. (1980). *Relationships between personality disorders, social disturbances, and physical disability following traumatic brain injury.* San Francisco: International Neuropsychological Society.

Lishman, W.A. (1968). Brain damage in relation to psychiatric disability after head injury. *British Journal of Psychiatry, 114,* 373–410.

Livingston, M.G., Brooks, D.N., & Bond, M.R. (1985). Patient outcome in the year following severe head injury and relative's psychiatric and social functioning. *Journal of Neurology, Neurosurgery, and Psychiatry, 48,* 876–881.

Mace, N.L., & Rabins, P.V. (1982). *The 36 hour day: A family guide to caring for a person with disease, related dementing illness and memory loss in later life.* Baltimore: Johns Hopkins University.

Mauss-Clum, N., & Ryan, M.R. (1981). Brain injury and the family. *Journal of Neurosurgical Nursing, 13,* 165–169.

Muir, C.A., Jacobs, H.E., & Martel, M. (1987, December). *Family training.* Paper presented at the Sixth Annual National Symposium, National Head Injury Foundation, San Diego.

Najenson, T., Groswasser, Z., Mendelson, L., & Hackett, P. (1980). Rehabilitation outcome of brain damaged patients after severe head injury. *International Rehabilitation Medicine, 2,* 17–22.

Oddy, M., Humphrey, M., & Uttley, D. (1978). Stresses upon the relatives of head-injured patients. *British Journal of Psychiatry, 133,* 507–513.

Panting, A., & Merry, P.H. (1972). The long term rehabilitation of severe head injuries with particular reference to the need for social and medical support for the patient's family. *Rehabilitation, 38,* 33–37.

Patterson, G.R. (1975). *Families: Applications of social learning to family life.* Champaign, IL: Research Press.

Romano, M.D. (1974). Family response to traumatic head injury. *Scandinavian Rehabilitation Medicine, 6,* 1–4.

Sbordone, R. (1983, August). *The emotional reaction of family members of head injured patients.* Paper presented at the International Traumatic Head Injury Conference, London.

Skinner, B.F. (1938). *The behavior of organisms.* New York: Appleton-Century-Crofts.

Skinner, B.F. (1953). *Science and human behavior.* New York: The Free Press.

Thomsen, I.V. (1974). The patient with severe head injury and his family. *Scandinavian Journal of Rehabilitation and Medicine, 6,* 180–183.

Thomsen, I.V. (1984). Late outcome of very severe blunt head trauma: A 10–15 year second follow-up. *Journal of Neurology, Neurosurgery and Psychiatry, 47,* 260–268.

Wood, R.L. (1987). *Brain injury rehabilitation: A neurobehavioral approach.* London: Croom Helm.

17

FAMILY AND SEXUALITY AFTER TRAUMATIC BRAIN INJURY

NATHAN D. ZASLER

JEFFREY S. KREUTZER

Significant sexual dysfunction is not uncommon after traumatic brain injury (TBI) and may affect the person's family as much, if not more than the individual. It is critical for rehabilitation professionals to have a basic understanding of the neuromedical and neuropsychological ramifications of traumatic brain injury on the person with TBI and family unit. In order to address sexuality issues most effectively, rehabilitation professionals must rely on a holistic approach to define the problematic areas, determine what changes can realistically be made, and work toward effecting those changes and accepting what cannot be changed. It is essential that this treatment approach be started early on in the rehabilitation process with both the person and family and continued throughout the continuum of care.

OVERVIEW OF SEXUAL
DYSFUNCTION AFTER TRAUMATIC BRAIN INJURY

In spite of the significant role that sexual satisfaction plays in contemporary society, there have been few studies that have examined the realm of sexuality after TBI. This is particularly surprising when one realizes the number of studies that have been published on both neuromedical and psychological aspects of traumatic brain injury.

Bond (1976) found no correlation between the duration of post-traumatic amnesia, level of physical disability, or cognitive impairment and level of sexual activity. Lishman (1973), in her classic article reviewing the neuropsychiatric sequelae of TBI, found that decreases in libido seemed to correlate with the severity of brain injury. Lezak (1978) as well as Sbordone (1984) noted that reports of sexual dysfunction after TBI seemed to be quite common. Rosenbaum and Najenson (1976), studying a small group of persons, found a drastic reduction in sexual relations, with no clearcut relationship between locus of injury and presence of sexual dysfunction. Weinstein and Kahn (1976) examined patterns of sexual dysfunction following brain injury and found that approximately 20% showed alterations in sexual behavior for at least 1 week during the study period. A study by Miller et al. (1986) described eight persons who became either hypersexual or homosexual following injury. Kosteljanetz et al. (1981) examined 19 males post-concussion and found a 58% incidence of sexual dysfunction in this small group. He also noted that the degree of dysfunction was highly correlated with the extent of intellectual impairment and cerebral atrophy by CAT scan.

Kreutzer and Zasler (1989) found that the majority of 21 males with brain injury reported negative changes in sexual behavior, including decreased libido, erectile function, and frequency of intercourse. There was correlation between affective disturbance and sexual dysfunction. Most subjects reported a good marital relationship despite problems in the realm of sexuality.

It becomes quickly apparent that there is an obvious trend in the data being generated even in light of the limited research in this area. The trend indicates that traumatic brain injury typically results in alterations in sexual behavior, as well as function, and most typically these changes are more pronounced with more severe injuries.

SEXUALITY AND DISABILITY

Sexuality is an excellent example of an integrative function, requiring the integration of physical, cognitive, and psycho-behavioral components in order to be adequately expressed. Rehabilitation professionals should be committed to addressing issues of sexuality as readily as they address issues related to mobility, self-care, and bowel and bladder management. A "double sensitivity" often exists regarding sexuality and disability on the part of the person with TBI, the family, and the health care professional (Chigier, 1980). Professionals and family members must overcome any and all emotional roadblocks that prevent them from accepting that a person with a brain injury can be and generally is a sexual being. All must learn to accept this fact, whether it be in terms of sexual rights, rehabilitation, or family/attendant counseling.

CONTROVERSIAL SEXUALITY ISSUES AFTER TBI

The rehabilitation health care professional is obliged to address certain issues related to sexuality that many might label as highly controversial. Among these topics are potential questions from both persons with TBI, spouses, and family regarding sex education and birth control, sexually transmitted disease, sexual abuse, issues of sexual release, masturbation, use of pornographic materials, and dating.

Birth control need only be addressed if it is truly a potential concern. Methods must be chosen only after fertility is established and the patient's physical and cognitive limitations clarified. Generally, patients who have been deemed competent and have the capability to understand and remember the ramifications of their actions are *probably* capable of being sexually active in a responsible manner. In light of the ever-present fear of AIDS (acquired immune deficiency syndrome) and other sexually transmitted diseases, both males and females should be instructed regarding the appropriate and timely use of condoms. Responsible decisions regarding sexual relations are critical for single and married persons with brain injury. Ongoing follow-up is essential to ensure that there is compliance with the program as well as satisfaction in the sex life as appropriate.

Health care professionals are obligated to ensure that if the person with TBI, a family member, an attendant, or an aquaintance is engaged in sexual misconduct, the proper authorities are informed. More radical methods of birth control, that is, sterilization, might be recommended for patients unable to make reliable and competent sexual decisions. If sexual abuse is suspected, the professional may be obligated to have the individual removed from the particular environment where it is occurring.

Alternatives for sexual release should be given for patients who are not sexually active for whatever reason. Masturbation should be encouraged as a form of sexual release as long as it is done in an appropriate environment. As necessary, the person with brain injury can be provided with additional sexual stimuli such as erotic reading material, pictures, or videotapes. There are and most likely will always be other alternative means of sexual release for anyone desirous of it and able to purchase it, that is, telephone sex services, sexual surrogates, and prostitution. The concept of sexual surrogates is quite controversial but intriguing nonetheless. Some health care professionals have advocated for the use of surrogates to help persons with TBI with proper psychosexual graces, as well as with attaining sexual satisfaction. Due to the present litigious nature of this society and Judeo-Christian moral and ethical beliefs, such solutions, although sound in principle (assuming the financial resources are available), may be perceived as too radical by most health care professionals, families, and society. Obviously, as noted previously, recommendations need to be made with the person's and family's moral, cultural, and educational background in mind.

Dating can be and generally is a very anxiety-provoking experience for persons with brain injury, particularly when they have more significant neurophysical or cognitive-behavioral deficits. Single persons should be encouraged, as appropriate, to pursue normal interactions with their peers of either gender. Typically, many of these individuals are unable, or at least think they are unable, to find a compatible companion of the opposite sex. Various recommendations can be provided to encourage reintegration into society and maximize the potential for resocialization. Attending social gatherings of head injury groups, churchs, synagogues, and local organizations is one alternative. Other more unique ideas include dating services for persons with disabilities (Garden, 1988) such as Handicapped Introductions (HI) and DateAble, which are national dating services providing individuals with disabilities the opportunity to meet each other.

On a less intimate basis, other unique programs such as the Partner's Program of Richmond (Morton, in press), hopefully a model to be used nationally, provide a starting point for resocialization by providing friendships (nonintimate) for persons with brain injury with volunteers without brain injury. This program, which is modeled after Big Brothers and Big Sisters, provides a starting point for the relearning of lost skills in the area of psychosocial and psycho-sexual conduct and may well be a stepping stone to the development of further social contacts and more intimate relationships.

SEXUAL PROBLEMS AND THE FAMILY

Sexual problems following traumatic brain injury can occur in the context of at least three types of family situations. First, persons with brain injury, typically adolescents or young adults, may be living with their parents. They may be unable to maintain sexual relationships established pre-injury and/or establish new relationships post-injury. Sexual problems for these individuals often center around finding a suitable partner as well as diminished physical capabilities. Second, a number of persons are able to maintain previously established relationships. These persons may be married, living with a significant other, or single and dating. Diminished frequency of intercourse and physical dysfunction may stem from emotional as well as physical problems encountered by either or both partners in the relationship. Third, sexual problems may arise between married partners, neither of whom has had an injury. Their sexual problems may be attributable to the negative consequences of head injury to their child. For example, parents may find themselves overwhelmed by the stresses associated with the demands of rehabilitation, guilt regarding causes of injury, maintaining a household, and the often difficult search for appropriate services. Sexual disinterest, diminished frequency of intercourse, or physical dysfunction may result.

Psychological as well as physical difficulties may contribute to sexual problems. In a limited number of cases, the person with the injury has a primarily physiological problem that results in orgasmic dysfunction. The individual may no longer be capable of achieving sexual satisfaction using previously successful techniques. In most cases, emotionally well-adjusted partners are able to adapt and compensate for physical problems. Sexual satisfaction remains achievable because both partners are emotionally stable and committed to maintaining their relationship. However, persons with brain injury usually have difficulty maintaining emotional stability. Those who served as their partners pre-injury also have difficulty maintaining emotional health post-injury. Grieving, adverse characterological changes resulting from the injury, and the stresses of caretaking seriously challenge emotional stability. Ambivalence or adversity toward maintaining a relationship often results. Notably, sexual difficulties in a majority of cases are primarily attributable to emotional and psychological problems.

The following three sections provide a discussion of sexual problems encountered by persons with head injury in each of three family situations: 1) the single individual living with parents; 2) the married individual living with the spouse; and 3) parents living together having a child with head injury. Each section contains a description of potential problems as well as suggestions for addressing and preventing sexual problems that are likely to occur.

Single Individuals Living with Parents

Epidemiologic research on traumatic brain injury indicates that a majority of persons with severe injury are single (e.g., Jacobs, 1988; Kozloff, 1987). In many cases, the effects of injury cause previously successful relationships to dissolve. Those who did not have a relationship prior to their injury often have difficulty establishing relationships post-injury. Adverse characterological, intellectual, and physical changes, as well as negative societal attitudes toward persons with disabilities contribute to difficulties establishing satisfying relationships. For those able to sustain relationships following injury, the effects of the injury and the diverse efforts required to actively participate in rehabilitation present formidable, long-term challenges to the maintenance of relationships.

There is little doubt that persons with head injury become more dependent on their families following injury (Jacobs, 1988). Research by Kozloff (1987) has indicated that social network density increases over time post-injury, with a corresponding decrease in the size of the network. In other words, persons with head injury become more socially isolated, have fewer friends, and rely more heavily on remaining support systems for emotional and physical needs. Kozloff found that most single people spent more time with their families partly because peers were apparently disinterested in maintaining previously established relationships. Thomsen (1974) reported similar post-injury changes in peer and family relationships.

Unfortunately, family members are often ill-prepared to assist the single person with brain injury in coping with sexual and social problems arising from injury. During adolescence, teenagers learn about sexual behavior and develop techniques for resolving sexual concerns through discussion with their peers. Occasionally, teenagers may discuss sexual concerns with an older sibling. On rare occasions, sexual concerns may be directed toward parents. Problem resolution becomes more difficult post-injury because persons with head injury most often do not have peer support systems for discussing sexual concerns. Furthermore, parents have little experience addressing sexual concerns with their children. Appropriate advice from peers or parents is difficult to obtain also because of ignorance regarding the effects of brain injury. Undoubtedly, the cognitive and emotional sequelae of brain injury complicate problems of sexual adjustment. Sexual adjustment is typically a challenge even for healthy adolescents and young adults.

Hesitancy to discuss sexual concerns with parents may reflect the person's beliefs that such a role is inappropriate for parents; concerns that parents may be critical; or deteriorations in the parent-child relationship, which may arise from perceived insensitivity, misunderstanding, and overprotectiveness. Parents may convey discomfort partly because of their inexperience in addressing their children's sexual matters, ignorance about means of problem resolution, and beliefs that sexuality should only be a concern for persons who are married. Parents may also express the opinion that sexual issues should be put off until the person is completely recovered both physically and cognitively.

Difficulties in establishing sexual relationships post-injury are attributable to a number of factors. Willingness to develop interpersonal and sexual relationships following brain injury is adversely affected by depression and lack of initiative. In some cases, depression and lack of initiative may stem from physiological and neurochemical changes in the nervous system. However, emotional and volitional changes may also arise as a reaction to the psycho-social consequences of injury. Loss of friends, cognitive abilities, work, and previously earned responsibilities and privileges contribute to grief and depression. Repeated failures also contribute to pessimism and diminished motivation. In a prospective study of psycho-sexual consequences of brain injury, Kreutzer and Zasler (1989) found increased depression, diminished sex drive, and reduced self-confidence in nearly two thirds of persons in their sample. Similarly, Mauss-Clum and Ryan (1981) found that a majority of patients with brain injury demonstrated depression (57%) and decreased initiative (53%).

Opportunities for meeting persons of the opposite sex can be limited by physical problems (e.g., fatigability, seizures); parental overprotectiveness; or the lack of transportation. For those unable to drive because of physical or financial problems, public transportation is often unavailable. Family members may be unwilling to provide transportation or the person with a head injury may feel uncomfortable adding transportation for socialization purposes to an already large list of parental responsibilities.

Those who have transportation available may be entirely self-conscious regarding their personal appearance and the reactions of others. Disfigurement from the injury, word-finding problems, difficulty attending in conversations involving more than one person, and cognitive deficits contribute to shyness and discomfort in public situations. Negative societal attitudes toward persons with disabilities also contribute to heightened tension in social situations. Persons who are insensitive may make crude comments or even ridicule the person with head injury. Many persons with head injury simply may choose to avoid the many anxieties likely to arise in interactions with strangers who may be insensitive, feeling more comfortable at home.

Those who are not self-conscious may have difficulty behaving appropriately in social situations because of cognitive impairments including poor self-awareness. Social facility is a complicated skill that requires good communication skills, the ability to empathize, an appropriate sense of humor, and memory for conversation. Persons with head injury may misconstrue the demands of a situation and misinterpret the reactions of others. Impatience, apprehensions arising from previous frustrations and failures, as well as incorrect interpretations of a partner's behavior may result in sexual advances that are far too premature. Such behavior may be interpreted by the intended partner as aggressive, insensitive, and anxiety-provoking.

For those who are able to establish intimate relationships with persons of the opposite sex, challenges to developing a mutually satisfying sexual relationship often arise. Performance anxiety, self-consciousness, fear of rejection, and recent inexperience may contribute to initial difficulties. Cognitive, physical, and communication impairments also contribute to difficulties attending to and satisfying the sexual needs of the partner.

The reader may feel overwhelmed after reviewing the list of potential obstacles to developing and maintaining sexual relationships following head trauma. Persons with head injury are often overwhelmed by these many obstacles. Fortunately, appropriate intervention by rehabilitation professionals can do much to relieve anxieties, improve performance, increase self-confidence, and diminish frustration levels.

Initial assessment begins with a thorough medical examination by an experienced physiatrist in conjunction with an interview with the person and family to address psycho-sexual and psycho-social issues. The major components of the General Rehabilitation Assessment Sexuality Profile (GRASP) include the sexual history, sexual physical examination, and clinical sexual diagnostic testing (Zasler & Horn, 1990). The physiatrist can provide appropriate referral and/or medical treatment for sexual dysfunction, enhancement of independent living skills, and pharmacologic treatment for amelioration of emotional disturbance. The physiatrist can also improve the person's sexual functioning by helping the individual reach maximum levels of independence through improved physical functioning and fitness.

Assessment by mental health professionals addresses the level of support provided by the family, knowledge about head injury, and attitudes toward the person's sexuality. In regard to the patient, the clinician should assess cognitive and interpersonal skills, degree of social involvement, and emotional status. A thorough neuropsychological examination helps to establish levels of cognitive, communicative, intellectual, and psycho-motor functioning. Furthermore, thorough examination of the person and interview with the family helps in the evaluation of executive functioning with respect to organization, initiation, self-awareness, planning, and problem-solving ability.

Most often, improved sexual satisfaction can best be achieved through participation in a holistic rehabilitation program that addresses the person's physical, medical, emotional, cognitive, and interpersonal needs as well. Because of interdependency among sexual and other skills, programs that address sexual functioning solely without considering related processes are likely to fail. In many cases, day rehabilitation and independent living programs offer the variety of services necessary to yield the greatest overall benefits in sexual as well as psycho-social functioning.

Consider the indirect and direct benefits to sexual functioning by implementation of the following set of interventions. Fatigability and cognitive dysfunction are reduced when the physician alters the person's seizure medication. A course of cognitive remediation therapy improves memory and attentional skills. The person is referred for a driving evaluation, subsequently participates in a specialized driving course, and ultimately receives a driver's license. A social skills program enhances communication skills and improves self-awareness. Referral to and participation in physical therapy improves ambulation and stamina. Participation in a supported employment program results in finding long-term employment following years of difficulty finding and maintaining jobs. Notably, these interventions are intended to increase independence and the person's sense of physical well-being. Indirectly, the benefits would likely include reduced depression, increased self-confidence, increased socialization, and improved social skills. Rehabilitation would ultimately benefit the person's ability to seek a partner, establish an intimate personal relationship, and achieve sexual satisfaction.

Mental health practitioners can directly benefit the patient and family by using a variety of techniques. A series of meetings held with family members can provide education regarding the overall effects of injury. Family members may need to acknowledge the importance of the person's sexual and emotional needs relative to other areas of rehabilitation. Parents may require help to acknowledge that persons with disabilities have sexual needs and desires that are similar to those of persons without disabilities. The clinician will be most effective by considering the family's religious and cultural beliefs in providing intervention and education. Parents may also need reminders that masturbation is normal and may be the person's only sexual outlet. Allowing the person appropriate opportunities for sexual expression often reduces the incidence of behaviors such as exhibitionism and sexually explicit verbal expressions, which are frequently labeled inappropriate.

Parents typically should not be encouraged to assume the primary role of sexual advisor to the person with head injury. Peers, older siblings, and the mental health professional can more appropriately assume this role. Furthermore, the clinician is encouraged to be cautious in discussing the person's sexuality with family members. Right to privacy should not be violated, and individual therapy sessions with the person are most appropriate for discussion of intimate concerns. Whenever possible during meetings including other family members, the therapist should obtain the person's permission to discuss material that may be perceived as personal.

Individual psychotherapy provides a safe environment for discussion of personal concerns. The availability of a trained therapist also provides parents with respite and reinforces the idea that they cannot be expected to meet their child's needs entirely. Therapy sessions to improve sexual, psychological, and interpersonal functioning may focus on developing relaxation strategies, improved problem-solving, and behavioral rehearsal for anxiety-arousing social/sexual situations. The therapist can provide support by acknowledging the client's struggle to improve, providing encouragement, and giving positive feedback for appropriate behaviors both inside and outside the therapy session. Clients must often be reminded of progress since their initial injury. Many persons with head injury inherently feel a sense of failure because they compare themselves to their pre-injury status. Reminders that sexual needs are normal, that society is often unfair to persons with disabilities, and reassurance that additional progress is possible with continued effort is frequently beneficial.

Discussion in individual therapy can focus on perceived failures in previous relationships, anxieties about sexual performance, and fears of rejection in attempts to establish a relationship. Confidence-building is an important therapeutic goal given the many failures often experienced by persons with head injury. Clients need help to accept that additional failures are possible and probable. Failures as well as successes are an inevitable consequence of trying. Both experiences offer a learning opportunity. The client also needs help to understand that persons without head injury also have difficulties establishing satisfactory relationships. In at least some cases, rejections by desired partners may not be a reflection specifically on the issue of head injury. Rejection of sexual advances may simply indicate that the relationship requires additional development and commitment.

In every case, clients should be encouraged to select partners with whom they have established a pattern of frequent, clear, and honest communication. Good communication helps avoid failures and rejections that may arise from misinterpretation of nonverbal messages. Partners who are patient, empathic, and accepting are likely to be sensitive to the client's special needs arising from injury. Clients should also be encouraged to communicate appropriately following perceived rejection from a potential partner they have known for some time. Discussion helps the client avoid reaching conclusions regarding personal behavior that are entirely unfounded. Angry words, a tantrum, or ignoring the other person inevitably hurts the client because these behaviors provide little or no opportunity for learning from the experience.

Ideally, individuals should be encouraged in and provided with opportunities for socialization with peers. Socialization allows the opportunity to develop friendships as well as dating and sexual relationships. Persons with head injury should be given a choice as to whether they wish to socialize with other persons having similar injuries. Some individuals feel safer within groups of persons having similar disabilities. Peer support groups offer a unique opportunity for sharing concerns as well as discussion of solutions to shared problems. Other clients may feel uncomfortable in groups of persons having disabilities. Religious and volunteer groups offer relatively comfortable alternative opportunities for socialization. Classes, intramural sports, social clubs, and groups of persons with shared hobbies also provide social opportunities.

Married Persons Living with Spouses

A minority of persons who sustain traumatic brain injury were married at the time of their injury. A smaller number were living with a significant other. Others were involved in steady dating relationships. These individuals develop a unique set of concerns in their efforts to maintain a satisfying relationship post-injury. Unfortunately, many of the relationships between single persons dissolve within the first year post-injury. Those who remain married face long-term challenges that threaten preservation of their emotional and sexual relationships.

The typical consequences of traumatic brain injury often affect the willingness and/or ability of both partners to engage in sexual activity. The partner without injury is most often a wife whose ability and desire for sexual satisfaction may be compromised by several stressful factors. Jacobs (1988) completed a survey of 142 families having persons with severe traumatic brain injury. His survey identified major sources of stress on family members and indicated that head injury had adverse effects on family systems years after injury. Despite their lack of formal training, family members were reportedly the primary source of therapy for many persons, due to the lack of services in the community. Ignorance about managing problems at home, and lack of available services contribute to the spouse's feelings of guilt, inadequacy, and being overwhelmed. In 28% of cases examined by Jacobs, family income was exhausted through payment for medical and rehabilitative services related to the injury. In approximately 37% of cases the person required constant supervision necessitated partly by the severity of the person's disability. In many cases uninjured family members left their jobs to assume home care activities.

Undoubtedly, the financial, physical, and emotional consequences of head trauma serve as major stressors to marital relationships and family activities. Priorities in relationships shift, with activities oriented toward stress reduction being assigned high priority relative to achievement of sexual satisfaction. Spouses without injury may exhaust their energy in attempts to find or provide services, maintain the smooth functioning of a household, and meet the emotional and physical needs of healthy children.

Role changes in the family arising from the injury can affect the willingness of spouses to engage in sexual activity. Pre-injury, marital relationships were likely to have involved equitable sharing of responsibilities among two persons in relatively normal adult roles. Following the injury, the partner with TBI is likely to have far fewer responsibilities and to become more dependent on the partner without injury. For example, the husband may be unable to work or resume household and child rearing responsibilities because of physical and cognitive impairments. Financially, the family may become entirely dependent on the wife's income. The wife may need to work longer hours to help pay medical bills and offset her husband's loss of income. Additionally, the wife may assume nearly all child rearing and household responsibilities. In her attempts to meet numerous additional responsibilities, the wife is likely to become both mentally and physically exhausted.

Typically, sexual relationships are likely to be most satisfying when both partners are able to assume adult roles. Many spouses report that their husband's have become more childlike following their injury. Husbands with injury are often described as behaving less maturely than the couple's children. Lezak (1978) has indicated that common characterological alterations subsequent to brain injury include self-centeredness and immaturity. Mauss-Clum and Ryan (1981), in their survey of family members, found that nearly 50% or more of persons with brain injury displayed childish behaviors including dependency, impatience, decreased self-control, self-centeredness, and inappropriate public behavior.

Because of physical disability, cognitive impairments, childishness, and poor self-awareness, wives often find themselves taking a parental role with the spouse with TBI. Restricting activities, giving regular feedback about appropriate and inappropriate behavior, providing assistance with activities of daily living, and ensuring that one's spouse follows the recommendations of professionals are responsibilities often assumed by spouses without injury. Reactions of rebellion and resentment demonstrated by the person with TBI who feels unnecessarily helped or restricted contribute to the spouse's apprehensions and feelings that her or his job is a thankless one. Notably, marital and sexual relationships are entered into on a voluntary basis. Unfortunately, many spouses report that they feel trapped (Mauss-Clum & Ryan, 1981).

Aggressive behaviors demonstrated by persons with head injury also diminish their ability to establish intimate relationships. For spouses without injury, previous feelings of affection and intimacy may be replaced by feelings of fear and resentment. Nearly one fourth of spouses surveyed by Mauss-Clum and Ryan (1981) reported that they had been verbally abused and threatened with physical violence. Brooks, Campsie, Symington, Beattie, and McKinlay (1986) followed a sample of 42 patients 5 years post-severe TBI. Relatives reported that a majority of persons were irritable and had a bad temper. Comparison of 5-year outcome data with information obtained at 1 year post-injury revealed that the number of persons with TBI who had threatened others with violence had increased with the passage of time, from 15% of the sample at 1 year to 54% at 5 years. Additionally, 20% of relatives had been assaulted on one or more occasions, and 31% of the persons with TBI had been in trouble with the law one or more times following injury.

Extreme and adverse personality changes arising from brain injury detract from the familiarity and intimacy that underlie a satisfying sexual relationship. Mauss-Clum and Ryan (1981) reported that many wives felt that they were married to a stranger. A number of wives also reported they felt as if they were married, but had no spouse. Obviously, spouses often miss the emotional support once provided by their partner.

As with single persons who have had a head injury, assessment focuses on medical factors, independent living skills, neuropsychological and emotional status, and communication skills. Partners should be interviewed regarding their pre-injury sexual adjustment, reasons for marriage, post-injury sources of stress, and individual beliefs about the value of quality of sexual satisfaction in their present relationship. Ideally, the client is able to participate in a holistic rehabilitation program that is oriented to improving overall levels of functioning, which directly and indirectly benefit the marital relationship.

The spouses without TBI benefit from education regarding the effects of injury as well as knowledge of behavior management strategies. Occasionally, spouses feel they must tolerate disinhibited and aggressive behaviors. They may offer excuses for the person such as, "He can't help himself; he's had a head injury." In these situations, spouses can be taught not to accept, but to help the person gain better control over aversive behaviors using simple behavior management strategies. The person must be treated as a responsible adult by being provided with consistent feedback and consequences for abusive or offensive behaviors.

The couple can also be helped by rehabilitation efforts directed toward improvement in daily living skills and equitable sharing of responsibilities. Shifting responsibilities closer to pre-injury levels also helps to re-establish former sexual roles. Unfortunately, problems with initiative, memory, or other cognitive impairments may interfere with the ability of the spouse with TBI to share in household responsibilities. However, as described by Kreutzer, Wehman, Morton, and Stonnington (1988), structuring daily activities by using checklists, and carrying out tasks routinely, at the same time in the same sequence every day, can help minimize the adverse effects of cognitive impairments.

Assisting clients in development and maintenance of good communication skills is perhaps the most important challenge for the mental health therapist. Previously effective means of communication may no longer be effective because of injury-related cognitive impairments and the presence of additional stressors. Frequent, direct communication allows spouses without TBI the important opportunity to indicate personal needs and frustrations. Communication regarding sexual issues is also vital to mutual satisfaction. Both spouses should be encouraged to discuss their sexual needs openly. Within this context, issues regarding intimacy and emotional needs should be discussed as well. Both partners should also share feedback about means of better meeting personal needs. Notably, persons with head injury often respond positively when they hear of the difficulties and frustrations encountered by their spouses in attempting to help them recover.

Unfortunately, some spouses prefer to bear the burden of caretaking alone, and act as "martyrs." The therapist may need to point out instances in which the "martyr" has chosen her or his role and rejected help. Spouses with injury need appropriate reminders that the injury has added to their partner's responsibilities and caused stress to both members of the marital dyad. Despite injury, couples should work as a team to overcome obstacles imposed by the injury and share responsibility as equally as possible. In other situations, the therapist helps the couple become aware of circular blaming behaviors, which interfere with effective problem-solving.

In cases of severe injury or crisis, individual psychotherapy sessions may be desirable. Individual sessions can help the spouse without injury to express feelings more freely. The therapist provides feedback regarding the spouse's actions, assists in problem-solving, and suggests solutions for recurrent problems. In many problem situations, there is no ideal solution. Frequently, spouses need reassurance that their frustrations arise from difficulties inherent in their situation, rather than from personal inadequacies. Spouses without injury experiencing severe emotional distress may require psychotropic medications to alleviate symptoms of depression and anxiety. Panting and Merry (1972) reported that 61% of relatives of persons with severe head injury had required tranquilizers or sleeping tablets to cope with the sequelae of injury. Mauss-Clum and Ryan (1981) have also reported a reliance on pharmacologic agents by relatives to facilitate post-injury emotional adjustment.

Following head injury, couples typically become socially isolated and the souse without injury may become entirely immersed in meeting the needs of the spouse with injury as well as children. Clinicians must encourage spouses to seek opportunities for respite and fulfill their own personal needs. The therapist provides "permission" and assurance to the spouse without injury by indicating that attention to personal needs allows development of stamina necessary to best meet the needs of the person with TBI and other family members. Additionally, attendance at head injury support meetings provides an opportunity for spouses to discuss mutual problems and solutions with other family members in similar situations. Spending time with friends and participating in social gatherings provides a chance to enjoy recreational pursuits and to focus on other topics besides head injury and rehabilitation.

Sexual Relationships of Parents Who Have Children with Brain Injuries

If the person with head trauma is a child, the sexual relationship of the parents may be negatively affected by a variety of stressors. In the absence of actual responsibility for the child's injury, parents often feel guilty. Gardner (1973) has suggested that guilt may help parents gain a greater sense of control, enabling them to reduce anxieties about the occurrence of a second head injury. Parents often become preoccupied with guilt. Personal needs may be sublimated entirely in an all-consuming effort to meet the needs of the child with TBI.

Consider the family in which a father and son were hit from behind by a speeding dump truck while stopped at a stop sign. The child was not wearing a seat belt; his head struck the windshield, resulting in a severe head injury. The father, who was wearing his seat belt, sustained minor injuries. Post-injury, the father's preoccupation with seeking services for his child with TBI was as much a consequence of guilt as responsibility. He neglected the needs of his wife and children without injury in this pursuit. The wife was overcome with anger toward the husband because of his perceived irresponsibility in not requiring the child to wear a seat belt. The wife became preoccupied with thoughts such as, "He would have been OK if his father had made him wear his seat belt," or "I would have made our son wear his seat belt." In this case, the father's preoccupation with guilt, exhaustion in his time-consuming search for services, and consequent neglect of his wife's emotional needs contributed to marital and sexual problems. Similarly, the wife's anger toward her husband, grieving for her child who was injured unnecessarily, and guilt about possible actions she could have taken to prevent the injury adversely affected the couple's relationship as well.

A variety of clinical interventions can help parents of children with head injury return to previous levels of sexual functioning. Initially, during the assessment process, clinicians should establish parental anxiety levels, sources of stress, belief systems regarding causes of injury, degree of involvement with the child's rehabilitation, parents' willingness to fulfill their own personal needs, and their sensitivity to those needs. History-taking allows the clinician to develop an accurate idea of pre-injury baseline levels of sexual functioning, which serves as a benchmark in establishing goals of intervention. Appropriate assessment allows the clinician to build a family intervention plan that enhances the quality of the parental relationship, reduces anxieties, identifies stressors, improves mutual problem-solving strategies, identifies areas where parental intervention is helpful or harmful, and ultimately benefits the couple's sexual relationship.

The clinician is encouraged to help relieve family members of guilt associated with the initial injury. Parents often need frequent assurance and reminders that the past cannot be changed and that dwelling on the past can only serve as an obstacle to achieving current goals. When appropriate, parents can also be reminded that they have always tried to act in the best interests of their child and that nobody intentionally contributed to the child's accident. The clinician can help parents recognize and avoid blaming behaviors and their adverse effect on anxiety levels and family teamwork.

In many cases, rehabilitation services for children are inadequate. Perhaps because fewer children than adults are injured, rehabilitation programs for children have lagged behind those for older persons. Parents often become frustrated in their efforts to find appropriate services, can easily become entirely immersed in the search for help, and may occasionally blame the lack of rehabilitation resources on their own inadequacy. Clinicians can help reduce family anxieties regarding the scarcity of services by acting as advocates, making families aware of available community resources, and making referrals. Frequent reassurance that parents are doing all that is possible can also help alleviate feelings of guilt and anxiety.

Parents are encouraged to view themselves as a team and are advised of the philosophy that teamwork is the most effective approach to rehabilitation. Parents often believe that personal needs must be sublimated entirely to meet the needs of the child with TBI. Lezak (1978, 1986) has encouraged clinicians to pressure family members to acknowledge personal needs. Parents may also require reminders that they can be more helpful to their child if they are emotionally and physically healthy. Encouragement to seek respite and spend quality time together often helps restore marital intimacy and the quality of sexual relationships. As an authority, the clinician relieves guilt about meeting personal needs by giving parents "permission" to do so. In some cases, "doctor's orders" may be necessary. Frank discussions with parents regarding individual sexual needs and priorities will also yield important benefits.

Family members often become overprotective and overinvolved in caring for the children with head injury. Of course, these behaviors detract from their ability to meet personal needs. Rehabilitation professionals can help parents to develop reasonable levels of concern and involvement in their child's recovery. Gordon (1975) has described the pitfalls of overprotectiveness and parents' fears about children making mistakes. He noted that parents are often overcontrolling due to their concerns about children's reaction to failure. They may believe they can preserve the children's psychological well-being by helping them avoid mistakes. Yet, Gordon has indicated that mistakes are an important part of the learning process. Children may learn as much or more from their failures as from their successes. Furthermore, overprotectiveness indirectly conveys to children that their parents perceive them as inadequate or incompetent. Appropriate levels of permissiveness convey acceptance. Gordon strongly suggests that parents allow their children to make mistakes, but be available to provide emotional support following failure when needed. By reducing levels of involvement to reasonable levels, parents can redirect their energies to meeting their interpersonal and sexual needs.

CONCLUSION

All attempts should be made to teach persons with TBI, partners, and other family members healthy sexual attitudes. As rehabilitationists, we must debunk the myth that disability excludes sexuality and that sexual intercourse culminating in orgasm is essential for sexual satisfaction. We must provide both the individual and the family with education regarding psychologic and physiologic aspects of brain injury and how these can adversely affect sexual function and sexuality. Reinforce the concept that the sexual problem(s) result(s) from the brain injury and is not a consequence of misdoing by the individual or family member. Be mature yet open in discussions with individuals and family members, and acknowledge the fact that sexuality is difficult for many people to discuss. Many persons may simply require the *rehabilitationist's* permission to discuss and acknowledge *their* sexual concerns before they open up. Professionals must help individuals and families identify what the problematic sexuality areas are, determine what changes can be made, work toward effecting those changes, and accept those that cannot be changed.

Sexuality and sexual satisfaction are extremely important parts of the overall experience of being alive and human and also of being in love. Rehabilitation professionals are encouraged to address sexuality issues with both persons with TBI and family members throughout the continuum of care, just as issues pertaining to other areas of function, such as mobility, self-care, or vocational reentry, are pursued. Only in this manner can rehabilitation efforts be truly fruitful and rewarding to individual, family members, and rehabilitation staff alike.

REFERENCES

Boller, F., & Frank, E. (1982). *Sexual dysfunction in neurological disorders.* New York: Raven Press.

Bond, M.R. (1976). Assessment of psychosocial outcome of severe head injury. *Acta Neurochirrurgica, 34,* 57–70.

Brooks, D.N., Campsie, L., Symington, C., Beattie, A., & McKinlay, W. (1986). The five year outcome of severe blunt head injury: A relative's view. *Journal of Neurology, Neurosurgery and Psychiatry, 49,* 764–770.

Chigier, E. (1980). Sexuality of physically disabled people. *Clinics in Obstetrics and Gynaecology, 7,* 325–343.

Garden, F. (1988, September). Dating services for the disabled: *Sexuality Update. Newsletter for the National Task Force on Sexuality and Disability, American Congress of Rehabilitation Medicine, 1,* 4.

Gardner, R.A. (1973). *The family book about minimal brain dysfunction.* New York: Jason Aronson.

Gordon, T. (1975). *Parent effectiveness training.* New York: The New American Library.

Horn, H.J., & Zasler, N.D. (1990). Neuroanatomy and neurophysiology of sexual function. *Journal of Head Trauma Rehabilitation 5*(2), 1–13.

Jacobs, H.E. (1988). The Los Angeles head injury survey: Procedures and initial findings. *Archives of Physical Medicine and Rehabilitation, 69,* 425–431.

Kosteljanetz, M., Jensen, T. S., Nørgård, B., Lunde, I., Jensen, P. B., & Johnsen, S. G. (1981). Sexual and hypothalamic dysfunction in the post-concussional syndrome. *Acta Neurologica Scandanavica, 63,* 169–180.

Kozloff, R. (1987). Networks of social support and the outcome from severe head injury. *Journal of Head Trauma Rehabilitation, 2*(3), 14–23.

Kreutzer, J.S., Wehman, P., Morton, M.V., & Stonnington, H. (1988). Supported employment and compensatory strategies for enhancing vocational outcome following traumatic brain injury. *Brain Injury, 2*(3), 205–224.

Kreutzer, J.S., & Zasler, N.D. (1989). Psychosexual consequences of traumatic brain injury. *Brain-Injury, 3*(2), 177–186.

Kreutzer, J.S., Zasler, N.D., Camplair, P.S., & Leininger, B.E. (1990). A practical guide to family intervention following adult traumatic brain injury. In J. Kreutzer & P. Wehman (Eds.), *Community integration following traumatic brain injury,* Baltimore: Paul H. Brookes Publishing Co.

Lezak, M.D. (1978). Living with the characterologically altered brain-injured patient. *Journal of Clinical Psychiatry, 39,* 592–598.

Lezak, M.D. (1986). Psychological implications of traumatic brain damage for the patient's family. *Rehabilitation Psychology, 31,* 241–250.

Lishman, W.A. (1973). The psychiatric sequelae of head injury: A review. *Psychological Medicine, 3,* 304–318.

Mauss-Clum, N., & Ryan, M. (1981). Brain injury and the family. *Journal of Neurosurgical Nursing, 13*(4), 165–169.

Miller, B. L., Cummings, J. L., McIntyre, H., Ebers, G., Grode, M. (1986). Hypersexuality or altered sexual preference following brain injury. *Journal of Neurology, Neurosurgery, and Psychology, 49,* 867–873.

Morton, M.V. (in press). *An experimental study to assess the effects of the community socialization program for individuals with moderate and severe traumatic brain injury.* Unpublished doctoral dissertation, Virginia Commonwealth University, Richmond.

Panting, A., & Merry, P. (1972). The long term rehabilitation of severe head injuries with particular reference to the need for social and medical support for the patient's family. *Journal of Rehabilitation, 38,* 33–37.

Price, J.R. (1988). Sexuality following traumatic brain injury. In M.E. Miner & K.A. Wagner (Eds.), *Neurotrauma treatment, rehabilitation, and related issues* (pp. 173–180). Boston: Butterworths.

Rosenbaum, M., & Najenson, T. (1976). Changes in life patterns and symptoms of low mood as reported by wives of severely brain injured soldiers. *Journal of Consulting and Clinical Psychology, 44,* 881–888.

Sbordone, R. J. (1984). Rehabilitative neuropsychological approach for severe traumatic brain-injured patients. *Professional Psychology Research & Practice, 15,* 165–175.

Thomsen, I.V. (1974). The patient with severe head injury and his family. *Journal of Rehabilitation Medicine, 6,* 180–183.

Weinstein, A., & Kahn, R.L. (1976). Patterns of sexual behavior following brain injury. *Psychiatry, 24,* 69–78.

Zasler, N.D., & Horn, L.J. (1990). Rehabilitative management of sexual dysfunction. *Journal of Head Trauma Rehabilitation, 5*(2), 14–24.

V

FAMILY INTERVENTION TECHNIQUES

Section V presents the resources and tools for family support. A sytems perspective provides information on self help, support by and for professionals, family therapy, social support, and individual advocacy. This approach does not focus on any one individual; rather, it focuses on the need for people to support one another to achieve true community for individuals, families, and other important people in their lives at any given time.

271

18

INTERDISCIPLINARY FAMILY EDUCATION IN HEAD INJURY REHABILITATION

MITCHELL ROSENTHAL
BRADLEY HUTCHINS

In the 1970s, families were often considered bystanders in the process of head injury rehabilitation, not well-informed as to the nature of brain injury, confused about the personality changes observed in their loved ones, and compelled to make important short- and long-term decisions with little security that their decision-making was appropriate. The 1980s have witnessed revolutionary changes in the types of services and programs available for persons with head injuries and new hopes for improved quality of life for them and their families (Rosenthal, 1989).

Past research efforts have been important in delineating the effects of traumatic head injury on the family system. Brooks, Campsie, Symington, Beattie, and McKinlay (1987) have shown that families' experience of burden caused by head injury remains until at least 7 years post-injury. In fact, in an earlier study Brooks and co-workers (1986) reported that, in a group of 39 families of people with head injury, the degree of burden shifted from a low to medium (at 1 year post-injury) to a medium to high level of burden (at 5 years post-injury). The burden experienced by families is perhaps exacerbated by the deterioration of their social network. Kozloff (1987) studied 37 families of people with brain injury and found that within 2 years post-injury, "the patient is dependent on his primary kin for financial, emotional and task-oriented support" (p. 20). Furthermore, families often feel as if they have not obtained adequate information about head injury and available services (Kozloff, 1987; Thomsen, 1974). It is, therefore, the authors' premise that the family that is overwhelmed by head injury fails to acquire or maintain social support and is inadequately informed about head injury. Lack of adequate knowledge about head injury often leads to suboptimal caregiver interaction with their relative with injury.

Today family education appears to be an integral part of the head injury rehabilitation process in virtually every inpatient rehabilitation program, yet very little has been written about this important aspect of intervention (Muir, Rosenthal, & Diehl, 1990). This chapter explores the basis for family education, its significance in the overall intervention plan, the processes inherent in model family education programs, and the manner in which family education may positively affect long-term outcome after traumatic head injury.

DEFINITION OF FAMILY EDUCATION IN REHABILITATION

In the rehabilitation setting, family education can be conceptualized as a process in which information about the nature of a disability and the pertinent rehabilitation are described in a manner so that families can apply it to help optimize outcomes. The information may be presented to individuals or groups, in a variety of formats: lecture or discussion, written materials, audiotape, videotape, and so forth. It is the authors' view that education provided by the physician, neuropsychologist, or social worker alone is inadequate to meet the educational needs of families in head injury rehabilitation. This is due to the many diverse physical, neurobehavioral, cognitive-communicative, and psycho-social difficulties that are often prevalent after severe head injury.

Family education, as an intervention strategy, overlaps with other techniques described in this volume (e.g., family therapy, support groups). Its significance in the rehabilitation process can be ascribed to several factors. First, it is probably the most pervasive form of family intervention; that is, many families will not accept or avail themselves of family counseling or peer support groups but will be more open to an educational approach. Second, it is an essential process for families to experience in all phases of rehabilitation if they are to adequately manage their relative at home or make informed decisions about future intervention programming.

TECHNIQUES USED IN FAMILY EDUCATION

Instructional Materials

An important source of education for many families is printed material specifically written in easily understood language and with figures and case illustrations to provide concrete examples of the principles that are described. Such materials are now abundant and cover diverse topics such as coma, return to work, neuroanatomy of head injury, medico-legal issues, case management, mild head injury, and so forth. In the early stages of acute care and rehabilitation, families are perplexed and emotionally overwhelmed by the changes they see in their relative. In most cases, families will acknowledge that their prior experience or knowledge of head injury was nil. Professionals should selectively guide families to materials appropriate to their concerns and the condition of their loved one. Many of these materials can be obtained directly from the National Head Injury Foundation (NHIF, 1989) or from one of its state chapters or affiliates.

Instructional Media

Many audiotapes or videotapes have been produced to illustrate the nature of head injury, residual consequences, rehabilitation options, and community services. This form of education is extremely valuable because it can provide an extremely clear picture of the process of recovery from head injury and a realistic portrait of the types of services that extend beyond the acute rehabilitation phase. For example, graphic presentations of a residential rehabilitation center may help demystify this type of program and influence families to consider such an option, if necessary. However, the professional is cautioned: not all of the commercially available tapes are suitable for viewing by all families. Some provide very graphic presentations of the mechanism of injury (e.g., automobile crashes) or focus more specifically on either very severe or mild head injury. It is also recommended that families view videotapes in the presence of professionals who discuss the content with them afterwards to assess their reactions and clarify any misinterpretations or provide additional information to supplement the video presentation.

Family Orientation

The most valuable asset a person with head injury can have is a supportive family. A coordinated family orientation and education program may facilitate advocacy and support from families of a person with a head injury. Family orientation to the rehabilitation facility and the head injury program begins prior to admission and continues through discharge.

When a person with a head injury is first admitted, the social worker meets with the family to discuss the rehabilitation program and the expectations of the family members. The family then meets with the physician, nurse, and other members of the interdisciplinary team. The family is then scheduled for a head injury orientation seminar. The initial objective of this seminar is to provide families with a general education about head injury, the recovery process, and the head injury program. Topics covered include head injury treatment, safety issues, seizure disorders, medication, and alcohol and drug interaction. The second objective is to create a forum for support among families of persons with head injuries. The group is led by a head injury clinician, with a guest speaker from a clinical specialty department.

Family Conferences

Family conferences with the interdisciplinary team are often scheduled within 10 days after admission. The primary focus is providing specific information and education to families regarding the person's status, severity of the head injury, resulting deficits, and potential recovery, from a medical, clinical, and functional viewpoint. With input from the person and family, functional rehabilitation goals are established by the team. Families are encouraged to express concerns and ask questions directly of members of the team. Additional family conferences are scheduled during the course of the rehabilitation stay depending upon the level of family involvement, the family's and the rehabilitation team's concerns, and the concerns of the person with the injury. A final family conference is scheduled just prior to the person's discharge from the inpatient rehabilitation program.

Family Education Days

For further facilitation of family education the family is scheduled for a day of rehabilitation. The family follows their relative to all scheduled therapy sessions and sessions with the primary nurse and physician. In addition to direct observation of the rehabilitation approach, the clinicians share specific intervention techniques, progress, impairments to progress, and suggestions for family members to assist in the follow-through of goals. This provides the family with an environment in which to seek discipline-specific answers to and suggestions for problems or behaviors that they may find confusing.

Day passes for the person to leave the facility to go on a visit provide another educational opportunity for the family of the person with a head injury. Prior to a day pass being approved (or, in some cases, an unsupervised but secure night pass where family members and the individual stay in an on-campus apartment within reach of nursing and medical supervision), a pass checklist of topics is discussed with the family by each member of the interdisciplinary team. Some items reviewed include management of medications, transferring the person, handling aggressive outbursts, feeding and swallowing precautions, and safety issues.

Family Education Groups

In many inpatient rehabilitation programs, structured family education groups have been established to provide a systematic approach to family education (Muir et al., 1990). These groups meet on a weekly or biweekly basis and cover a wide range of topics, usually beginning with neuroanatomy and medical aspects of head injury and ending with discharge planning and community reintegration. Typically, members of the interdisciplinary team are invited to selected sessions to present topics pertinent to their expertise such as cognitive rehabilitation, mobility training, vocational rehabilitation, and so forth. These groups, often composed of 8–12 family members, provide not only an opportunity to gain specific information, presented by lecture, discussion, and media presentation, but also a source of emotional support and a vehicle for family networking. Thereby families can share their own frustrations and solutions to various problems encountered during their own unique experience with head injury.

ROLE OF THE INTERDISCIPLINARY TEAM MEMBERS IN FAMILY EDUCATION

Fundamental to quality care of the person with injury is a well-integrated interdisciplinary team. This is also true in family education. Each member of the interdisciplinary team is essential in providing the family with education regarding head injury rehabilitation. The team is often led by a physician with a specialization in physical medicine and rehabilitation (physiatry) who has extensive experience in the management of head injury.

The physician develops, prescribes, and oversees the management, goals, and outcome of rehabilitation. The physician educates the family with respect to the pathology, mechanics, prognosis, and complications associated with head injury. Effects of medications prescribed are monitored for their impact on seizure control, spasticity, memory, agitation, and sexuality.

The nursing staff coordinates all of the nursing care needs. Working closely with the physician, the nursing staff attends to the well-being and medical condition of the person with head injury. The nursing staff will conduct many medical education classes for family members focusing on management of medications and the bowel/bladder, as well as other safety issues.

Speech-language pathology staff focus on improving the understanding of impairments of speech and language expression, auditory and reading comprehension, cognitive communication, and written and gestural communication. Specifically, the speech-language pathologist differentiates between a head injury communication disorder and aphasia. Although these two diagnoses are not entirely independent of each other, the speech-language pathologist's educational activities focus on cognitive-communication deficits, which include topic maintenance, verbosity, attention, memory, pragmatics, problem-solving, and so forth. Education also focuses on providing and increasing the family awareness of the most effective means of communicating with the person. Management of swallowing disorders, along with augmentative communication systems education, is provided to families who may require these services.

Social services staff work closely with the family to provide support during their emotional adjustment to the person's head injury. Additionally, social work educates the family about potential discharge plans, follow-up care, and community contacts and support groups. Included is assistance in helping families understand insurance benefits and help in completing any necessary documents.

Education provided by the occupational therapy staff for families of persons with head injury focuses on improving the person's independence with daily living tasks. Although the person may have the coordination to complete these activities, education as to visuospatial deficits, memory impairments, and other safety-related issues includes detailed explanations.

The vocational counseling staff begins family education early on in the person's recovery process. Most families are unfamiliar with vocational services. Initial contacts with the family are focused on education as to what this service is and what it can offer to the person and family. For the individual, these services often include employer contacts, videotaped job performance analysis, supported employment, and onsite job coaches. Depending upon the projected discharge goal, the vocational counselor will provide the family with a better understanding of disability benefits, supported employment, educational supervision, and community/state resources available to assist the person following discharge from the acute rehabilitation setting.

Pastoral care staff minister to families depending on their expressed need. Frequently, multiple members of the family or friends have been injured or died as a result of an accident. Education and ministry to needs concerning adjustment, grief, ascription of blame, and loss associated with head injury are the focus of the pastoral care department.

Physical therapy focuses on educating the family to the fact that although the person can perform the functional task of ambulation, he or she may be and often is unsafe because of cognitive deficits. If the person has associated orthopedic or sensori-motor involvement, education also focuses on weight bearing, brace management, coordination, spasticity, and balance and how these interfere with the person's gait.

The psychologist specializing in neuropsychology provides several important services for families. First, the psychologist who performs an in-depth neuropsychological evaluation should provide specific feedback to the family as to their relative's performance on relevant tests, and how observed deficits in such areas as memory, judgment, reasoning, and so forth are related to specific loci of brain injury as well as to pre-injury deficits in cognition and behavior. This information should be provided in functional terms so that the family understands how specific neurobehavioral deficits may be manifested in everyday life and how they may be managed. The psychologist also helps the family in their adjustment to the head injury and associated loss they may be experiencing. During the individual's stay, the psychologist provides the family with education regarding psychological/emotional issues and provides counseling with many members of the family system (spouse, children, siblings) to facilitate maximal understanding and adaptation.

Information regarding leisure skills and activities that are both therapeutic and motivating to the person are taught to families through the therapeutic recreation department. Additional information is provided by the therapeutic recreation department regarding accessible restaurants and leisure activities available to the person and family following discharge.

FAMILY REACTIONS

Though many families respond positively and appreciate the educational efforts made by the interdisciplinary team, some families have a negative reaction. Certain types of information can be difficult to accept, for example, disappointing prognostic statements, altered cognitive or behavioral status as reflected by the neuropsychological examination, or the need for 24-hour supervision. It is therefore not uncommon for a given family to reject the information provided by a certain health care practitioner or the entire team and seek out second and third opinions. Though this may be an entirely appropriate reaction from the family, it may cause considerable disruption in ongoing treatment if it occurs on a daily basis. In such cases, it would be highly advisable to have a family conference early on in inpatient rehabilitation to develop a mutually agreeable set of goals and rehabilitation strategies, and periodic follow-up meetings to monitor family understanding and acceptance. However, if a family consistently rejects the philosophical approach of the family's rehabilitation program, options for other facilities or providers should be presented to the family. Though it is difficult, rehabilitation team members must respect the uniqueness of each family and their own method of adapting to their relative's head injury. Defensive staff reaction may only reinforce a family's unwillingness to hear certain information. Finally, it may be helpful to refer a resistant family to the local support group of the NHIF to receive some peer counseling, support, and advice.

A MODEL FAMILY EDUCATION PROGRAM

To develop a strong and effective family education program, the following seven-step process is essential:

1. Review existing educational programs. It is helpful to select unfamiliar educational programs to put the reviewer in the role of a family member. Assess the programs' strengths and weaknesses.
2. Interview individuals with head injuries and their families. Ask them what they find confusing about the program and what information they would find helpful.

3. Interview other interdisciplinary team members to determine what questions they have or what questions they are asked by their clients and the family members regarding the rehabilitation program.
4. Select the teaching aids appropriate to facilitate maximum communication. Provide families with both static and dynamic information. A combination of visual, printed, and audio information is the most effective means of education.
5. Make the information package clear, concise, and well-organized; it should be presented in a supportive manner. Oral information presented by the professional should make no assumptions of prior knowledge by the family. Printed and video information should be produced professionally.
6. Conduct a discharge interview; it is an important but frequently omitted step in a family education program. Ask for both general and specific information regarding the program. Information acquired from families during the discharge interview is necessary to strengthen the family education program.
7. Follow-up on family outcomes; this helps verify the effectiveness of the family education program. Documentation of positive client outcomes and follow-through on techniques taught that may directly result in increased quality of care is crucial.

Following is an example of a family intervention education program developed specifically to educate families of persons with swallowing disorders (dysphagia). (For a more complete description of this program, see Hutchins, 1989.)

The dysphagia family intervention program takes approximately 30 minutes to present, with time allotted throughout for questions and answers. Both the client and family are present during the program. Presentation to the individual family unit allows for very individualized information regarding the specific aspects of the individual's dysphagia. The program is divided into three phases: a 10-minute videotape, a review of the person's videofluoroscopic study, and presentation of printed materials.

In *Phase 1*, a 10-minute videotape explains the swallowing evaluation and intervention program. The videotape includes explanation and examples of the referral process, case review, clinical bedside evaluation, and the videofluoroscopic examination. The necessity of the videofluoroscopic examination and information gained are discussed. The videotape shows various examples of normal and abnormal swallowing patterns. Highlighted frame enhancements are used to direct the family's attention to the text and vital structures. Dysphagia treatment techniques and compensatory strategies are explained and demonstrated. These strategies include: attention to food consistency and amount, adjusted positioning, attention to safety, attention to rate of swallowing, liquid wash, multiple swallows, and so forth.

In *Phase 2* the speech-language pathologist plays the individual's actual recorded swallow from the videofluoroscopic evaluation. Because of the speed of the oropharyngeal swallow, the tape player's freeze frame and slow motion features are used. The bedside clinical swallowing results are also presented at this time. Finally, the speech/language pathologist comments on the severity of the client's dysphagia.

Phase 3 includes the distribution of a preprinted informational booklet completed for each person with a head injury and family. The information was developed to allow maximum flexibility and individualization. Each page provides the person's family with diagrams and a list of alternative interventions that are appropriate for the client. Topics covered include: general information on swallowing, major videofluoroscopic findings and clinical evaluation results, dietary restrictions and guidelines, compensatory techniques for use during feeding/swallowing, therapy, questions and answers, and terminology.

CASE STUDY

An unrestrained passenger sustained a traumatic brain injury resulting in bilateral damage and a subdural hematoma over the parasagital region of the brain. Five months post-injury the person was readmitted to the rehabilitation unit specializing in head injury. Educational activities focused on understanding head injury, long-term effects, issues of recovery, and discharge planning. After meeting with the social worker, primary nurse, and physician, the family was referred to the head injury family education group. At the biweekly meetings the family learned about the nature of head injury, ambulation and safety concerns, various stages of head injury recovery, cognitive deficits with a communication emphasis, bowel and bladder management, medications, long-term needs, and behavioral management techniques. The family took an active role in the rehabilitation program, attending numerous family education days and reading and participating in all educational classes offered. They attended therapy with their relative, talked with the clinician, and participated in goal-setting, progress monitoring, and functional follow-up of the intervention goals outside of therapy. The family participated in team conferences and provided feedback to the clinician, nurse, and medical staff relating to the effectiveness of the rehabilitation program. Discharge planning done in conjunction with the family included options such as a nursing home, residential head injury programs, government institutions, and supervised home care with a day treatment program. Due to the extent of the family education, the family had realistic extended-care expectations and was able to successfully take the person home and arrange daily supervision and a head injury day treatment program.

CONCLUSION

Though the effectiveness of family education in head injury rehabilitation has not yet been examined in a rigorous research design, clinicians, facilities, and most important, families, have attested to the inherent values in such efforts. A family system experiencing a head injury is traumatized and often feels helpless. Organized, comprehensive family education programs can provide families with the knowledge base to feel more secure in their interactions with their relatives and plan more realistically for the future. Much progress has been made in the development of educational materials and in the refinement of educational practices. However, the need still exists to provide continuing education throughout the continuum of care in order to aid in lessening the burden felt by family members and improve ultimate outcome.

REFERENCES

Brooks, D.N., Campsie, L., Symington, C., Beattie, A., & McKinlay, W. (1986). The five year outcome of severe blunt head injury: A relative's view. *Journal of Neurology, Neurosurgery and Psychiatry, 49*, 764–770.

Brooks, D.N., Campsie, L., Symington, C., Beattie, A., & McKinlay, W. (1987). The effects of severe head injury on patient and relative within seven years of injury. *Journal of Head Trauma Rehabilitation, 2*(3), 1–13.

Hutchins, B.F. (1989). Establishing a dysphagia family intervention program for head injured patients. *Journal of Head Trauma Rehabilitation, 4*(4), 64–72.

Kozloff, R. (1987). Networks of social support and the outcome from severe head injury. *Journal of Head Trauma Rehabilitation, 2*(3), 14–23.

Muir, C.A., Rosenthal, M., & Diehl, L. (1990). Methods of family intervention. In M. Rosenthal, E.R. Griffith, M.R. Bond, & J.D. Miller (Eds.), *Rehabilitation of the adult and child with traumatic brain injury* (pp. 433–448). Philadelphia: F.A. Davis.

National Head Injury Foundation. (1989). *Catalog of educational materials.* Southborough, MA: Author.

Rosenthal, M. (1989). Trends in head injury rehabilitation and research: The past decade and future challenges. In M. Miner, & K. Wagner (Eds.), *Neurotrauma* (Vol. 3, pp. 195–207). Boston: Butterworths.

Thomsen, I.V. (1974). The patient with severe head injury and his family. *Scandinavian Journal of Rehabilitation Medicine, 6*, 180.

19

FAMILY THERAPY AS APPLIED TO HEAD INJURY

JOHN J. ZARSKI
ROBERTA DEPOMPEI

Each family is like a diamond, with many facets. You can't possibly know them all. (Anonymous)

Consider the following scenario. The family of an 18-year-old son with head injury is having problems controlling his angry outbursts and verbal abuse of other family members. The son's speech therapist has recommended family therapy, and the family is now assembled in the therapist's office for its initial meeting. Following a brief period of social interaction, the therapist poses the question, "How can I be of help?" A family's common response is: "Well, I don't know why we are all here. The problem is John." This is a legitimate statement, and it requires a response that will validate the family's feelings, engage the members in the therapy, and remove the need for an identified client. An effective response requires knowledge and understanding about family functioning, skill in working with families, and most important, a perception that focuses on the family, not solely an individual member. The main objectives of this chapter are to provide a brief introduction to the field of family therapy as well as suggestions for when family therapy may be indicated for families with a member with head injury and to provide strategies and interventions for working with these families, including a case example.

The authors are indebted to Linda Pannell Zarski for her helpful comments on drafts of this chapter.

FAMILY THERAPY

Family therapy is a rapidly growing field that has become the intervention of choice for a wide range of problems, including problems associated with families whose members have health-related concerns such as cerebral palsy, asthma, cerebral-vascular accident, cancer, and head injury. In the context of the statement, "Why are we all here? It's John's problem," family therapy is an approach to helping the member with head injury as well as other family members explore areas of concern and conflict in an environment of accommodation so that no individual feels singled out as the problem or responsible for any family crisis. Family therapy is often indicated in the later stages of the rehabilitation process, after the person with head injury has returned home and the demands and problems of everyday living begin to exceed the coping mechanisms available to the family. Usually all family members attend the sessions, although numerous combinations of members involving dyads or triads may be arranged depending upon the presenting concerns. In practice, it is common for the entire family to begin rehabilitation together, after which subsystems of the family (e.g., the parents and the member with a head injury, the siblings) are selected for special attention (Glick & Kessler, 1974).

An important initial decision facing the family therapist is whether to include the person with head injury in the sessions. In regard to this concern, Rosenthal and Muir (1983) point out that family therapists should exercise caution before involving the person with head injury since this individual must be able to participate in a meaningful way. Through our experience in working with families, we have come to believe that severity of injury is not a reason to exclude the person from therapy. If the therapist has reason to believe the person can learn and profit from the experience, family therapy can be a meaningful intervention for the person with head injury and other family members, although it certainly will not solve all problems for all families.

Several additional points deserve mention. Family therapy may be indicated under other circumstances as well. Family therapy may be helpful when the severity of the head injury requires transfer to a nursing home or intensive rehabilitation facility and the person is not expected to return home. It may also be indicated in the weeks or months following the trauma, during which time the person may be in a coma or be receiving hospital rehabilitation. However, in these latter instances, an intensive form of family therapy, that is, family crisis intervention, is recommended (Figley & McCubbin, 1983; Pittman, 1987). A major focus of family crisis intervention is the emphasis on supporting family members in their struggle to deal with the injury, as contrasted to the more traditional family therapy with an emphasis on change and growth. The remainder of this chapter centers on family therapy for families in which the member with head injury will be returning home following a period of hospitalization and rehabilitation.

INDICATIONS AND CONTRAINDICATIONS

Generally speaking, family therapy may be indicated when it is important to clarify and resolve relationship problems in the family (Hoffman, 1981). For example, family members may begin to blame themselves or their member with head injury for disruption in the family, resulting in conflict between family members. Also, family therapy may be indicated at separation or individuation points in the family. It may be especially useful when the person with head injury wants to return to school or seek independent living. Furthermore, family therapy may be helpful if family members begin to withdraw from contacts outside the home, choosing instead to form a protective net around the person.

Some therapists question the value of family therapy where there are severe, chronic physical and/or mental deficits, maladaptive behavior patterns, multiple problems, high-risk (Block & LaPerriere, 1973), or openly violent behavior problems (Ackerman, 1970). Rollin (1987) suggests that the quality and degree of the cognitive-emotional-communicative deficit in the person may be reason to question the value of family therapy. This is a separate issue that is covered under the Degree of Impairment section of this chapter.

Nevertheless, when family therapy is indicated, it is imperative that therapists be given direction. It is imperative that they understand not only what impact the head injury has on the family, but also the phases of the recovery process and the importance of matching appropriate strategies and interventions for each phase, each family type, and the degree of injury.

In the words of Frank Pittman (1984), "Technique without direction is bad enough in coloratura sopranos; in therapists and surgeons it can be disastrous" (p. 39). While Pittman's observation is relevant for family therapy in general, it is especially pertinent for therapists working with families with a member who has experienced a head injury. As discussed in Chapters 7 and 8, disruptions in family relationships, shifting social roles within the family, and an increase in stressors are likely following the head trauma. Experiences such as the daily burden of care, uncertainty about the future, hope for the return of the "pre-injury person," and certain life cycle disruptions are not uncommon. Each of these stressors makes effective intervention with the family of a person with head injury a most complex, difficult, and challenging task.

Although each specific head injury has its own unique neurophysiology and medical treatment needs, Klonoff and Prigatano (1987) and Rosenthal and Muir (1983) indicate that there are many commonalities in terms of what impact the injury has on the family. For example, most families will pass through predictable phases following the rehabilitation period. There is a time of realignment, followed by an adjustment sequence, followed by a reintegration of the person into the family unit. In some cases, however, families may develop altered self-perceptions of both the person with head injury and others in the family system. These altered perceptions result in major obstacles and an inability to make the transition through one or more of these stages. The role of the family therapist is to help the family negotiate these transitional points so that a new repertoire of behaviors and, consequently, new self-perceptions will evolve. Keeping in mind the cognitive-communicative impairments of the person, the family therapist can base intervention strategies on goals formulated in the assessment phase (see Chapter 4). In order for the therapy to be successful, the intervention must address the phase of the recovery process that the family has reached and the degree of impairment of the person with the injury.

The following sections suggest specific therapeutic goals for each phase of the recovery process, describe typical interventions for accomplishing these goals, present a case example illustrating a family therapy approach, and conclude with special considerations for family therapists who desire to work with these families.

FAMILY INTERVENTION MATRIX

Figure 9 is a highly simplified family intervention matrix that pairs important family variables (phase of the recovery process with level of family functioning, the person's degree of impairment) with therapeutic strategies and possible systems intervention techniques. Similar to the way that a parent teaches a child about color by beginning with the basic colors, and then moving to combinations to create more colors, therapists must be taught about the basics (degree of impairment, phase of recovery, and level of family functioning) before considering strategies for intervention.

DEGREE OF IMPAIRMENT

Assessment of the different levels of neurological, psychological, social, physical, and cognitive-communicative functions and impairment can be a difficult and demanding task. For various functions there are standardized and observational protocols to identify appropriate functional levels in a real-life situation (Adamovitch, Henderson, & Auerbach, 1985; Cochran, 1988; Hagen, Malkmus, & Durham, 1979; Sohlberg & Mateer, 1989). It is imperative that the family therapist have familiarity with these protocols so a judgment can be made regarding the inclusion of the person with head injury in the therapy or regarding the usefulness of a particular strategy or intervention with the family. In this chapter, the terms minor, moderate, and severe head injury are used to define three categories of behaviors of the person that might be observed by the family therapist. Although these categories should prove useful to the therapist unfamiliar with persons with head injury, it is important

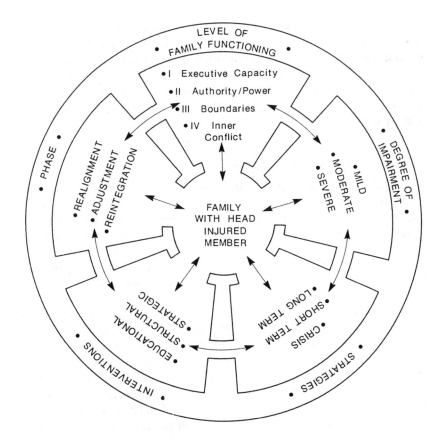

Figure 9. Family intervention matrix.

that the final decision for including the person in the family therapy session be made on the basis of the therapist's knowledge of appropriate functional levels of the person as they are revealed in the context of the family (McCay, 1986; Prigatano, 1987; Rosenthal, 1989; Ylvisaker & Gobble, 1987).

Category I: Mild Head Injury

Individuals with mild head injury are often unable to identify what is different about themselves, and they report a general feeling of "losing their minds" or loss of control. The deficits these individuals experience and describe are often not apparent to an outside observer. For example, there is self-doubt, sometimes referred to as a "shaken sense of self" (McCay, 1986). Other deficits include a lack of organizational skills and problem-solving skills, depression, denial, and problems with concentration and information processing. Some of these individuals are unable to continue in school or work, and usually they do not know why. Families, peers, and employers have difficulty understanding that anything could be different about these individuals because they "seem to look just fine." In family sessions, these persons may be withdrawn, angry, or sullen. Younger children may exhibit a variety of behaviors typically associated with attention deficit disorders or learning disabilities with or without hyperactivity.

Category II: Moderate Head Injury

Individuals with moderate head injuries may demonstrate motor impairments, which commonly include motor weakness and visual impairment, although physical recovery is often good. Cognitive-communicative impairments of memory, concentration, pragmatic language skills, and problem-solving are more apparent. There is obvious delay in processing information. New learning is extremely difficult. Control of emotional outbursts and inappropriate language is sometimes a problem. Self-sufficiency at home, in the community, and on the job is often impaired, and different behaviors are noticeable to family members, peers, and employers. Persons with moderate head injury report loss of jobs, friends, and support systems. They indicate they are alone, depressed, and unable to move on with their lives. Families have concerns over this changed family member and how to adapt to, accommodate, or change his or her behavioral differences. In family therapy sessions, these individuals may be slow to respond, requiring patience on the therapist's part, but the session provides an opportunity for the therapist to model desirable responses to the person for other family members. If these individuals have experienced a closed head injury to the frontal lobes, they may demonstrate childish behavior, social disinhibition, and inappropriate aggressive behavior (Rosenthal & Muir, 1983). When these behaviors are present, the therapist faces the difficult challenge of helping the family cope with the reality of living together.

Category III: Severe Head Injury

Persons with severe head injury demonstrate severe impairment in physical abilities, cognitive-communicative skills, and emotional and social behaviors. These individuals have spent long periods of time in hospitals and rehabilitation settings. Families are faced with the prospect of years of rehabilitation and with individuals who may need custodial care for a lifetime. When family therapy is indicated and the person with head injury is present, it is helpful for the family therapist to work with a co-therapist, usually a speech-language pathologist, to ensure that the therapeutic environment promotes adaptive and functional behaviors.

PHASES IN THE RECOVERY PROCESS

There is a growing literature on the stages families and individuals pass through following a normal or catastrophic event (Bepko & Krestan, 1985; McCubbin & Figley, 1983; Moravetz & Walker, 1984). Family therapists may find identification of the following three phases helpful in their understanding of what impact head injury has on the family system in the period following hospital discharge.

In *Phase 1*, the realignment, the family is beginning to respond to the multiple changes that occurred during the time the person was in a rehabilitation setting. According to Rollin (1987), it is during this stage that family members begin to recognize their helplessness and frustration. Family functioning (rules, boundaries, roles, and communication channels) is strained, and members may refuse to acknowledge the presence of problems. For example they may insist that once the person comes home, there will no longer be any communicative problems (DePompei & Zarski, 1989). From a family therapy perspective, the most important characteristic of this phase as it relates to the therapeutic process is the family's perception of reality (Minuchin & Fishman, 1981). During this time, the family faces the need to accept the reality of living with a person with head injury. Individual issues are usually emphasized, and problems may appear as, for example, fighting between siblings, the fighting plunging a parent deeper into depression, or angry outbursts between a parent and a child with head injury, the outburst being an expression of the rage originating from the feeling that the injury "should never have happened." An important part of the therapy at this phase is the therapeutic triangle, consisting of the family, the person with head injury, and the therapist (Doherty & Baird, 1983, 1987). The task of the therapist is to form a team with the family system without becoming part of the system. If the therapist's connection with the family is too tight or enmeshed, the therapist may have difficulties confronting family issues. If the therapist becomes frustrated with or disengaged from the family, the family may decide to terminate rehabilitation prematurely.

Phase 2, the adjustment, refers to the movement toward resolution and adaptation. Family members may continue to struggle with role adjustments characteristic of Phase 1. However, in Phase 2, the family has developed appropriate coping mechanisms to deal with the person's physical/medical needs, and the person has begun to establish a new social life in the context of the changed reality. Problems at this phase usually focus on the fear that the person will regress to old behaviors or that parent(s) may be reluctant to encourage the now fully capable individual to live independently or in a community-type arrangement. In cases involving a person with severe head injury, the problem may center on the lack of new skills or social life or behaviors that are unacceptable to the family. Family therapy typically consists of work with dyads (mother/person with injury, father/person with injury) or subsystems (parental, marital, or sibling).

Phase 3, the reintegration phase, is the family's successful transition to an appropriate fit between family developmental tasks and the need for closeness or disengagement. By Rolland's (1984) definition, head injury can be considered a constant-course illness in which the biological course stabilizes following the initial trauma. The individual or family is faced with a semipermanent change that is stable or predictable over a considerable time span. Except in cases of severe incapacitation, a constant-course illness provides the family with the opportunity to stabilize to the extent that the person's interactions with the family and the family life cycles allow (Combrinck-Graham, 1985). Important family therapy interventions at this phase typically center on individuals and the extended family. Typically, role reallocations have occurred, and the member with special needs is no longer competing with others for potentially scarce family resources. An important caveat for family therapists is that families are not expected to move through these phases in any set pattern. Each family's recovery is individualized, and no definitive time span can be assigned or anticipated (Figley & McCubbin, 1983).

LEVELS OF FAMILY FUNCTIONING

Chapter 9 reviewed empirical and clinical methods for assessing families. The purpose of this section is to discuss a highly simplified approach for understanding levels of family functioning that will facilitate the therapist's selection of intervention. The following model is an adaptation of Weltner's (1985) matchmaking approach for choosing the appropriate therapy for families at various levels of pathology. Weltner suggests that families may operate at four different levels. At *Level 1,* therapists are concerned with the family's ability to deal with life and death issues. The main focus is on whether an executive capacity exists that is sufficient to manage needs for food, shelter, medical care, and minimal maintenance. Important issues in *Level 2* families focus on authority and limits. The stability of the family system may be in jeopardy since the executive subsystem may be unable to respond with sufficient control to the person with head injury or other family members. *Level 3* families appear to be working and have developed some effective coping patterns. Problems that do develop with these families usually center on boundary issues, especially around the person with head injury and extended family. *Level 4* families have established a broad range of effective coping patterns and have demonstrated competence in adapting to the needs of the person. Therapeutic issues with these families center on insight, inner conflict, or a more sensitive awareness of the relational world.

STRATEGIES AND INTERVENTION

Strategies and interventions provide the family therapist with the opportunity to use the palette of basic colors and create a new color appropriate for the family picture. Based upon Weltner's levels of family functioning, family therapists may select from a variety of strategies to address crisis situations or to focus on short- or long-term goals and interventions related to educational, structural, and strategic models of therapy. Strategies include a therapist's attempts to focus on strengths, not problems; clarification and resolution of the trauma; and generational individuation. Intervention techniques range from providing accurate information about head injury to complex therapeutic moves involving restructuring, symptom resolution, and changing the family's perception of reality. (See Table 3 for additional examples of strategies and accompanying interventions.)

CASE EXAMPLE—GINGER

The following case example is presented to illustrate the above framework for working with families and their member with a head injury:

Ginger was 11 years old when she was injured in the school parking lot. She was hit by a school bus that was backing up. Previously she was enrolled in the school's gifted program and was involved in athletics through basketball and softball.

Ginger spent 4 months in the hospital and a rehabilitation facility. She has recovered physically except for a mild right side weakness. She has poor memory and cognitive-communicative impairments, which interfere with new learning, recall, and problem-solving. Her speech is slowed and hesitant. Word finding continues to be a problem for her. She missed 6 months of school but was placed, at her parents' request, in the seventh grade with her class.

Ginger lives at home with her parents, Harold, a lawyer, and Marion, a third grade teacher. Her older brother, Jeff, 19, has moved back home from college this semester to help "however he is needed." He is taking several classes at the local university. Her older sister, Nancy, 16, has given up her part-time job so that she can be available to help Ginger with her homework and to assist with the housework so her mother will have more time with Ginger. She is uncertain about out-of-state college plans that she was making.

Ginger has a tutor, at her parents' request, who works with her 1/2 hour before school, during lunch, and for 1 hour after school. She is also tutored 3 hours on Saturdays. Teachers report that Ginger is a C student and that learning new material is difficult and time-consuming for her. They have recommended less classroom time with fewer subjects for the current year. Her parents would not sign the IEP for fewer classroom obligations for the current year. Ginger's behavior in the classroom has deteriorated, with out-

Table 3. Family-focused strategies and interventions

Level of family functioning	Strategies	Interventions
I. Focus on executive capacity	• Education—teaching family members ways to recognize needs of other members • Reframing strengths and weaknesses	• Teach skills • Network • Assign tasks • Restructure to focus on problem resolution
II. Focus on authority and power	• Modification of unacceptable social behaviors • Reduction of power-confrontation episodes	• Work with alliances, coalitions, and roles • Use written behavioral contracts • Focus on behaviors of person with head injury as opposed to possible dysfunctional relationship between parents
III. Focus on boundaries	• Recognition that pre-injury personality is not there and will not return • Reliance on new communication patterns rather than old sequences	• Actualize transactional patterns • Mark boundaries • Challenge family structure through unbalancing • Highlight triangulation supporting severe symptomatology
IV. Focus on inner conflict and intimacy	• Insight • Future goals • Alteration of expectations for role of the person with head injury in the family	• Challenge family reality through cognitive constructs • Use creative strategies • Family sculpture • Imagery work

bursts occurring several times a week. She also complains of headaches and stomachaches.

Her parents will not allow her to attend Girl Scouts or to go on the class trip to camp for 1 week in the spring. They express concern that no one will watch Ginger closely enough and that she may fall or be injured. They are also worried that she may be incontinent and embarrass herself. They have denied her the opportunity to be in gym class or to participate on the basketball team because they feel it would be embarrassing for her. Her physician has recommended that she participate in any athletic activities that she chooses.

Ginger has been invited to friends' houses. She is allowed to go but not to stay overnight. Ginger's friends are beginning to shy away from her and say that she acts like a baby. They feel she does not talk with them as she used to and that her silly behavior in class is unacceptable. She has received fewer invitations from her friends in recent months. Her older brother and sister have filled in by taking her to movies and to sporting events with them. The parents feel that their friends are not supporting them and that Ginger's friends are mean to have deserted her. They express anger that their family and friends do not understand their dedication to bringing their very bright child back to her old standard of development. They state that once she is back to her old intellectual self, the athletic abilities and friends will come back.

After a consultation with her physician and school counselor, the family agreed to participate in family therapy sessions. In the initial session the therapist noted family transactional patterns associated with an enmeshed family system. Parents spoke for their children, the children looked at their mother before responding, and Ginger spent most of the session clinging to her mother or father, all of these behaviors suggesting the family was functioning at Level III, with boundary problems the predominant theme.

Ginger appeared to have moderate head injury. She presented with inappropriate social skills; that is, she leaned her head on her mother's shoulder, sat on her lap, had problems processing information, had word finding problems, and lacked concrete-level reasoning skills. The family seemed to be operating at the realignment stage of the recovery process. The family was refusing to acknowledge the presence of problems and difficulties in relation to the sibling subsystem that was emerging. The family members were experiencing difficulty accepting Ginger's social skills. Her sister Nancy seemed disinterested and seemed to reject Ginger, and her brother seemed like a pseudo-parent, being highly protective of his sister. Initial goals centered on: 1) education relative to Ginger's limitations to help family members understand Ginger's deficits so that family rules could be changed, 2) modification of Ginger's unacceptable social behaviors, 3) readjustment of roles for family members, and 4) delineating family boundaries so as to allow Ginger the opportunity to engage in activities that would enhance her recovery.

The theme of enmeshment was highlighted in session three:

Therapist: Tell me, Ginger, do you like basketball?
Ginger: (Pause) Uh, huh.
Mother: But it really isn't possible now.
Therapist: Ginger, when was the last time you played?
Ginger: (pause) Not, (pause) not since last month or so.
Mother: She hasn't played since last year. She's not physically ready, I don't think. Do you, Harold (father)?

Father: Well sometimes I wish things were different. She was pretty athletic.
Therapist: Ginger, you are 12 years old, yet at times your parents treat you
    like a 4-year-old. They're very protective of you.
Nancy: That's the truth!

In this session, the therapist selected the theme of enmeshment in the
family and worked through helping Ginger to confront the parents on their
protective behaviors, which were limiting Ginger's recovery. Although Ginger's chronological age is 12, she is functioning at about age 8 due to cognitive-communicative impairments, but her parents are responding to her as if
she were a 4-year-old. Ideally, the therapist would like to support Ginger in
her efforts to challenge her mother, but at this early stage in the therapy the
therapist decided to form a coalition with Nancy regarding the parents' protective stance. With the family functioning at Level III and boundary problems
the predominant concern, the therapist started by challenging the family reality regarding Ginger. The therapist then began to send therapeutic messages
that allow family members, especially the parents, to experience Ginger in a
new way, in this session, as more capable.

With this particular family, the therapist will use family therapy techniques to support Ginger's ability to initiate actions and differentiate herself
from her mother. For example, reframing may be used to alter labels and
experiences to present a more positive view of reality. Ginger's silly or clinging behaviors may be represented as her attempt to be different from the other
family members, sort of the family's teddy bear. This strategy will help
Ginger communicate her feelings and gain greater self-esteem. Another example involving boundary issues could focus on the dynamic in which family
members interrupt each other or the parents answer questions for their children. The therapist might delineate the boundary by noting it and asking the
parent if he or she is always so helpful and then double checking the answer
with the child or spouse. Other stock phrases that serve this purpose include:
"You take his voice," and "If she answers for you, you do not have to talk"
(Minuchin & Fishman, 1981). However, before initiating any interventions
for Ginger, it would be helpful for the family therapist to consult with a
speech-language pathologist to understand Ginger's appropriate expressive
level. Future sessions will focus on her siblings and their feelings of anger and
resentment resulting from the loss of parental attention and changes in plans
for college.

SPECIAL CONSIDERATIONS

Although generally acknowledging the family as an important variable in the
recovery process of a person with head injury, the traditional medical model
has not actively employed the family as partners in the recovery process.

Family therapists must be aware of the same problem and must be able to interact, in a knowledgeable way, with physicians, social workers, rehabilitation specialists, and other health care workers providing services to persons with head injury and their families.

CONCLUSION

The authors believe that family therapy may be beneficial to families regardless of whether the member with head injury attends the sessions. However, family therapists need to follow certain guidelines when including the person in the therapy sessions (see Figure 10). By using the approaches presented in this chapter, it is expected that family therapists who work with persons with head injuries and their families can most effectively alter and

---

1. Treat the person as an adult or with regard to whatever other appropriate chronological age level.
2. Be sure to maintain the person's attention to the discussion in the session. Short sessions may be necessary in order to maintain interest and assure adequate participation.
3. Redirect attention rather than confronting the lack of it.
4. Plan to repeat and restate more often than usual.
5. Remember that persons with head injury can often verbalize what task should be done, but may be unable to perform the task due to poor recall or lack of self-initiation.
6. Understand that generalization of a solution for one situation to a second similar situation may not occur.
7. Know that poor memory will influence what the person recalls from session to session. Take time to recall the results and decisions from the last session before beginning the next.
8. Allow the use of any compensatory strategies necessary, for example, writing down lists, tape recorders, maps, reminder cards for appointments, notebooks.
9. Understand that denial is often a serious problem and needs attention within the session.
10. Realize that vile language, inappropriate sexual behavior, lack of empathy for others in the family, causing embarrassment for the family, poor personal hygiene, and self-centeredness are behaviors that may not yet be under the person's control.
11. Allow the person a chance to express ideas without others in the family speaking for him or her, even when speech and language problems exist.
12. Remember that frequent cueing and rehearsal for new information is essential.

Figure 10. Guidelines for including a member with head injury in family therapy sessions.

improve family capabilities and recovery. Just as it is impossible to completely understand the many facets of a diamond's beauty, family therapists will not uncover the multitude of factors that enable families to deal with their situation. Family therapists can only strive to maximize the difference that family therapy can make in people's lives.

REFERENCES

Ackerman, N.W. (Ed.). (1970). *Family therapy in transition*. New York: Little, Brown.

Adamovitch, B., Henderson, J., & Auerbach, S. (1981). *Cognitive rehabilitation of closed head injury patients*. San Diego: College-Hill.

Bepko, C., & Krestan, J.A. (1985). *The responsibility trap: A blueprint for treating the alcoholic family*. New York: The Free Press.

Block, D.A., & LaPerriere, K. (1973). Techniques of family therapy: A conceptual frame. In D.A. Block (Ed.), *Techniques of family psychotherapy: A primer*. New York: Grune & Stratton.

Cochran, W. (1988). *Rehabilitation of the traumatically head injured*. Carbondale, IL: Regional Rehabilitation Continuing Education Program, Region V.

Combrinck-Graham, L. (1985). A developmental model for family systems. *Family Process, 24*, 139–150.

DePompei, R., & Zarski, J.J. (1989). Families, head injury, and cognitive-communicative impairments: Issues for family counseling. *Topics in Language Disorders, 9*, 78–89.

Doherty, W.J., & Baird, M.A. (1983). *Family therapy and family medicine: Toward the primary care of families*. New York: Guilford Press.

Doherty, W.J., & Baird, M.A. (1987). *Family-centered medical care: A clinical casework*. New York: Guilford Press.

Figley, C.R., & McCubbin, H.I. (1983). *Stress and the family: Volume II: Coping with catastrophe*. New York: Brunner/Mazel.

Glick, I.E., & Kessler, D.R. (1974). *Marital and family therapy*. New York: Grune & Stratton.

Hagen, C., Malkmus, D., & Durham, P. (1979). *Levels of cognitive functioning. Rehabilitation of the head injured adult*. Downey, CA: Professional Staff Association.

Hoffman, L. (1981). *Foundations of family therapy: A conceptual framework for systems change*. New York: Basic Books.

Klonoff, P., & Prigatano, G. (1987). Reactions of family members and clinical intervention after traumatic brain injury. In M. Ylvisaker & E.M. Gobble (Eds.), *Community re-entry for head-injured adults*. Boston: College-Hill.

McCay, T. (1986). *The unseen injury. Minor head injury: An introduction for professionals*. Framingham, MA: National Head Injury Foundation.

McCubbin, H.I., & Figley, C.R. (1983). *Stress and the family, Volume I: Coping with normative transitions*. New York: Brunner/Mazel.

Minuchin, S., & Fishman, H.C. (1981). *Family therapy techniques*. Cambridge: Harvard University Press.

Moravetz, A., & Walker, G. (1984). *Brief therapy with single-parent families*. New York: Brunner/Mazel.

Pittman, F.S. (1987). *Turning points: Treating families in transition and crisis*. New York: W.W. Norton.

Prigatano, G. (1987). Neuropsychological deficits, personality variables and outcome. In M. Ylvisaker & E.M. Gobble (Eds.), *Community re-entry for head injured adults* (pp. 1–24). Boston: College-Hill.

Rolland, J.S. (1984). Toward a psychosocial typology of chronic and life-threatening illness. *Family Systems Medicine, 2,* 245–263.

Rollin, W. (1987). *The psychology of communication disorders in individuals and their families.* Englewood Cliffs, NJ: Prentice-Hall.

Rosenthal, M. (1989). *Rehabilitation of the head injured adult.* Philadelphia: F.A. Davis.

Rosenthal, M., & Muir, C. (1983). Methods of family intervention. In M. Rosenthal, E. Griffith, M. Bond, & J.D. Miller (Eds.), *Rehabilitation of the head-injured adult.* Philadelphia: F.A. Davis.

Sohlberg, M.M., & Mateer, C.A. (1989). The assessment of cognitive-communicative functions in head injury. *Topics in Language Disorders, 9,* 15–33.

Weltner, J.S. (1985). Matchmaking: Choosing the appropriate therapy for families at various levels of pathology. In M.P. Mirkin & S.L. Koman (Eds.), *Handbook of adolescents and family therapy* (pp. 39–50). New York: Gardner Press.

Ylvisaker, M., & Gobble, E.M. (1987). *Community re-entry for head-injured adults.* Boston: College-Hill.

20

FAMILY SUPPORT

JANET M. WILLIAMS

In a study investigating the relationship between parents' future planning for their children with disabilities and family functioning and stress, one researcher found that of 57 families, only 8.8% found professionals useful in forming strategies for coping with stress of future planning (Brotherson, 1985). Positive reframing (21.1%), turning to family and friends (17.5%), and turning to religion (12.3%) were the most frequently used coping strategies. Not only was help from professionals rated fifth out of 10 strategies presented, it was rated equal to the use of alcohol, cigarettes, and television. Short of providing all families with alcohol, cigarettes, and televisions, what can professionals learn about supporting families based upon the results of such a study and what is already known about families?

1. In most cases families turn to professionals only when necessary because assistance is not available from their present social networks (Dunst, Trivette, Gordon, & Pletcher, 1989).
2. Professional support should reinforce the inherent strengths that already exist in family coping strategies in addition to developing those that are needed.
3. Personal social networks are more available to families than professional support over the long-term future (Jacobs, 1988).
4. Professionals should learn strategies to support families in gaining access to social support networks.

This chapter defines social support, describes the need for social support for families who have experienced head injury, presents an example of a family situation that lacks social support, and offers four social support strategies through which families can receive help. The four strategies include family-to-family programs, self-help groups, family outreach and advocacy and community networking. Presentation of each strategy includes a commentary on the family example presented earlier detailing ways in which the specific social support model could have enhanced the family's ability to deal with the experience of head injury. In addition, suggestions for professional involvement in each model will be offered. The chapter concludes with a look at future implications for professionals and families in making social support an integrated part of the lives of people with head injuries and their families.

The chapter is based upon three basic assumptions about families. First, families are already competent or have the capacity to become competent (Dunst, Trivette, Gordon, & Pletcher, 1989). Second, a person who has experienced a head injury is part of a family. Therefore, the use of the word "family" includes the person who has experienced head injury. Third, social support should exist in collaboration with professional support, not supplant professional support. The reader should keep these assumptions in mind throughout this chapter.

DEFINITION OF SOCIAL SUPPORT

Caplan and Killilea (1976) define social support as "attachments among individuals, or between individuals and groups that serve to promote competence in dealing with short-term crisis and life transitions as well as longterm stress." Dunst et al. (1989) considers social support to be a multidimensional construct that includes physical and instrumental assistance, attitude transmission, resource and information sharing, as well as emotional and psychological assistance. Both definitions of social support can be found in communities, which DeJong, Batavia, and Williams (1990) define as a whole network of friendships, schools, religious organizations, self-help groups, and various businesses and civic organizations. McKnight (1987) further defines community as the place where social attachments and interactions defined by Caplan and Killilea can be carried out. In short, social support is the support provided in communities through attachments or interactions with other people that help families increase their competency to meet challenges. Professionals play a vital role in social support, not as "experts" who "fix" families, but as supporters who enable families to reach the competency needed to seek out resources and meet challenges.

THE NEED FOR SOCIAL SUPPORT

There are four basic reasons why families need social support after head injury. First, the American family is changing in ways never before noted in its history (Vincent & Salisbury, 1988). The traditional nuclear family who lived in extended kinship bonds is not as readily available as it was in the past. Smaller families, family members living farther apart from one another, institutions that often take on some roles families have traditionally held, and the high cost of professional intervention (DeJong et al., 1990) force families to look to the community for support.

Second, families dealing with head injury experience difficulties across the entire life cycle in the eight areas presented in Chapter 8 by Williams, which include cognitive and social problems, lack of information, lack of services, uncertainty of the future, financial problems, role changes, social isolation, and prolonged caretaking. Professional support is not always available, nor is it always the most effective intervention for these difficulties. For many individuals, family and community support remain essential on a long-term basis (Beals, Mathews, Elkins, & Jacobs, 1990).

Third, intervention team members often do not know enough about the person's life history, or environment after discharge to predict or provide for the future (Beals et al., 1990). Given the fact that many people are between the ages of 16 and 35 when they experience a head injury, and after a head injury they have an average life expectancy, an intervention team is part of a person's life for only a comparatively short period of time. Conversely, family and friends are with a person before, during, and after a head injury and often live in the same community that the person will return to. The community is the logical place for people with and without disabilities to find support.

Fourth, families need social support to bridge the gaps in a person's life. For example, when a person returns home from rehabilitation, social support is necessary while the family is trying to gain access to new service delivery systems. Service systems they may look to after specific head injury rehabilitation, like schools and vocational rehabilitation agencies, often do not know enough about head injury to effectively support the person alone (Savage, 1985). Seldom do people return home from rehabilitation on a Friday and report to a supported work site on Monday. Long periods of time may pass before an individual is able to make the connection between one system and another. Additionally, the services that these agencies do provide only support a part of the person's life, not always addressing the family functions affected by all members' needs, as presented in Chapter 6.

FAMILY EXAMPLE

The Randall family's experience illustrates a common situation that families encounter after a member experiences a head injury:

Ruth Randall received the telephone call at 2 A.M. Julie had been in a car accident and the hospital would say no more. Ruth rushed to the hospital to find that her 17-year-old daughter was in critical condition and might not live. Julie's father, Pete, arrived at the hospital shortly after Ruth, with his new wife. All three sat in the waiting room all night. Julie's older twin brothers returned from college to wait.

Days passed and it was determined that Julie would live. Friends and family sent well wishes and flowers. They also spent a lot of time at the hospital with Ruth. Several people mentioned head injury to the family who really were not sure what that meant. They assumed that her brain would heal and she would resume her life as before.

During the 4th week of her hospital stay, the doctor told the family that Julie was "medically stable" and they should move her to a rehabilitation hospital. It was apparent to the family that Julie needed further treatment; they wanted the best. The social worker approached the family with a brochure from a specialized rehabilitation hospital some 300 miles away. When the family asked if there was anything closer, the social worker said she would check. A representative from the rehabilitation hospital came the next day to talk to the family. She assured them that the program was the best, and the quality of care Julie would receive there would far outweigh any concern the family might have about the distance. The family gave the rehabilitation hospital representative their insurance information and waited. The social worker told them she had not had a chance to check on other rehabilitation programs. Julie was moved to the rehabilitation program 300 miles away. Family and friends could not believe that the nearest facility was 300 miles away but resolved that Ruth was a bright woman and must know what she was doing.

At first, Ruth took a leave from her job and went to stay near Julie. After a month, the rehabilitation team suggested that Julie might "do better" if her mother was not there every day. Finances were tight so Ruth decided to return home and to work. Time passed, and after 2 years the family's weekly trips became semi-monthly and monthly. Julie still received cards and well wishes from friends but few people came to visit. The family received updates from the hospital but were not clear on what would happen next.

What happened next was as unpredictable to the family as everything before it. Julie's insurance company decided that she was not making enough progress in rehabilitation and they would no longer pay for services. The rehabilitation hospital called Ruth to tell her that Julie would have to leave in 3 weeks. They suggested that Ruth come a week early to learn more about how to care for Julie. She was still using a wheelchair and had some behavior problems, both of which were foreign to Ruth. Ruth spent time with each therapist and thought things might be okay; they made it all look so easy. There was a going away party on the last day, the physical therapist transferred Julie into the car, and off they went. The first few weeks after Julie's return were a nightmare. She was in a strange environment with no structure. Many friends and family came to visit, but most went away shaking their heads.

STRATEGIES FOR SOCIAL SUPPORT

In examining strategies for social support, it is important to understand the link families have to their social environment and understand ways in which the social environment may provide support to families. Through family-to-family programs, family outreach, self-help groups, family advocacy organizations, and community networking, families are beginning to use community resources in a way that allows them to receive social support. The following sections review the different programs, discuss their use, and apply them to the Randall family, and discuss ways in which professionals can facilitate social support.

Family-to-Family Programs

Family-to-family programs are based upon the concept of experiential knowledge, using a person's actual experience, which is unique yet similar to the experience of others who have the same problem (Borkman, 1976). The approach is pragmatic rather than scientific or theoretical, oriented to the here and now, and is holistic rather than segmented. In a family-to-family program, a family who has experience with head injury offers support and information to other families dealing with head injury for the first time.

Beth O'Brien was able to benefit from experiential knowledge:

> Meeting other people who had already experienced what I was going through was enormously helpful to me. Meeting Jean Bush, for instance, was a major breakthrough. Jean and her husband Gerry also have a son who has experienced head injury. . . . The information I began to receive became a lifeline. I knew I wasn't alone. (O'Brien, 1987, p. 424)

Marty Beaver received similar support from another spouse of a man with a head injury.

> Ever since John's accident I had wanted so much to meet another wife and mother who was in a similar situation. I felt it would be good to be able to share some of my feelings with someone who really understood. After 3 years I met Opal, who more than met my expectations. Her understanding, role modeling, and support have meant so much to me over the last 9 years. (Marty Beaver, spouse)

Family-to-family has been shown to be one of the most helpful supports that can be offered (Winch & Christoph, 1988). Only another family can say, "I have been there and I know what you are feeling" (Borkman, 1976). Families find offering one-to-one support to be a way in which they can help other families and also help themselves. There is mutual reward.

The purpose of the program is not to provide counseling or supplant professional assistance (Iscoe & Bordelon, 1985). The program aims to provide emotional support and information from one family member to a member of a different family. Not only do parents become involved in family-to-family programs, but matches are made between siblings, spouses, children of people with head injuries, and between people who have experienced head injuries themselves. Families are often grateful to meet other people soon after a person experiences a head injury. Marty Beaver and Opal could have provided even more support to one another if they had met 3 years earlier.

The family-to-family program formalizes the matching process so that families can meet other families as soon after an injury as possible. In many situations, a formalized training program can be set up for families who want to provide family-to-family help, allowing families to learn the most supportive techniques. Training also helps families to know when they are emotionally ready to provide such support. Ongoing sessions provide updates and brainstorming after the program has started.

Cultivation of referral sources and a systematized referral process are crucial to a successful family-to-family program. Referrals come directly from a head nurse or social worker in an intensive care unit. With permission of the family who is in the hospital, the call is made and a trained family member is often available within 48 hours. Matches are made based upon a variety of criteria including severity of the injury, age of the person injured, and where the person lives. Often, the family member offering support simply gives the family an information packet and telephone number. The new family is encouraged to call as their questions arise. This is an unintrusive aid.

The family-to-family program also has great benefit to families at various points along the way after a head injury. For example, as a family decides on what rehabilitation hospital to choose, it is helpful to talk to other families who have used it. If the rehabilitation team has recommended a new procedure to a family, it is helpful for the family to talk with a family with experience with the procedure. Also it is helpful to the family whose member with a head injury is returning home to talk with a family who has already negotiated that milestone. Families can always offer helpful insights from the decisions they made or wish they had made in handling their situations.

There are many points in the Randall family's experience where they could have benefited from the family-to-family program. In the initial days, the feelings of isolation and the lack of information could have been decreased by another family. Having someone to sit with them in the intensive care unit waiting room to validate their feelings and confirm having had the same experience early on would have let them know that they were not alone in their fear and uncertainty. As the Randalls began to search for rehabilitation they might have learned of other options and been able to make a better informed decision. While in the rehabilitation setting, the family may have been able to give and receive support with another family who lived a long way from the program, learning new strategies to cope. As the move home approached, Ruth might have been able to prepare the family more had she been matched with a family who had already experienced the move home. These are but a few possible ways in which family matches could have helped the Randalls gain some degree of assurance and control in dealing with intervention systems.

There are several ways that professionals can be involved in family-to-family programs. First, professionals can always keep in mind the possibility of matching families each time they meet and work with family members who are likely to benefit. Second, professionals can serve in an advisory capacity to family-to-family programs. Involvement in training, grant writing, and referral are but a few possible roles. Third, professionals can encourage other professionals to make referrals to family-to-family programs to help increase the credibility of the service. By relating success stories and providing education about the role of families in the program, professionals can help dispell fears about nonprofessional support.

A word of caution about family-to-family programs: in the author's opinion, successful family-to-family programs offer families a sense of control, predictability, and opportunity. They should be family-centered, not physically centered in rehabilitation programs. Professionals should support families in keeping the family focus intact.

Self-Help Groups

A group setting for families can provide a highly supportive environment in which families can share feelings and explore alternative ways of coping with difficult situations (Winch & Christoph, 1988). Stewart (1989), in describing social support, suggests five areas that are helpful in understanding the effectiveness of self-help groups as social support: attribution, coping, equity, loneliness, and social comparison. *Attribution* is a family's search for meaning in the experience of a threatening event and attempt at mastering the situation. The web of pain and fear that overwhelms the family is enormous, and the family soon needs to find meaning in the event (why us?) and master the situation (why can't you tell us?). *Coping* is the family's ability to draw from their environment the resources that will allow them to manage specific external and internal demands. The constant need to cope forces families to continually draw upon the same resources of family and friends for prolonged periods of time. *Equity* suggests that there is a desire to maintain equity in exchanges in relationships. Over time, families begin to question their own ability to make decisions and offer help to their family member because so many experts are available to provide help. In addition, they find few opportunities in which they can give back to professionals all that professionals gave to them. *Loneliness* is a subjective experience resulting from a perceived deficiency in social relationships or relational benefits. As families travel through systems that are unfamiliar to their personal network of family and friends, the journey can become lonely. *Social comparison* is the tendency for people to evaluate themselves and their situation, through comparisons with those that are similar. Seeing that another situation is worse can be comforting to families in dealing with their own situation.

All five areas have great importance in consideration of the role and function of self-help groups. Families, including persons with head injury, find that they can develop mastery and find meaning in their situation, develop coping strategies, have mutual and reciprocal relationships, find new social relationships to ease loneliness, and meet other people in similar situations who help them realize that their own situation could be worse.

Maureen Campbell-Korves relates her experience in a self-help group:

> By August of 1983 when the first head injury support group meeting for the New York City region was held, I was desperate. I wanted—and needed—this meeting so badly. . . . I found people going through pain on all levels and I found hope. I have met wonderful people willing to share what they went through and how they are coping with their ordeals. (Maureen Campbell-Korves, person with a head injury)

There are various philosophies of the best approaches to developing and maintaining self-help groups (Jacobs & Goodman, 1989; Williams, 1987). Generally, the group should be held away from a hospital setting, at a time most convenient for the members and should be led by an individual with similar experiences. Many families will not attend meetings in a hospital or rehabilitation setting because they do not want to return to that setting. If the family is beyond the rehabilitation phase, the hospital may remind them of previous struggles and situations. The best time to hold the meeting, the site of the meeting, and the format of the meeting are determined through a survey of all members and potential members. Leadership comes from the group itself. If the group requests a professional, they should strive to phase the person out over time to allow for more group cohesion and control. This is especially true for people with head injuries who may want to focus on issues of control and autonomy. The presence of someone who has not experienced a head injury may inhibit their discussion and create inhibition to individual growth.

The Randall family would have benefited greatly from a self-help group. Ruth Randall might have found meaning in her situation, found the resources she needed to help her cope with the overwhelming tasks involved in caring for Julie, and found opportunities to overcome the loneliness of being a single parent of a child with a disability. Pete might have benefited by learning more about head injury, thereby understanding how to interact further with Julie and perhaps include her in his new family. Julie's brothers might have been able to talk with other siblings with a similar experience and learn that their guilt over the situation is not uncommon. Julie might have been able to communicate her frustration to others with the same feelings.

Generally there are four possible roles for the professional in self-help groups: providing referrals, serving as guest speaker, serving as group advisor, and creating a new group. As mentioned previously, professionals are often crucial in helping to start the group. It is important to clarify the professional's role in the group. A common pitfall for professionals is to continue to play the traditional role of leader. This may promote ongoing dependence on the professional while also stifling the members' own sense of responsibility and ownership, which spark the energy and dynamics of self-help groups.

Family Outreach and Advocacy

After a person experiences a head injury, the person's social network increases in density over time, with a corresponding decrease in the size of the network (Kozloff, 1987). Social influence is most likely to be positive when it comes from people with whom the person has encouraging social experiences, that is, members of the person's social network (Clark, 1983). By their nature, many head injury rehabilitation programs will not be able to provide the close personal relationships families need for several reasons. First, families are sent through a continuum of services, seldom having time to establish long-term and lasting relationships with professionals or other families in the setting. Families often know that the stay is temporary, and they may not want to invest in personal relationships that they may also perceive to be temporary. Second, if a family must travel great distances to see their relative, focusing on maintaining social ties while also devoting energy to the person's rehabilitation program is difficult. Third, the very nature of rehabilitation still often focuses on the individual with the head injury to the exclusion of the family. If the rehabilitation focuses on short-term goals of individual habilitation, the long-term circumstances families face over the life cycle may not be addressed.

A family outreach program for families supports the family's long-term social needs while understanding their immediate social needs. For example, a family may be able to create a vision of what the final outcome of their experience may be while discussing what social support will be needed to reach it. Knowing that families may experience social isolation and loss of support from extended family and friends, professionals can begin early to help the family maintain these important ties. One family, as they began to realize that the rehabilitation process was going to take months rather than days, tried to create strategies to keep all of their extended family and friends up-to-date on the progress of the person with a head injury. One family member took all of the cards and notes the member with injury had received early on after the injury and created a family mailing list. In the early days, the family wrote monthly updates in the form of a newsletter on her progress. The newsletter included a description of her typical day and notes on how much she appreciated the mail she received. As time passed, the family sent the updates every 3 months and included messages from the person with injury. They found that their interaction with friends became easier over time because people began to understand the consequences of the head injury. For example, extended family and friends understood that an increase in range of motion in her arms was significant because it could lead to being able to move her wheelchair or feed herself. The rehabilitation team also received the updates which enabled them to understand how the family perceived the situation. Rather than offering generic support, friends offered creative options for support. When the person was ready to return home, the family sent an update and list of items and supports they needed. They were happily surprised to find that all of the people who said they wanted to help came through at the time of discharge from rehabilitation. This is one of many creative outreach strategies useful in dealing with stressors that the family anticipates facing over time.

The development of family advocacy groups is an important factor in the overall development of support for people with head injuries and their families. The growth of the National Head Injury Foundation (NHIF) and its state affiliates is indicative of the ability of family advocacy to help families reach beyond their own personal situations in dealing with head injury. Marty Beaver relates her experience:

> It was during this time that I learned of the National Head Injury Foundation (NHIF), a newly formed organization for persons with head injuries and their families. I sent in my membership and shared my trials of lack of resources and understanding. I attended a conference on head injury and, after meeting Marilyn Price Spivack, the founder, came back to Georgia with the commitment to begin an NHIF chapter. I was soon put in touch with two other family members who shared my frustrations. Together we started the Georgia Head Injury Foundation (GHIF). . . . When not working full time, caring for two children, or visiting my husband, I was talking to individuals and groups and sending out information about head injury and its consequences. (Marty Beaver, spouse)

There are many issues that draw families into involvement with advocacy organizations. For the most part families seek to make changes in a system that did not provide what they needed at crucial times. Some families choose drinking and driving as an important issue, others choose seat belt laws or the development of community-based services. The desire to make changes in the system and the desire to give back what the system gave to them provide the motivation to make important contributions to the resources of other families and to professionals.

Both outreach and advocacy would have benefited the entire Randall family. If Ruth had been involved in updating people on Julie's situation, the rehabilitation team would have better understood the areas in which she needed information. Unfortunately, time passed and the gap in Ruth's knowledge widened because she was soon at a loss as to what questions she should ask. If friends and family had understood the amount of time and care Julie was going to need when she returned home, they might have rallied to support Ruth. In the area of advocacy, Pete or Julie's brothers might have become involved in advocating for services closer to home. As time passes they may want to become involved in supporting the development of respite programs for Julie.

As in self-help groups, professionals can serve several roles in family outreach and advocacy. In family outreach, professionals can work to support families in problem-solving by talking with them about their options and choices. Instead of doing for the family, the professional supports the family to do for themselves. In advocacy groups, professionals work side-by-side with families. Family and professional roles should only be distinguished when the experience of either perspective is specifically called for. For example, in legislative testimony, the personal experience of a family member is critical in demonstrating the experience of head injury. Likewise, when one family member needs support from another, it is the similar personal experience that makes the interaction special. In other situations such as in organizing a conference or holding a fundraiser, there is no need to distinguish the roles of the family and the professional. The different talents that individuals can bring to advocacy groups help make their combined effort effective.

Community Networking

Regardless of the severity of a person's head injury or of the personality or coping abilities of the family, the most important determinant of reintegration for most families is the availability of supportive resources in the community (Seligman & Darling, 1989). O'Brien (1989) defines this community as the environment in which a person who depends on services lives, learns, works, and plays. Other crucial elements of reintegration are the activities that fill a person's day, whom the person encounters, and where the person appropriately should go. Probably most important after the experience of head injury, is perception of the individual by himself or herself and by others. If every day after therapy a person returns to a custodial institution without any other aspect of community life, head injury begins to define the person. If the person lives in the community, participating in activities with all other community members, head injury becomes only one aspect of the person's life. The person and family begin to understand the person as a contributing community member.

To enhance a person's capacity to be a contributing member of a community, Dunst et al. (1989) define five strategies to enhance social support. First, it is necessary to identify existing natural ties as well as untapped resources. The existing ties may include people the person worked with in the past, school friends, or family members. New resources can be identified through the person's current interests. Second, the identification of resources should be needs-based, be conducted by the family, and have a consumer orientation. If a family says that they need laundry detergent to help them do the laundry and thus deal with the increase in laundry, they should be provided with laundry detergent, not counseling to discuss why they are having a hard time doing the laundry. Third, a major emphasis should be placed upon building on family capabilities as a way of strengthening family functioning. Too often people tend to see only those families that cannot manage well and tend to miss the families that are coping well and do not attract attention. Fourth, the exchange of resources should occur among individuals who come together around shared interests and common causes. And fifth, professionals who work with families should not mobilize resources on behalf of the families; rather, they should create opportunities for families to become better able to do so for themselves.

Now that the Randall family is in the community, a program to enhance and build relationships is crucial. Developing a circle of friends that consists of people concerned about Julie would help to enable her to participate in the community and understand herself not as a "head injured person," but as a person who has experienced head injury. Friends who were close with Julie before the accident can be brought into her circle to understand the unique challenges she faces as a result of the head injury. New friends may be members of her house of worship or a community group. By identifying Julie's current interests, new people in her life can be discovered.

A program that truly seeks to build on community ties provides a provocative and challenging role for professionals. Professionals do not serve in the traditional role of "paid" counselor or therapist, rather they bring their unique skills to the circle as a friend or volunteer as do other circle members. For example, a person who works as a counselor by profession may choose to be friends with a person with a head injury and offer skills that support the person. At the same time, they have stepped out of the role of "professional" and can truly have a friendship with the person.

Of course this raises many questions about when the professional role ends and the personal role begins. Can professionals be friends with people who were formerly clients in rehabilitation? Can professionals interact with families in a way that promotes friendship? If we are not able to challenge the traditional patient-professional or family-professional role in ways that promote relationships that are supportive to everyone in the community, we risk losing the meaning of what community is all about. That is not to say that all professionals want to be friends with *all* people who were once patients in families they have known, or vice versa, but are we limiting opportunities for growth if we say that this can *never* happen?

SUMMARY

All families seek a sense of control, predictability, and opportunity to maintain a sense of balance. When a member of the family experiences a head injury, any sense of control and predictability is gone for the immediate future. Families require a strong social support network to gain the mastery and predictability they need. Traditionally, families have been forced to rely on professional support during rehabilitation and social support when professional support stops. Social support should be mobilized with professional support immediately after a head injury through the use of family-to-family programs, self-help groups, family outreach and advocacy, as well as community networking. As families acquire the skills to mobilize resources, they will begin to create their own social support. It is the social support that families enlist throughout their experience that will encourage them toward successful outcomes.

REFERENCES

Beals, M.P., Mathews, R.M., Elkins, S.R., & Jacobs, H.E. (1990). Locating community resources. *Journal of Head Trauma Rehabilitation, 5*(1), 31–39.
Borkman, T. (1976). Experiential knowledge: A new concept for the analysis of self-help groups. *Social Service Review, September,* 445–456.
Brotherson, M.J. (1985). *Planning for adult futures: Parents' self report of future planning and its relationship to family functioning and stress with sons and daughters who are disabled.* Unpublished doctoral dissertation, University of Kansas, Lawrence.
Caplan, G., & Killilea, M. (1976). *Support systems and mutual help.* New York: Grune & Stratton.
Clark, M. (1983). Reactions to aid in communal and exchange relationships. In J.D. Fisher, A. Nadler, & B.M. DePaulo (Eds.), *New directions in helping: Volume 1: Recipient reactions to aid* (pp. 281–304). New York: Academic Press.
DeJong, G., Batavia, A.I., & Williams, J.M. (1990). Who is responsible for the life-long well-being of a person with a head injury? *Journal of Head Trauma Rehabilitation, 5*(1), 9–12.
Dunst, C.J., Trivette, C.M., Gordon, N.J., & Pletcher, L.L. (1989). Building and mobilizing informal family support networks. In G.H.S. Singer & L.K. Irvin (Eds.), *Support for caregiving families* (pp. 121–141). Baltimore: Paul H. Brookes Publishing Co.
Iscoe, L., & Bordelon, K. (1985). Pilot parents: Peer support for parents of handicapped children, *Children's Health Care, 14*(2), 103–109.
Jacobs, M.K., & Goodman, G. (1989). Psychology and self-help groups. *American Psychologist, 44*(3), 536–545.
Kozloff, R. (1987). Networks of social support and the outcome of severe head injury. *Journal of Head Trauma Rehabilitation, 2*(3), 14–23.
McKnight, J. (1987, Winter). Regenerating community. *Social Policy,* 54–58.
O'Brien, B. (1987). A letter to professionals who work with head injured people. In M. Ylvisaker & E.M. Gobble (Eds.), *Community re-entry for head injured adults* (pp. 421–430). Boston: College-Hill.
O'Brien, J. (1989). *What's worth working for? Leadership for better quality human services.* Lithonia, GA: Responsive Systems Associates.
Savage, R.C. (1985). *A survey of traumatically brain injured children within school-based special education programs.* Available from the Head Injury/Stroke Independence Project, Rutland, VT.

Seligman, M., & Darling, R.B. (1989). *Ordinary families special children: A systems approach to childhood disability.* New York: The Guilford Press.

Stewart, M. (1989). Social support: Diverse theoretical perspectives. *Social Science and Medicine, 28*(12), 1275–1282.

Vincent, L., & Salisbury, C.L. (1988). Changing economic and social influences on family involvement, *TE CSE, 8*(1), 48–59.

Williams, J.M. (1987). *Head injury support groups.* Available from Southborough, MA: National Head Injury Foundation.

Winch, A.E., & Christoph, J.M. (1988). Parent-to-parent links: Building networks for parents of hospitalized children. *Children's Health Care, 17*(2), 93–97.

21

THE NATIONAL HEAD INJURY FOUNDATION

ITS ROLE AND RESOURCES

HEIDI HANSEN MCCRORY

The mission of the National Head Injury Foundation (NHIF) is to improve the quality of life of people with head injuries and their families and to develop and support programs in injury prevention. In 1980, people with head injuries and their families across the United States in Missouri, Indiana, and Massachusetts among other places were gathering to confront the challenges that they were facing. Experiencing firsthand the frustration resulting from lack of services, support, and information, and motivated to find and develop these resources, people with head injuries, their families, and professionals began to address the needs. The commitment and dedication of these individuals, along with Marilyn Price Spivack and Martin Spivack, who founded the national office in their home in Framingham, Massachusetts, resulted in the birth of a national organization and movement.

From these very modest beginnings, the National Head Injury Foundation has grown into a network of state and local organizations. The NHIF has evolved and expanded its resources in four key areas: support for people with head injuries and their families, advocacy, public and professional education, and prevention.

SUPPORT FOR
PEOPLE WITH HEAD INJURIES AND THEIR FAMILIES

Since the NHIF's inception, providing assistance and support to people with head injuries and their families has been a top priority. At the time of the NHIF's creation, the resources for family members dealing with the consequences of traumatic head injury were extremely limited. In 1980 only a handful of specialized head injury rehabilitation programs existed and no support groups for the individual or the family were in operation. By 1989, the NHIF network included some 44 state associations and affiliates and over 350 local chapters and support groups. Individuals who contact the NHIF at the national, state, or local level receive information and guidance about resources in their geographic area and/or information related to their specific needs, such as information on rehabilitation programs, support groups for the individual and the family, state and local assistance programs, and community and other services.

The national office of the NHIF maintains a toll-free helpline with the express purpose of providing more immediate access for persons with head injuries and their families. With a telephone call to the NHIF, a family or individual can speak with an information and resources specialist who will provide referral to educational information such as articles, books, journals, and videotapes; suggest a number of specialized head injury rehabilitation programs that meet geographical/therapeutic needs of the caller; and provide guidelines for what the individual should look for when selecting a program.

In addition, the NHIF publishes the *National Directory of Head Injury Rehabilitation Services,* which offers information on various private, nonprofit, and government organizations that may be of assistance to the individual. The 1989 edition of the directory includes program listings for 12 categories of rehabilitation: acute rehabilitation, subacute rehabilitation, transitional living, lifelong living, homecare, day treatment, independent living, coma treatment, behavior disorders, education, respite/recreation, and employment. Each listing contains the name, address, telephone number, contact person, appropriate ages, and accreditation (i.e., JCAHO—Joint Commission on Accreditations of Hospital Organizations, and CARF—Commission on Accreditation of Rehabilitation Facilities) for that program. The directory also includes a specialty services section with information on programs featuring driver education, evaluation, respirator dependence, Spanish language translation, substance abuse, visual impairment, pediatrics, and adolescent concerns. A supplemental glossary, guidelines for selecting a rehabilitation program, and coma assessment scales complete the directory.

Another wisely used resource of the NHIF is its *Catalogue of Educational Materials,* featuring over 100 articles and tapes pertaining to head injury. Articles, audiotapes, and videotapes are categorized by an assortment of topics. Although the majority of articles are suitable for nonprofessionals as well as professionals, the more technical articles are clearly identified. The newest of the NHIF information pieces includes the Tailored Information Packets (TIPs)—four-page monographs—covering advocacy, community resources, legal aspects of TBI, first person accounts, and general questions about head injury and prevention.

The role and resources of the state associations and local chapters of NHIF closely mirror those of the national office, with some differences. State and local groups support information and resource clearinghouses and libraries, albeit on a smaller scale; several associations publish state-specific resource directories and catalogues; and many produce quality handbooks and other materials. In contrast to the national office of the Foundation, state associations and local chapters are involved more directly with individuals and families through support groups, family-to-family networks, state toll-free helplines, direct service recreation programs, case management, and so forth. The national office clearly serves as a flagship in the areas of public policy, public awareness, and professional and public education, while the state and local groups focus more specifically on the immediate, direct contact with the individual or family.

Organizationally, the NHIF has established a Survivors' Council to include people with head injuries in a more visible and active role in the Foundation's operation and representation. The Council has functioned as a formal committee for policy-making and activity recommendations to the NHIF, in addition to serving as a more informal network of support for its members.

EDUCATION

A second key focus area for the National Head Injury Foundation is education—of professionals, families, and the general public. The NHIF sponsors a number of national conferences each year including a national symposium, advocacy and training conference, trial lawyers' seminar, and other educational events. The NHIF National Symposium is generally directed towards the professional or clinician working in head injury, for example, physical, occupational, and speech therapists, case managers, neuropsychologists, educators, and nurses. A second NHIF national conference, usually held in the spring, focuses on education for NHIF state association leaders and members. This conference is generally held in Washington, D.C. and also emphasizes national advocacy with congressional representatives. A third national seminar targets trial lawyers who handle head injury cases. The Trial Lawyers Conference generally provides lawyers with an overview of head injury, specifics on handling the head injury case, individuals with head injury as witnesses, minor head injury, and other related legal topics.

At the state and local levels, hundreds of conferences are conducted each year to educate medical and legal professionals, educators, families, public policy makers, individuals with head injury, and others on the issues of treatment, rehabilitation, education, advocacy, and many more topics of interest to people with head injuries, their families, and professionals in the field.

Furthermore, the NHIF has an elaborate structure of professional committees and task forces targeting a myriad of concern areas from special education to substance abuse to medical research. The special education task force and substance abuse task force have produced two outstanding publications respectively: *An Educator's Manual* and the *Substance Abuse Task Force White Paper*.

In addition to conferences, the Foundation plays an active role in educating the general public on head injury and the scope of the problem of head injury. This is accomplished through a combination of programs including radio and television public service announcements, newspaper and magazine articles, posters, brochures, and similar promotional and educational materials. State and local chapters are also actively engaged in public education through special events, workshops, media relations, publicity, advertising, and other methods. The national office offers a *Guide to Community Relations* manual as an educational resource for interested state and local chapters and individuals.

PREVENTION

One area in which the NHIF and its state organizations have conducted very active education programs is the prevention of head injury. Although involved in a variety of prevention issues—helmets, safety belts, drunken driving, pedestrian safety, and air bags—the Foundation currently is most active in focusing on safety belts and bicycle helmets. In 1989 the NHIF joined with the American Academy of Pediatrics and the Bicycle Federation of America to form the HEADSMART coalition to increase the use of bicycle helmets, particularly among young children. The NHIF's campaign has included the production and distribution of brochures, coloring booklets, posters, and community guides. In addition, television and radio public service announcements were produced and distributed along with a variety of other press materials. On the community level, NHIF state and local offices have conducted helmet giveaways; promoted helmet use at schools, health fairs, and bicycle rodeos; assisted youth organizations with bicycle helmet activities; and worked with other health and safety organizations on legislative and public policy issues.

Long active in the automobile safety arena, the NHIF has, in the late 1980s, joined with other safety organizations to promote safety belt use through school and community programs, newspaper articles, radio and television programs, public service announcements, other media promotions, and safety belt laws and federally-mandated passive restraints (air bags and automatic safety belts). The Foundation has worked nationally through cooperative agreements and grants with and from numerous private companies, nonprofit associations, and government agencies, most notably the National Highway Traffic Safety Administration of the Department of Transportation, the Centers for Disease Control, and Traffic Safety Now, Inc. Both the national, state, and local offices have materials, manuals, community guides, and other resources to assist with a variety of prevention programs.

ADVOCACY

Perhaps the greatest and most widely recognized of the Foundation's efforts have been in the area of advocacy. The national, state, and local groups of the NHIF have had a hand, not only in the establishment of public policy, federal funding, and cooperative interagency agreements, but also in the motivation, mobilization, and training of grassroots volunteers. At the time of the NHIF's inception, public policy makers and federal, state, and local agency representatives were, for the most part, ignorant about head injury and the needs of people with head injuries and their families. The NHIF, mostly through grassroots efforts of letter writing and personal visits, has drastically altered the attitudes of the various levels of government and has been responsible for the creation of the bulk of legislation and policies affecting service delivery for people with head injuries.

In May of 1985, the NHIF established a cooperative agreement with the Office of Special Education and Rehabilitative Services (OSERS), the Rehabilitation Services Administration (RSA), the National Institute on Disability and Rehabilitation Research (NIDRR), the Office of Special Education Programs (OSED), and the National Association of State Directors of Special Education. Commonly called the OSERS Agreement, its purpose was, and continues to be, ensuring the delivery of appropriate services to persons with head injury, at the national, state, and local levels. Originally drafted at the national level, this cooperative agreement or similar agreements have been replicated in over 25 states. In addition, the Foundation has worked through the years with a variety of other disability organizations to develop and support various government and legislative initiatives such as the extension of the Rehabilitation Act of 1973, which has resulted in increased opportunities for supported employment; extension of the Developmental Disabilities Assistance and Bill of Rights Act to empower individuals with disabilities to decide their own future; and recognition of head injury by the Social Security Disability Administration (SSDA), the National Institute on Mental Health (NIMH), and other organizations.

One of the most concrete examples of the Foundation's advocacy efforts is the increased levels of federal funding for research into a broad spectrum of head injury issues. Marilyn Price Spivack and numerous other families, individuals, and professionals have testified before a variety of congressional committees including the United States Senate and United States House Appropriations Committees. As a result, many federal agencies have expanded their funding for a number of medical, rehabilitation, public education, and training research projects, including a $300,000, 2-year public education grant to the NHIF from the National Institute on Disability and Rehabilitation Research.

Finally, the work of the NHIF and other head injury related groups resulted in the establishment in 1988 of an Interagency Task Force with representatives from 28 federal agencies including the National Institute on Disability Rehabilitation and Research, the Social Security Disability Administration, the National Highway Traffic Safety Administration, Health Care Financing Administration (HCFA), and the National Institute of Neurological Disorders and Stroke. The Task Force released its findings and recommendations in the summer of 1989. The report called for establishment of a comprehensive system of care with increased attention and funding for the entire spectrum of head injury issues—prevention, emergency medical and trauma care, acute medical care and rehabilitation, extended and lifelong rehabilitation, and community resources.

Of great importance at the state level, the NHIF network has joined with other public health agencies, emergency medical services, trauma centers, and state and local private health officials and organizations to develop and establish statewide head injury registries in 16 states. These registries are critical to the collection of data regarding the incidence of head injury in a given area, the cause of the injuries, medical outcomes, funding, and so forth.

Unquestionably, the mission of the NHIF is to educate and motivate individuals and organizations concerned with the head injury issue. Not only has the organization focused on advocacy within the public policy arena, but it has also put great emphasis on the advocacy skills of the individual. Much of the NHIF's information, resources and educational conferences are focused on the individual or family as advocate. An underlying theme in all of the NHIF's efforts—materials, conferences, and support groups, and so forth—has been training the family or person with head injury in self advocacy, to work within existing service delivery and social structures to ensure that the individual receives the appropriate care and intervention. Fulfilling this role as motivator and educator has been the Foundation's greatest service and will be its legacy.

The National Head Injury Foundation and the individuals it represents has been one of the most significant, if not the primary catalyst for change in the awareness, services, and policies that affect all people involved with head injury. The increased exposure and understanding of head injury across all segments of this society and the extraordinary growth of the NHIF is proof of its influence and importance.

INDEX

Page numbers followed by "*t*" indicate tables.